Children's Palliative Care in Africa

Edited by

Dr Justin Amery

Supported by

The Diana, Princess of Wales Memorial Fund

OXFORD
UNIVERSITY PRESS

OXFORD

UNIVERSITY PRESS

Great Clarendon Street, Oxford OX2 6DP

Oxford University Press is a department of the University of Oxford.
It furthers the University's objective of excellence in research, scholarship,
and education by publishing worldwide in

Oxford New York

Auckland Cape Town Dar es Salaam Hong Kong Karachi
Kuala Lumpur Madrid Melbourne Mexico City Nairobi
New Delhi Shanghai Taipei Toronto

With offices in

Argentina Austria Brazil Chile Czech Republic France Greece
Guatemala Hungary Italy Japan Poland Portugal Singapore
South Korea Switzerland Thailand Turkey Ukraine Vietnam

Oxford is a registered trade mark of Oxford University Press
in the UK and in certain other countries

Published in the United States
by Oxford University Press Inc., New York

© Oxford University Press, 2009

The moral rights of the author have been asserted
Database right Oxford University Press (maker)

First published by Oxford University Press 2009

British Library Cataloguing in Publication Data

Data available

Library of Congress Cataloging in Publication Data

Data available

Typeset in Minion by Cepha Imaging Private Ltd., Bangalore, India
Printed in Great Britain
on acid-free paper by
CPI Antony Rowe, Chippenham, Wiltshire

ISBN 978–0–19–956–7966

1 3 5 7 9 10 8 6 4 2

There can be no keener revelation of a society's soul than the way in which it treats its children.

Nelson Mandela

This book is dedicated to my wonderful family: Karen, Mikey, Mair, Rhiannon, Florence and Tende

Foreword by Elton John

In 1990, an 18-year-old American haemophiliac named Ryan White died of an AIDS-related illness. He had been diagnosed with HIV aged 11. At the time, AIDS was seen as a deeply stigmatised 'gay disease'. Ryan and his family were regularly subjected to abuse and excluded from community life. Their astounding acceptance, even forgiveness of this treatment was truly humbling. Because of Ryan, I realised there was so much more I could and should be doing in the fight against AIDS and this was the inspiration behind establishing The Elton John AIDS Foundation.

We have come a long way since then. Ryan White became a national icon in America and the Ryan White Care Act is still responsible for the largest number of HIV/AIDS programmes in the USA. My Foundation has become one of the twenty largest HIV/AIDS charities in the world. Last year alone, we supported nearly 30,000 children to go on antiretroviral treatment.

If Ryan were sick today, we would know so much more about how to help him – medically and emotionally. However, we still could not 'cure' Ryan's HIV/AIDS and that is why this book is so important. Of course health promotion, disease prevention and curative approaches remain our goal, but this cannot be at the expense of palliative care. Indeed in my view, the two are largely inseparable, and the need is truly mind-boggling. Worldwide, nearly 11 million under-fives are dying every year. Most of them are living in developing countries, with more than four million of these deaths in sub-Saharan Africa, where child mortality rates are running at an average rate of 172 deaths per 1,000 babies born (compared with 9 per 1,000 in developed regions).

For many economic, political, cultural and sociological reasons, palliation and symptom relief remain the only realistic treatment options for the majority of these children. Our duty is to make sure it is as good as it can be. One of the things Ryan's illness taught me is that sick children are not simply 'small sick adults', and children's palliative care needs to reflect this. Helping very sick or dying children to understand what is happening to them, and working with them to overcome the physical, psychological, social and spiritual challenges that come with impending death, is achievable, easily affordable, and highly rewarding even in the poorest settings with the least resources.

However, to practice children's palliative care, health workers do need to gain some additional knowledge, skills, support and confidence. Unfortunately, in resource-poor settings, it is very rare for health workers to receive any training in children's palliative care. Research has shown that, not surprisingly, health workers feel particularly lacking in confidence and competence in children's palliative care and tend to avoid these issues in practice – to the significant detriment of children who continue to suffer needlessly as a result. However, the research also suggests that health professionals in Africa (and across the world) see a great need for children's palliative care, highly value further training in it and find it extremely rewarding, empowering and satisfying when they try it for themselves.

For these reasons I applaud the publication of this book, which sets out with understanding and tenderness the specific palliative care needs of children. It can support thousands of health workers to better care for children for whom there is no immediate cure; can give them pride and clarity in their role and can make life better for millions of children around the world.

Ryan would have approved.

Contents

The authors *xiii*

Acknowledgements *xix*

List of abbreviations *xxi*

1 Introduction *1*

Section 1: **The basics of children's palliative care**

2 Communicating with children and their families *11*
Justin Amery, Gillian Chowns, Julia Downing, Eunice Guranganga,
Linda Ganca and Susie Lapwood

3 Play and development *37*
Sue Boucher and Justin Amery

4 Assessment and management planning *79*
Caroline Rose and Justin Amery

Section 2: **Symptom control in children's palliative care**

5 Pain *97*
Justin Amery, Michelle Meiring, Renee Albertyn and Sat Jassal

6 Respiratory symptoms *125*
Justin Amery and Michelle Meiring

7 Feeding and hydration problems *133*
Justin Amery

8 Gastrointestinal symptoms *155*
Justin Amery, Michelle Meiring and Caroline Rose

9 Neurological symptoms *171*
Justin Amery, Susie Lapwood and Michelle Meiring

10 Skin problems *189*
Justin Amery and Michelle Meiring

11 Urinary symptoms *201*
Justin Amery and Michelle Meiring

12 HIV/AIDS *207*
Justin Amery, Jenny Sengooba, Ivy Kasiyre and Michelle Meiring

Section 3: **Holistic care**

13 Psychosocial and family care *227*
Justin Amery, Nkosazana Ngidi, Caroline Rose, Collette Cunningham,
Carla Horne and Linda Ganca

14 Pre-bereavement and bereavement *249*
Justin Amery, Collette Cunningham, Nkosazana Ngidi, Eunice Garanganga,
Carla Horne and Jenny Ssengooba

15 Spirituality *271*
Justin Amery, Eunice Garanganga and Carla Horne

16 Palliative care for adolescents *289*
Justin Amery, Julia Downing and Collette Cunningham

17 Ethics and law *305*
Justin Amery, Joan Marston and Nkosazana Ngidi

Section 4: **Bringing it all together – caring at the end of life**

18 Caring for children at the end of life *327*
Michelle Meiring and Justin Amery

Section 5: **Caring for yourself**

19 Caring for yourself *351*
Justin Amery, Mary Bunn, Susie Lapwood and Gillian Chowns

Section 6: **Children's palliative care formulary for Africa**

20 Formulary *377*
Justin Amery and Sat Jassal

Further reading *411*

Index *415*

The authors

Renee Albertyn is a researcher in the department of Paediatric Surgery at the Red Cross Children's Hospital in Cape Town, South Africa. In addition, she is also clinically involved in the Pain Management Unit of hospital. In 2002, Renee obtained her PhD degree from the University of Cape Town Medical School in Pain Management and Assessment Strategies. She developed a Burn Pain and Anxiety Scale for children (BOPAS), which led to her PhD degree. Renee is involved in ongoing research and conducts weekly lectures on hospital palliative care to medical students. She regularly gives talks on her subject both locally and abroad. Renee has extensive experience and vast knowledge on the evaluation, assessment and management of pain in children.

Justin Amery was Medical Director at Helen House (the world's first children's hospice) from 1995 until 2005. He also helped design and develop one of the world's first hospices for young adults, Douglas House, where he was founding Medical Director. In 2006, he moved to Hospice Africa Uganda where he took over as Clinical Director, setting up a new Children's Palliative Care service, coordinating the Distance Learning Diploma Course in Palliative Care and developing a new post-graduate certificate course in children's palliative care. He has authored and contributed widely to texts, original articles and reports in children's palliative care. His research interest is education and training for health workers in children's palliative care. He is currently working on the Diana Fund project to develop new CPC services in Africa, and also with Great Ormond Street Children's Hospital in London.

Sue Boucher is a qualified teacher with over 30 years of experience in early childhood education as an educator, head of department and school principal. She is a published author of teaching manuals and teaching aids as well as 12 children's reading books, including one about Sunflower House, a children's hospice in Bloemfontein, South Africa. Author of the handbook *Promoting Early Childhood Development within Paediatric Palliative Care* and co-author of *A Toolkit for Children's Palliative Care Programmes in Africa*. Since December 2007, she has held the position of International Information Officer for the International Children's Palliative Care Network (ICPCN). At every opportunity, she tries to use her position in the children's palliative care movement to emphasize not only the value and importance of play, but also the constitutional right of every child to be given opportunities to play and the educational stimulation that will ensure their development to the best of their potential.

Mary Bunn (MB, BChir, DTM&H(London), MRCGP) completed MPhil part 1 in Palliative Medicine by distance learning from University of Cape Town and currently working towards part 2. Mary worked for 2 years in a rural area of the Gambia as a junior doctor before training in General Practice in the UK. She moved to Malawi in 2005 to work as Medical Director of a paediatric palliative care service attached to Queen Elizabeth Central Hospital, Blantyre – a large government hospital with over 200 paediatric beds, including a paediatric oncology unit. The palliative care unit offers in-patient and out-patient care and home visits to patients with a wide range of life-limiting and life-threatening illnesses including cancer, AIDS, cardiac disease and severe neurological sequelae from cerebral malaria and meningitis. Mary is also involved in medical student training. She has a husband who is a paediatrician and four school age children, all of them enjoy the beautiful mountains, lake and people of Malawi.

Gillian Chowns began her social work career in a Children's Department in the United Kingdom, continued in Social Services Departments and then moved into the NHS and palliative care in the late 90s. As a specialist palliative care social worker with the East Berks Macmillan Palliative Care team, her remit was to support the children of seriously ill parents. She has also taught at primary, secondary and tertiary levels and was until recently a Senior Lecturer in Palliative Care at Oxford Brookes University. Her research interests are focussed on pre-bereavement work with children and families and on palliative care education in resource-poor settings. She has lived and worked in Africa for various periods and has taught on the Oxford Brookes/Nairobi Hospice Diploma in Palliative Care. Dr Chowns has contributed chapters to several books on palliative care and a chapter in Reason and Bradbury's Handbook of Action Research (2nd edition). She is currently a Visiting Fellow at the University of Southampton.

Collette Cunningham (M.A. Public Policy & Management, B.A. Dev. Studies, H.Dip. Education, R.N. R.M). A nurse by profession, she has a vast and varied experience in children's palliative care. She has worked in Rwanda, Burundi, DRC, Kenya and Zambia improving the quality of life through palliative care programmes especially for children. Her work has involved curriculum development and teaching palliative care to health care professionals in resource-limited settings. She has also been involved in the development of palliative care policy and guidelines especially for the use of oral morphine in resource-limited settings. She has been a co-author and editor of several publications that includes Psychosocial Counseling of HIV+ Children and Adolescents (2008, ANECCA, CRS, AIDSRelief). Her particular area of expertise has been that of helping health care professionals to communicate bad news and to communicate with children who have life-threatening illnesses. This expertise has contributed in the writing of this textbook. She has recently taken up a position with the Irish Hospice Foundation.

Julia Downing is the Deputy Executive Director of the African Palliative Care Association (APCA) and is an experienced palliative care nurse and educationalist, with a PhD that evaluated palliative care training in rural Uganda. She has been working within palliative care for 16 years, with the last seven being in Uganda where she was the Director of the Mildmay International Study Centre before joining APCA. Her work in palliative care in Africa has been for both children and adults. She is experienced in presenting at conferences and writing for publication, and is on the editorial board of the International Journal of Palliative Nursing (IJPN) and is co-editor of the PCAU Journal of Palliative Care. Dr Downing is a member of the Palliative Care Country Team in Uganda, serves on the Boards of several international NGOs in Africa, is the Vice-President of the Palliative Care Association of Uganda and is an Honorary Research Fellow with the Department of Palliative Care, Policy and Rehabilitation, at King's College London, England. She was also the recipient of the IJPN's Development Award in 2006.

Linda Ganca (Dip.Sec.Ed-Unitra; BSocSc(Social Work)Hons-UCT) is a social work tutor with the HPCA. She qualified as a teacher in 1977 and taught at Ikhwezi Lokusa school for the physically disabled children in Umthatha-Eastern Cape. She studied social work in 1996 and then worked for 3 years at St. Josephs Childrens Home which is closely linked with Red Cross Hospital and then at St. Lukes Hospice(Gugulethu) for another 3 years. She joined HPCA in March 2006 as a Social Work Palliative Care Tutor. She currently runs training outreach to institutions caring for children, training staff in Paediatric Palliative Care. She also works with Health Care Facilities through the South African Department of Health (training staff in Interdisciplinary Team (IDT) approaches to palliative care), schools training teachers and learners in bereavement support). She trains social workers and medical students in palliative care. She currently is a research assistant in the cohort study on the Impact/Response of ARTs on patients with a CD4 count <50 (research site – St. Lukes, Lentegeur).

Eunice Garanganga (RN, BSCC, Dip Palliative Care, Palliative Care Nursing Certificate, Dip. Midwifery) is currently studying for a masters' degree with a focus on palliative care for children. She is on the Board of Directors for African Palliative Care Association, a member of the working group that developed the African Palliative Care Outcome Scale and a team member of the WHO Palliative Care Initiative Zimbabwe. She has over 26 years of experience in health care, having worked in hospice and palliative care since 1986. In 1991, she 'head and led' a palliative care Nursing Department which saw Island Hospice developing a strong nursing basis and its emerging role as a leader in the training of health personnel in the public, private and NGO sectors in the newly established discipline of palliative medicine in Zimbabwe. At present she is working as a Palliative Care Technical Adviser at Hospice and Palliative Care Association of Zimbabwe, a national body that promotes and supports palliative care providers in Zimbabwe.

Carla Horne is currently working with Family Health International providing technical support in palliative care programs for their offices in Africa and the Caribbean. Previously she lived and worked in Zimbabwe where she was fortunate enough to become the Director of Island Hospice Service and founding Director of the Hospice and Palliative Care Association of Zimbabwe. With a Master's Degree in psychology, she has found palliative care and its interdisciplinary approach a rich and meaningful area that has become her passion in providing care for human services, particularly for those infected and affected by HIV in resource-limited settings.

Sat Jassal is a general practitioner and medical director of Rainbows Children's Hospice in Loughborough, Leicestershire, and has worked in children's palliative care for 15 years. He has written and edited the Rainbows Children's Hospice Symptom Control, is an editor of PaedPalLit an abstract journal and has written the chapter on team working in the Oxford Textbook of Paediatric Palliative Care for Children. He is currently co-writing the Oxford Handbook of Paediatric Palliative Medicine. He co-chairs the education and training subgroup of the British Society of Paediatric Palliative Medicine and Association of Children's Hospice Doctors. He has a very tolerant wife and two even more tolerant children.

Ivy Kasirye (MBChB, MMed Paediatrics) is Head of the Paediatric Clinic at The Mildmay Centre, Uganda. She supervises a team of Paediatricians and Medical officers and is responsible for the day-to-day running of the Paediatric outpatient clinic. The Mildmay Centre for HIV/AIDS Care and Training is an international non-governmental organization run by Mildmay International, which is based in London, UK, and operates in Africa and Eastern Europe. Dr Kasirye has 3 years experience in Paediatric HIV clinical care, as well as training of local and international medical students and health workers in Paediatric HIV and Paediatric Palliative Care both at the Mildmay centre and in Zimbabwe. Dr Kasirye graduated with an MBChB from Makerere University, Kampala, Uganda, in 1998. Between 2000 and 2005, she was a resident in the Department of Paediatrics at the San Matteo Polyclinic of Pavia and graduated from the University of Pavia, with a Master of Medicine in Paediatrics in 2005. She immediately returned to Uganda where she started her career in Paediatric HIV care.

Susie Lapwood (MA (Cantab), BM BCh (Oxon), MRCGP, DFSRH, Dip Pall Med (Dist)), is lead Doctor, Helen and Douglas House Hospices for Children and Young Adults, Oxford, UK. She is also External Examiner, Cardiff Diploma and Masters in Palliative Medicine (Paediatrics), co-chairs the Education and Training Working Party for the British Society of Paediatric Palliative Medicine and Association of Children's Hospice Doctors. She is a paediatric contributor (lead assistant editor) for Palliative Care Formulary 4th edition (Editors in Chief Robert Twycross and

Andrew Wilcock, Palliative Drugs. Com, in preparation) and is also a GP and GP appraiser. Susie has worked in children's palliative care since 1998, latterly (with the opening of Douglas House), including the palliative care of young adults. Beyond her clinical role, she has particular interests in facilitating professional development, education and training for doctors working in the field of palliative care of children and young adults.

Joan Marston is presently the children's palliative care manager for the Hospice and Palliative Care Association of South Africa (HPCA). She used to be the advocacy manager at HPCA. She is a nurse by background and has been involved in Hospice and palliative care for about 20 years, first as a hospice volunteer, and then as a nurse and CEO of a hospice. Ten years ago she established the St. Nicholas children's hospice programme, which is probably the first children's palliative care service in Africa. She has been involved in starting the International Children's Palliative Care Network (ICPCN) and is its current Chair. Her special interest is getting into the hospitals children's palliative care, bereavement issues and education.

Michelle Meiring, MBChB (Pret), FCPaeds (SA), MMED Paeds (Wits), graduated from University of Pretoria in 1994 and did her internship at McCord Hospital in Durban, and then specializing in Paediatrics at the University of the Witwatersrand graduated in 2002 (FCPaeds). She has worked predominantly in the field of Paediatric HIV and Palliative Care and started her career as a consultant working in the Paediatric HIV Clinic at the Chris Hani Baragwanath Hospital in Soweto. In 2003, she co-founded the Children's Homes Outreach Medical Programme (CHOMP), since renamed the Bigshoes Foundation (www.bigshoes.org.za) that assists in improving the medical and palliative care of HIV-affected orphaned and abandoned children in the Johannesburg and Durban children's homes. During this time she completed a Masters Degree in Paediatrics through research exploring the impact of HIV on the children's homes. Also in 2003 (in partnership with Hospice Witwatersrand), she helped to set up a small children's hospice in Houghton, Johannesburg. In 2004, she was part of a steering committee that facilitated the recognition of palliative care as a discipline within the Department of Family Medicine at the University of the Witwatersrand. During 2004 and 2005, she worked as part of a team led by the Hospice and Palliative Care Association of South Africa (HPCA) to design a short course for professionals on aspects of paediatric palliative care. In 2006, Dr Meiring started the first hospital-based Paediatric Palliative Care team in South Africa, providing a bedside consultative service to three academic hospitals in Johannesburg. In 2007, the Bigshoes/Hospice partnership opened a second children's hospice in Soweto. A third children's hospice in Durban is being set up in partnership with McCord Hospital, recognizing that the hospice model of care could only benefit a small number of children. In 2008, Dr Meiring was appointed the Paediatric Director of the Gauteng Palliative Care Centre of Excellence based in Chris Hani Baragwanath hospital in Soweto. Dr Meiring also represents the Paediatric discipline on the board of the newly established Palliative Care Society of South Africa and is involved in setting up the South African Children's Palliative Care Network.

Nkosazana Ngidi is a married mother of three children aged 25, 19 and 18 years. She graduated from the University of Zululand with a BA (Social Work) and holds a Diploma in Speech and Hearing Therapy (University of the Witwatersrand. She also has post-graduate qualifications in Process Work Psychology (Oregon-Portland, USA), Marketing Management (Certificate, University of SA) and a Development Facilitation (Diploma, CDT, Johannesburg). She has 22 years experience in clinical, development and social work education in a variety of settings from child welfare, disability, employee wellness programme as well as Social Work student supervision at university. She became involved in palliative care in October 1996 at Highway hospice as a Development Social Worker as well as part time Regional Hospice Mentor in 2005. She is currently the National Education and Research Manager for Hospice Palliative Care Association.

Caroline Rose is a nurse from London, UK. Since qualifying she has worked in the areas of cancer and palliative care nursing. Caroline spent 2007–2008 working at Hospice Africa, Uganda, helping to set up and implement children's palliative care services in Kampala and around Uganda. Currently Caroline is working in South West London as a community paediatric palliative care nurse specialist.

Jennifer Ssenbooga is the Clinical Director of Hospice Africa Uganda, and previously, for 7 years, was lead doctor at the Mildmay Paediatric Care Centre (formally Jajja's Home) which deals with intensive rehabilitation of children with HIV/AIDS. She is also involved in training – particularly primary caregivers for the children, plus medical students and doctors from around the region. She has also done several courses in HIV/AIDS children's care and is currently completing her Masters in PH in Pretoria, with a focus on children.

Acknowledgements

Hospice Africa Uganda – for their support, encouragement and inspiration. What an inspiration!

The Diana Princess of Wales Memorial Fund – for sharing the vision, for financial support and for pushing us on.

The Hospice and Palliative Care Association of South Africa – for bringing us all together.

The African Palliative Care Association – for developing the links and for the sponsorship.

Sat Jassal – for generously allowing us to use the Rainbows Guide and for all the work he has put into Children's Palliative Care over the years.

My fellow authors – for their input, their thoughts and the fun.

List of abbreviations

5HT3	Serotonin 3
AFB	Acid-Fast Bacilli
AIDS	Acquired immune deficiency syndrome
ART	Antiretroviral therapy
ARV	Antiretroviral drugs
AZT	Zidovudine
BCG	Bacille calmette-guerin
bid, bd	Twice daily
BMI	Body mass index
CD4	Cluster of differentiation 4
CHW	Community health worker
CMV	Cytomegalovirus
CNS	Central nervous system
COPD	Chronic obstructive pulmonary disease
cP450	Cytochrome P450 isoenzymes
CPC	Children's palliative care
CSF	Cerebrospinal Fluid
CSI	Continuous Subcutaneous Infusion
CT	Computerized Tomography
CTZ	Chemoreceptor Trigger Zone
CTZ	Cotrimoxazole
DNA	Deoxyribonucleic acid
DOT	Directly observed therapy
EBV	Epstein barr virus
EC	Enteric coated
EEG	Electroencephalograph
EOL	End of life
FBC	Full blood count
FBO	Faith-based organization
GI	Gastrointestinal
GIT	Gastrointestinal Tract
H, hr	Hour
HAART	Highly active antiretroviral therapy
HBV	Hepatitis B virus
HCW	Health care worker
HIV	Human immunodeficiency virus
HPV	Human papilloma virus
HSV	Herpes simplex virus
ICP	Intracranial pressure
ICPCN	International children's palliative care network
IM	Intramuscular
IRIS	Immune reconstitution inflammatory syndrome
IU	International units
IV	Intravenous
KS	Kaposi's sarcoma
LIP	Lymphoid interstitial pneumonitis
LRTI	Lower respiratory tract infection
MAC	*Mycobacterium Avium* complex
MAI	*Mycobacterium Avium* intracellulare
min	Minute
MOH	Ministry of health
MRI	Magnetic resonance imaging
MTCT	Mother-to-child transmission
Na	Sodium
NGO	Non-Governmental Organization
NNRTI	Non-nucleoside reverse transcriptase inhibitors
NRTI	Nucleoside reverse transcriptase inhibitors
NSAID	Nonsteroidal anti-inflammatory drug
od	Once daily
OI	Opportunistic Infection
ORS	Oral rehydration salts
OVC	Orphans and vulnerable children
P450	Cytochrome P450 Isoenzymes
PCA	Patient-controlled anesthesia
pCO2	Partial CO2 pressure
PCP	*Pneumocystis Carinii* pneumonia
PGL	Persistent generalized lymphadenopathy
PI	Protease inhibitor
PLHA	People living with HIV/AIDS
PLWHA	People living with HIV/AIDS
PML	Progressive multifocal leukoencephalopathy
PMTCT	Prevention of mother-to-child transmission

PO	By mouth (*Per Os*)	SSRI	Selective serotonin reuptake inhibitors
PPE	Papular pruritic eruption	STI	Sexually transmitted infection
PR	By rectum	TB	Tuberculosis
PRN	As needed	TCA	Tricyclic antidepressant
Q	Every	tds	Three times daily
qHS	At bedtime	TENS	Trans-cutaneous electrical nerve stimulation
qod	Every other day		
QOL	Quality of life	TLC	Total lymphocyte count
RDA	Recommended daily allowance	UNAIDS	United Nations Joint Programme On HIV/AIDS
RSV	Respiratory syncytial virus		
RT	Reverse transcriptase	UNICEF	United Nations Children's Fund
SC	Subcutaneously	VC	Vomiting center
SCI	Subcutaneous infusion	VCT	Voluntary counseling and testing
SL	Sublingually	WHO	World Health Organization
SSA	Sub-Saharan Africa	wk	Week

Chapter 1

Introduction

Welcome to the world of children's palliative care. In our view, there is no discipline more rewarding, challenging or interesting. Arguably, there is nothing more satisfying to a health professional than relieving a child's pain and distress. Across the world, with rates of childhood illness, bereavement and death ever higher, this simple skill is required more than ever. And nowhere is the problem greater or the need higher than in Africa, where HIV/AIDS has made a bad situation much, much worse. Sadly, health workers are often nervous about working with dying children. Sometimes they fear the child's distress, sometimes they fear their own reactions and sometimes they fear feeling a sense of 'failure' for being unable to 'cure' the child. The good news is that, while of course children's palliative care can be challenging, with that challenge comes a profound satisfaction and sense of achievement. What is more, children's palliative care is surprisingly easy to learn and simple to practice. This textbook aims to show you how. Please read on!

1.1 Why do we need children's palliative care in Africa?

In Africa, it is often said that palliative care is 'salvage work' and not worth investing precious time and money into. But even a moment's thought shows this to be nonsense. Our role as health workers is primarily to relieve suffering and to protect life. Of course, in children's palliative care, children have diseases that can no longer be cured. In that sense, children's palliative care cannot claim to protect the quantity of a child's life. But children's palliative care can claim to protect the quality of a child's life, and of course to relieve suffering. There can be few things more important or more valuable in life than to relieve the suffering of a child and to help the child live the life they have as fully as possible.

1.1.1 Some facts and figures

All health workers in Africa know fully well the scale of the problem they face. The figures are so enormous that they are barely comprehensible. In practice, most of us would give up if we focused too much on the enormity of the challenge. Instead, most of us cope by focusing on the child and family in front of us, and then the next and the next.

However, in an introduction to a book like this, it wouldn't be right not to make an attempt to state the size of the task. So here are a few facts and figures:

- Today, nearly all child deaths occur in developing countries, almost half of them in Africa[1].
- In Sub-Saharan Africa, 16% of children born alive die before their 5th birthday (compared to 1.7% in the West), and 14 countries in Africa have seen their child mortality rates actually worsen in the last 10 years[2].
- AIDS and cancer are the two commonest incurable childhood diseases in Africa, with HIV/AIDS directly responsible for up to 60% of child deaths in Africa where more than 400,000 children under 15 died of AIDS in 2003 alone[3].
- Children infected with HIV/AIDS in Uganda have a mortality rate of 54%[4].

- Fifteen million children under 18 have been orphaned as a result of AIDS. Around 11.6 million of these children live in sub-Saharan Africa. It is projected that by 2010, the number of children orphaned by AIDS will increase to more than 25 million. In countries badly affected by the epidemic such as Zambia and Botswana, it is estimated that 20% of children under 17 are orphans – most of whom have lost one or both parents to AIDS[5].

- Each year, there are approximately 166,000 children under 15 diagnosed with cancer worldwide. Eighty-four per cent of cases are diagnosed in the developing world. Each year, there are at least 80,000 deaths from cancer in children under 15. Worldwide, 90% of these deaths occur in the developing world[6].

- The incidence of cancer is increasing as the threat from other diseases is decreasing, due to the additional burden of HIV-associated cancers.

- The majority of African children live in countries where the survival gains of the past have been wiped out, largely as a result of the HIV/AIDS epidemic.

- About 90% of all HIV/AIDS and malaria deaths in children in developing countries occur in Africa, where 23% of the world's births and 42% of the world's child deaths are observed[7].

- The immense surge of HIV/AIDS mortality in children in recent years means that HIV/AIDS is now responsible for 332,000 child deaths in Africa, nearly 8% of all child deaths in the region[8].

- Around 80% of the children dying in Africa die at home without seeing a health care provider[9].

- Severely malnourished children are eight times more likely to die before their fifth birthday as against those who are well nourished. Malnutrition is a contributing factor in around half of all child deaths[10].

- In countries like the UK and USA, survival rates are particularly high – more than 7 out of 10 children are still alive 5 years after diagnosis. In the developing world, however, the majority of children with cancer are either not diagnosed, or are denied life-saving treatment. In India, for example, more than 10,700 children die of cancer each year, compared to less than 350 children in the UK[11].

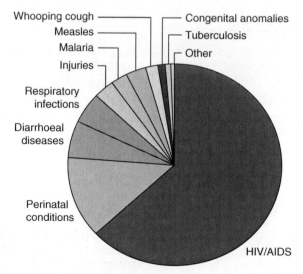

Fig. 1.1 Causes of child deaths in Africa[12].

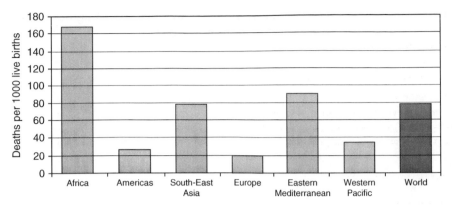

Fig. 1.2 Child mortality across the world[13].

1.2 **Why do we need a special book for children's palliative care in Africa?**

Some people might ask why we need another palliative care textbook. After all, there are now numerous general palliative care texts available, and even some focused on Africa. There are also now a few books specializing in children's palliative care. These are good questions, but we think the answer is clear. African children's palliative care is different to children's palliative care elsewhere. And African children's palliative care is different to adult palliative care in Africa. These differences are significant and not covered elsewhere.

1.2.1 **Differences between Children's and Adult palliative care**

While there is significant overlap between adult and children's palliative care, there are also significant differences. Communication with children tends to be more difficult than with adults. The pharmacokinetics and pharmacodynamics of drugs with children differ from those with adults. Children's understanding of death and dying differs from that of adults, so different psychotherapeutic approaches need to be adopted. The ethical dilemmas vary, as children (by law) cannot give consent, although they can often have very major roles to play in dilemmas requiring consensual agreement amongst child, family and professionals. Children are particularly fearful of separation from family, friends, home and school, and so children's palliative care services have to take care to 'normalize' the lives of children with life-limiting illnesses as much as possible. The families of dying children have a different role than the families of dying adults, and therefore their experiences of bereavement differ. There are subtly different challenges facing professionals dealing with dying children, and these require well-structured support and development systems. Children tend to have a broader range of people involved in their care, and so team-working and an understanding of team dynamics is especially important.

1.2.2 **Differences between African and Western children's palliative care**

Children's palliative care in Africa presents very different challenges to those in the West. There is simply no comparison between the number of children requiring children's palliative care in Africa and those in the West. This is, of course, largely down to HIV and AIDS. In my first day at Hospice Africa Uganda, I saw more children with HIV/AIDS than I had in my previous 12 years working at a children's hospice in the UK.

Then, of course, there are massive differences in the physical and human resources available to children with life-limiting illnesses in Africa. Here, it is common for children to die simply for want of a few cents to buy simple antibiotics or to remain in pain for want of simple pain-killers. Curative treatment in the African setting is frequently not a viable option. Chemotherapy is expensive and usually needs to be given by trained staff. Chemotherapy and ARTs require monitoring of organ function and treatment response. Services are often unevenly distributed. Travelling within Africa is difficult and expensive. Children often present late due to the lack of knowledge about disease and lack of affordability and access to services.

Even when children do present in time to be cured from HIV/AIDS or cancers, they may not be due to the significant problems with the capacity of health services. Health care professionals frequently have no palliative care training, let alone children's palliative care training, so terminally ill children are often placed in inappropriate acute care facilities. While the advent of ARTs has been a tremendously good thing for Africa, they place a huge demand on a heavily overburdened health service, and so palliative care is competing for a slice of even less capacity. Drugs and consumables are difficult to access and assure. The drug treatments for cancer and AIDS are expensive, complex and toxic, and often cause more symptoms than they solve. The regimes are often complex and children's formulations often unavailable, making it more likely that those children will default and relapse.

In our experience, there are significant similarities between Western and African approaches to children. The vast majority of parents and families we have met in both cultures want their child to be happy, healthy, pain-free and thriving. However, there are, of course, ways in which cultures vary which impact on how children's palliative care is planned and delivered in Africa. Traditional African family structures and dynamics differ from those in the West, although in many areas these traditional structures are breaking down, creating more challenges for children with life-limiting illnesses. Children's rights are a live issue in Africa, and issues of child's consent and child protection must be addressed in the palliative care context.

As in all cultures, there are complex psychosocial issues, belief systems and rituals surrounding death and dying in Africa, some of which can mitigate against good palliative care. Children with HIV/AIDS and cancers are often stigmatized, which can lead to failure to engage with health care services. Parents may suffer with guilt associated with mother-to-child-transmission of HIV. Ancestral beliefs and cultural norms often dictate that 'everything must be done' to cure a child, even when the condition is hopeless, thereby delaying palliative intervention. It is common for several family members to be sick or dying, and so families may emotionally withdraw in the face of these enormous psychosocial and financial pressures, thereby missing out on health services.

For all these reasons, palliation and symptom relief are the only realistic option for most African children with advanced cancers and AIDS. This is the situation in most Sub-Saharan African countries. The importance of children's palliative care in the developing world has been highlighted by the World Health Organisation, WHO[14].

1.3 A suggested 'African Children's Palliative Care Charter'

Of course, children's palliative care in Africa faces some considerable challenges – financial, logistical, social and political to name a few. But we must not allow ourselves to be disheartened. Let us set the bar high, so as to ensure we do the best we can. In the UK, which was the first country to develop children's palliative care, there is an organization called the Association of Children's Palliative Care (ACT), and when it was founded, a charter defining the ideal scenario for children was written. The International Children's Palliative Care Network (ICPCN) (a worldwide network of agencies working with children and young people with life-limiting conditions)[15] has adapted the original ACT Charter[16], but amended to be more appropriate for African and other world settings.

1.3.1 The International Children's Palliative Care Network charter of rights for life-limited and life-threatened children

- Every child should expect individualized, culturally and age appropriate palliative care as defined by the World Health Organisation (WHO)[17]. The specific needs of adolescents and young people shall be addressed and planned for.

- Palliative care for the child and family shall begin at the time of diagnosis and continue alongside any curative treatments throughout the child's illness, during death and in bereavement. The aim of palliative care shall be to relieve suffering and promote the quality of life.

- The child's parents or legal guardians shall be acknowledged as the primary caregivers and recognized as full partners in all care and decisions involving their child.

- Every child shall be encouraged to participate in decisions affecting his or her care, according to age and understanding.

- A sensitive but honest approach will be the basis of all communication with the child and the child's family. They shall be treated with dignity and given privacy irrespective of physical or intellectual capacity.

- Every child or young person shall have access to education and wherever possible be provided with opportunities to play, access leisure opportunities, interact with siblings and friends and participate in normal childhood activities.

- The child and the family shall be given the opportunity to consult with a paediatric specialist with particular knowledge of the child's condition where possible, and shall remain under the care of a paediatrician.

- The child and the family shall be entitled to a named and accessible key worker whose task is to build, co-ordinate and maintain appropriate support systems which should include a multi-disciplinary care team and appropriate community resources.

- The child's home shall remain the centre of care whenever possible. Treatment outside of this home shall be in a child-centred environment by staff and volunteers, trained in palliative care of children.

- Every child and family member, including siblings, shall receive culturally appropriate, clinical, emotional, psychosocial and spiritual support in order to meet their particular needs. Bereavement support for the child's family shall be available for as long as it is required.

1.4 How to use this book

This book is aimed primarily at health workers in the African context. It may well also be of use to health workers in other resource-poor settings and of course, to health workers in the West who wish to know more about aspects of children's palliative care in Africa.

The book tries to strike a balance between theory and practice but, where there is a choice to be made, the book focuses on practice first and foremost. We therefore hope that this book will be easy to use in actual day-to-day practice: as a guide and as an aide memoir.

For that reason, we have tried to limit the amount of the text and to use key-points, bullet points and tables as often as possible. The index and content pages should make it simple for readers to jump straight to the relevant section. We have included references to evidence or supporting texts where we can, so readers will be able to pursue particular lines of enquiry that might interest them. Where evidence is not available, we have given advice from our own experience, recognizing that anecdotal evidence needs to be handled with care.

The book has also tried to strike a balance between action and reflection. The bulk of the text explains in clear terms what to do, how and when. In other words, it focuses on action. However, we have also included case studies and 'questions for you' (to which we don't provide answers) to help readers to reflect a little more on their own practice and to think about how they might improve on their practice.

1.5 **Questions for you**

◆ Take a moment to think about all of the children you have seen who have life-limiting illnesses. Is there more you could have done to help relieve their suffering?

Undoubtedly the answer to this must be yes: none of us is perfect!

As a health professional working in Africa, no doubt you are constantly frustrated by huge demands, limited resources, poor working environments and personal exhaustion. This book cannot change the resource constraints within which you operate. Despite all of these problems, however, we can all do more. A more important question therefore might be this:

◆ With better knowledge, training and confidence, is there more you could do to help children suffering with life-limiting illnesses in the future?

We are fairly confident that the answer to this will be yes. We can all improve what we do and how we perform. The only thing limiting this is ourselves – and more importantly the limits on our own capacity, knowledge and confidence. This book is designed to help you build all three.

◆ Did you know that there are simple and common-sense ways that can boost your resilience and build your capacity? There are, and this book includes some of them (see Chapter 19 – 'Caring for yourself').

◆ Is there more you could learn about the theory of children's palliative care? If so, this book will help you build your knowledge base. It is packed with useful, relevant and accessible information to help you understand more about children's palliative care.

◆ Do you feel confident about putting that knowledge into practice? We all know that we can have all the theoretical knowledge in the world, but it won't help anyone unless we apply that knowledge in our day-to-day practice. This book includes case scenarios and questions for you to reflect on, with the aim of helping you apply your newly acquired knowledge to your day-to-day practice.

Welcome again to the world of children's palliative care. Our hope as authors is that this book gives you the capacity, knowledge and confidence to take part – right here and right now.

Good luck.

Notes

1   World Health report (2003) – *Shaping the Future*. WHO Geneva. Available at: www.who.int/whr/2003/chapter1/en/index2.html

2   UN 'Millennium Development Goals Indicators Database' (2007)

3   WHO Global Health Report (2003). Global Health: today's challenges, Chapter 1.

4   Newell, M.L., Brahmbhatt, H. & Ghys, P.D. (2004). Child mortality and HIV infection in Africa: A review. *AIDS. 18*(2), S27–34.

5   UNAIDS (2008). *Report on the global HIV/AIDS Epidemic*, WHO Library. UNAIDS/08.25E/JC151OE. ISBN 9789291737116.

6   Cancer Research UK: Cancer Worldwide – The global picture. Available at http://info.cancerresearchuk.org/cancerstats/geographic/world.

7   WHO Global Health Report (2003). Global Health: Today's challenges, Chapter 1.

8   WHO Global Health Report 2003: Chapter 1: Global Health: today's challenges.

9   Department for International Development (DFID) Online at www.dfid.gov.uk/mdg/childmortality-factsheet

10 Department for International Development (DFID) www.dfid.gov.uk/mdg/childmortalityfactsheet

11 Children in developing world bear the burden of cancer, Cancer Research UK. Press Release 14.2.03

12 World Health report (2003). *Shaping the Future*. WHO Geneva. Available at www.who.int/whr/2003/chapter1/en/index2.html

13 World Health report (2003). *Shaping the Future*. WHO Geneva. www.who.int/whr/2003/chapter1/en/index2.html

14 The World Health Organisation, '*Cancer Pain Relief and Palliative Care in Children*' WHO ISBN-13 9789241545129.

15 See www.icpcn.org.og

16 The Association for Children's Palliative Care. Online at http://www.act.org.uk/dmdocuments/act_charter.pdf

17 Palliative Care for Children (2002). Found at http://www.who.int/cancer/palliative/definition/en/

Section 1

The basics of children's palliative care

In this first section, we will offer guidance on the core skills of children's palliative care. These are

(1) communicating with children,

(2) playing with children and

(3) assessing and developing holistic management plans for children.

Chapter 2

Communicating with children and their families

Justin Amery, Gillian Chowns,
Julia Downing, Eunice Garanganga,
Linda Ganca and Susie Lapwood

Key points

- Children speak three languages: body language, play language and spoken language.
- Just because you haven't spoken it, it doesn't mean you haven't expressed it.
- Communication usually happens when and where the child wants it, so be prepared for a tricky question or conversation when you least expect it.
- Talk does not solve all problems, but without talk we are limited in our ability to help.
- The best way to find out what a child understands and believes is to ask the child.
- Never underestimate a child: the evidence is that children usually know and understand a great deal more than parents or health workers think.
- Children who have long-term life-limiting illness generally go through various stages of understanding of illness, death and dying, but the most important factor in a child's understanding is the child's own experience.
- Breaking bad news is very hard, so practise beforehand. Armies train for battle, actors rehearse before they go on stage and we too should prepare ourselves in advance.
- It is immoral, unethical, and legally culpable for a health worker to withhold the truth from children and families who want to hear it.
- You should always be honest with a child and never make promises that you cannot keep.
- The wishes of the parents and the child may not always be the same.
- Communication is a team issue: dysfunctional teams cause dysfunctional communication which causes dysfunctional children's palliative care.

2.1 Introduction

In our experience and in the studies carried out both in UK[1] and Africa[2–4], communicating with children in a children's palliative care situation is one of the greatest educational needs of health workers in this field. It is an area that all involved in palliative care with children find hard (including social workers, nurses, doctors, teachers, religious leaders, parents and the community), and often try to avoid. That is a shame because it is one of the most rewarding and satisfying parts of children's palliative care. Hopefully, this chapter will help.

2.2 **Why do we need to communicate in children's palliative care?**

Contrary to the belief of many, good communication skills are learnable[5]. There is plenty of evidence that communicating honestly and openly with the child and family is beneficial[6] and there are many reasons why communication is so important in children's palliative care. Here, are just a few of them:

+ Talk does not solve all problems, but without talk we are even more limited in our ability to help.

+ Not talking about something doesn't mean that we aren't communicating; avoidance in itself is a message.

+ By talking we may discover what children know and do not know (and probably that they already know there is a problem[7]), and then we can help by providing needed information, comfort and understanding.

+ There is no evidence that unwanted communication is harmful[8].

+ Children and parents tend to protect each other from being upset by avoiding difficult discussions. This means that at times the child can become emotionally isolated.

+ Good communication helps children to become involved in their own care management[9] and improves adherence to treatment[10].

+ Open communication with children and their families improves professional job satisfaction and reduces burnout.

+ We may well need to put right what fellow professionals have done wrong[11].

+ And (of course) communication helps us to elicit useful information so that we can diagnose problems and develop management plans.

2.3 **Children's understanding of illness, death and dying**

2.3.1 **Basic theory**

There are many theories about how children develop and about how that development affects their understanding. Further information can be found in Chapter 3: Play and development. However, the theories do not always agree with one another, and the detail is beyond the pragmatic, down-to-earth approach of this book. For those who are interested, descriptions of the major theories are included in the reference section[12–16].

What is important to realize is that children's understandings of health, illness, death and dying go through stages. These stages are related to chronological age, but note this relationship is highly variable. Perhaps what is even more important is that the stage of a child's understanding also depends heavily on their own experiences. In Africa, where exposure to disease, death and dying is much greater than elsewhere, children have a lot of experience.

A summary of children's perceptions of death and possible interventions is included in Table 2.1 below. However, the key messages that you do need to know are as follows:

+ The best way to find out what a child understands and believes is to ask the child himself!

+ Children's understanding of themselves, other people and the world around them varies as they get older. This has an important effect on how children perceive illness, death, and bereavement. You need to understand what the child understands and try to see the world through their eyes. Once you can do that, children's palliative care becomes a whole lot easier.

◆ No one child is exactly the same as another, and children develop faster the more experience they have. That means children who have experience of illness, death and dying will probably understand a great deal more than their peers who do not[17].

◆ Never underestimate a child: the evidence is that children usually know and understand a great deal more than parents or health workers think.

2.3.2 Children's perceptions of death and possible interventions[18–20]

Table 2.1 Children's perceptions of death

Perception of death	How to help the child
1–3 years	
Equate death with sleeping and expect people who have died to wake up. Fear separation from parent/caregiver.	Keep the child's daily routine as unchanged as possible. Make time each day to hold, talk to and comfort the child.
3–4 years	
Children of this age do not accept death as final and think of it as a temporary separation. Children may believe that they are in some way responsible for the death because of powerful imaginations (magical thinking). Perhaps, if they wish hard enough, the dead person will come back.	Explain clearly why the person died: 'X died because she was not well. It had nothing to do with you, with something that you did or didn't do'.
5–8 years	
Begin to accept death as final and view it as separation from loved ones. They have a great fear of a sick parent dying and of being abandoned. They worry about their own death.	Reassure the child that minor illnesses and injuries can be treated. Reassure the child that it is okay to cry, to feel angry, sad or frightened when someone dies. Reassure them that they are not responsible for the death. Allow the child to cry and talk about the loss; write a daily journal; draw pictures of how he or she feels; pray; compile a picture album of the loved one.
8–10 years	
Children learn that all living things must die. Interest in the mystery of death grows.	Answer questions as fully as possible. Do not discourage normal curiosity about death. Acknowledge the child's feelings. Allow the child to cry and talk about the loss; write a daily journal; draw pictures of how he or she feels; pray; compile a picture album of the loved one.
9–11 years	
React strongly to death. Interested in what happens after death. Death is accepted as a part of life.	Answer questions fully. Acknowledge and explore the child's feelings. Interventions may include: talking about memories; writing a daily journal; drawing pictures of how he or she feels; pray; compiling a picture album of the loved one.

2.3.3 **Children's understanding of illness, death and dying**

As we have already emphasized, the most important factor in a child's understanding of illness, death and dying is the child's own experience. A child who has been sick for some time will have a far more advanced understanding of health and illness than healthy children of his or her own age. Within Africa even the healthy child will have experience of illness, death and dying far above children of his/her age in other societies. In palliative care, this applies to the majority of children we see.

Children who have long-term life-limiting illness generally go through various stages of understanding. These are[21]:

- I am sick
- I am sick but I am going to get better
- I am going to keep on getting sick but I will still get better each time I am sick
- I am going to keep on getting sick and I won't get better
- I am going to die.

As a general rule, you can be fairly confident that dying children mostly[22]:

- can understand that they have a serious illness by the age of 3
- can understand that their illness is getting worse even if no one tells them
- interpret death as an inappropriate topic for adults
- conversely interpret death as a safe topic for other children who are eager to share information
- learn to safely discuss their illness away from parents
- are very frightened of separation, particularly from their family, but also from friends and from school
- are frightened of pain
- may view illness and death primarily in terms of separation and pain
- won't really appreciate the differences between curative and palliative approaches.[23]

Young children (pre-school):

- may confuse death with sleep and don't understand that death is forever and[24]
- will not understand abstract concepts of death such as eternal life, heaven, etc.

Children between the ages of 5 and 9 years:

- are still very frightened of separation and by 6 years will usually understand that death means separation from the person who has died, lack of movement from the deceased and that it does not change back to normal
- are still frightened of pain
- may begin to understand that if they have a long-term illness they may not get better
- may continue to talk about what they will do when they grow up
- may be able to talk about what they feel
- may begin to develop some abstract ideas such as 'good' and 'bad'
- may start believing that somehow he/she may have deserved or willed the illness or death to happen
- by 6 years many children will also be aware of how the body changes after death

- may have a well-formed concept of death before the age of 10
- may have very varied beliefs about God, heaven, ghosts, spirits and life after death – but these tend to be imaginary rather than concrete.

Children over 10 years of age:

- will usually have a clear idea that they have a serious illness even if they have not been told
- may keep silent about what they know if adults are also silent and do not encourage open communication
- may begin to ask more 'difficult' questions, as they begin to realize the severity of their illness.

2.4 Mind your language: speaking to children

You wouldn't try to speak to someone who does not speak or understand your mother tongue well, without adapting your language to make it easier for him to understand you. Ideally, if you could, you would speak in his language. If you think in those terms about speaking to children, you won't go too far wrong.

Children speak three languages (listed in the order in which they learn them):

- Body language
- Play language
- Spoken language.

Therefore, if you want to speak to children, particularly young children, you need to get proficient in all three.

2.4.1 Body language

When seeing children in a children's palliative care setting, we need to watch the child's body language carefully. How does the child enter the room? How does the child sit in the chair? Who are they sitting close to? Is the child's body tense or relaxed? Is their body posture changing in response to any of the topics discussed? However, it is important to be aware that sick children do not always respond in the way that you would expect them to, for example just because a child is laying still it does not mean that they are not in pain.

Remember also that children are excellent readers of body language. In fact they learn body language far sooner than verbal language. They will be assessing you and reading you as soon as they see you. They will watch carefully how you interact with their family, and vice versa. If they don't like what they see, they will make it hard for you when you come to examine them. So, be aware of your own body language and what it might be conveying to the child. Smile, make yourself smaller, respect their space and be as non-threatening as you can be.

2.4.2 Language of play

> Adults talk and children play

All children play, although you may find that you need to give 'permission' to children to play in a health care setting (where they may be ill at ease). Through play, children communicate what is in their hearts and minds. Children *show* you rather than tell you about their life.

If you have your own children, or relatives who are children, or you know friends who will lend you their children, have a go at letting them play with you.

It sounds easy, but adults tend to find it very hard because we have great difficulty in letting go and allowing the child to take charge. Remember, children are the experts in play, and adults are the novices. In fact, simply by sitting down next to a child and waiting, rather than trying to work things out by set rules, play magically happens. Children do it naturally, as they are the masters. All we have to do is watch and follow.

Of course play varies from culture to culture, but play itself is universal. In our experience, the most universal things are music, drawing and imaginary games. Chapter 3, Play and development, goes into a lot more detail about the importance of play in children's palliative care. However, for now, some useful ways of communicating with children are as follows[25]:

- If you can, try and keep a drum and some crayons handy.
- Drawing pictures side by side is not only an incredibly powerful tool for communication and trust-building, it is actually great fun.
- We have yet to come across children that don't enjoy singing.
- Storytelling is a good way to help children. Traditional stories and plays can be acted out, and children can be given the opportunity to finish the story and express themselves.
- Children may like to write poems or songs. In particular, this may appeal to the older children and adolescents.

2.4.3 Spoken language

This is the language that adults most frequently speak, but remember that it is not the first language of very small children, and even older children may prefer to converse in other ways. Therefore, try and imagine you are speaking to someone from a different country, a different culture and with a different mother tongue. That will help you filter out jargon and cultural presuppositions from your own language. However, as children get older, you will find that spoken language gradually becomes their language of choice and you will naturally find spoken communication easier.

2.4.4 Barriers to communication with children

While it is not always easy to build good communicative relationships with children, it is quite easy to upset them. But, if you mess it up, *don't be put off*. Saying sorry and asking for another chance tells children that you respect them, and may even put you in a better position than you started from. Children are usually incredibly forgiving and prepared to give you a second chance (and a third, fourth, fifth etc.).

However, you will make life a lot easier for yourself if you avoid the following:

- Appearing judgemental
- Being patronizing
- Interrupting
- Second guessing what they are trying to say
- Using a commanding voice or tone
- Comparing children with adults
- Showing displeasure with them
- Not keeping your word

- Arguing with children
- Making promises that you can't or may not be able to keep.

2.4.5 Helpful hints for effective communication with children

Communication with children can be enhanced through following a few simple guidelines[26]:

- Ensuring confidentiality.
- Showing respect, listening and attending to everything that they have to say.
- Allowing them to explore issues within their own context and letting them be involved in decision-making as appropriate.
- Getting down to the same level as the child, i.e. being eye to eye.
- Asking questions in response to the child's questions in order to clarify understanding and the meaning behind some questions. For example, to the question 'Am I dying?' you may respond 'What makes you think that?' or something similar.

Box 2.1 Barriers to communication

Think about the last time you saw a child as a patient. Was it possible to ensure confidentiality? Was the room that you were in 'child friendly'? Did you try and put the child at ease and try to speak to the child directly?

2.5 Why do we find it so difficult to communicate with children in children's palliative care?

In the authors' experiences and research in both the UK and Africa[27,28], health professionals consistently rate this as the area that causes them the most anxiety and where they feel least confident or competent. When we break this down further, one specific fear is of being asked difficult questions or getting stuck in difficult conversations about death, dying and the hereafter.

More of that is given later. However, let's first reflect on some societal, cultural, patient and health worker factors that might inhibit effective communication with children.

2.5.1 Societal factors

In Western society, childhood death is now rare. For example, in the USA, in 1900, 30% of all deaths occurred in children less than 5 years of age compared to just 1.4% in 1999. Infant mortality dropped from approximately 100 deaths per 1,000 live births in 1915 (the first year for which data to calculate an infant mortality rate were available) to 29.2 deaths per 1,000 births in 1950 and 7.1 per 1,000 in 1999[29].

People therefore have fewer encounters with childhood death and Aries suggests that this has led to the lack of experience, fear and unrealistic expectations[30]. In the African context, although there is a lack of evidence, it seems reasonable to assume that this does not apply to the same degree, as child mortality even prior to the AIDS epidemic was much higher than in the West, and also traditional death ceremonies usually involve much closer contact with the body than in the West. However, there is still a knowledge gap regarding the effect that societal attitudes about childhood death have on communication in the African context. Also, although death may be more commonplace within the African setting, it may not be discussed with children due to societal norms and/or taboos.

2.5.2 **Cultural factors**

We are more and more aware that cultural factors play a major role in how we view health, illness and dying[31,32]. Health beliefs and practices vary considerably around the world. We often tend to assume that children share the same culture as their families; however, whilst this might be the case, we should not always assume it to be. In fact, it may be fair to say that children never live in exactly the same culture as their parents. After all, 'child-world' is a very different place to 'adult world'. If you ever doubt this, check out what children draw or write about when describing their families, or observe the way a child watches the world by giving them free rein with your camera for an hour or two. You may well be surprised by what you find.

In many cultures in Africa talking about death and dying is seen as taboo (see Chapter 14 'Pre-bereavement and bereavement'). Some feel that it suggests an expression of a hidden wish that the person should die. Others feel that discussing a person's death may lead to a withdrawal of hope and thereby a hastening of death. However for the child, they will be questioning and wanting to know more and the truth around death, especially deaths within the family or friends. It is important to recognize questions children may have and address these in an honest and age appropriate manner. As the child grows into adolescence, this may involve questioning the various beliefs and practises that they grew up with. Cultural factors have a great influence on how children respond to death and dying in their adult lives, and they need to be given the freedom to explore these as they grow up.

Our cultures are precious and we all treasure and feel protective of our own. But culture is not a fixed thing. Rather it is a fluid, organic and evolving thing which means different things to different people at different times. Sometimes we have to protect our own cultures, and sometimes we have to challenge them. What we should never do is to use our cultures as an excuse for avoiding doing the right thing.

2.5.3 **Patient factors**

Children and their families might hold back for various reasons including a belief that 'nothing can be done', for fear of burdening carers or because they wish to appear strong. In our experience, children tend to under-report their problems, partly because they fear going to hospital and/or painful procedures, partly because they have got used to living with fear and (perhaps most importantly) partly because they know that difficult discussions can upset their parents, and they do not want to see their parents upset or unhappy. Of course also, some children, especially very young ones, may not have the ability to communicate what they are feeling in words, although of course they try to find other ways.

Occasionally, different carers will be seen with the patient on each visit, and this can cause challenges in communication with the family and child. Likewise, sometimes a sick or dying child may be being cared for by another child which can also cause challenges in communicating the care and treatment plan for the sick child.

2.5.4 **Health worker factors**

These are the factors over which we have most control, and therefore, the most responsibility. When you have read through this section, stand in front of a mirror and ask yourself which factors may apply to you.

2.5.4.1 **Making assumptions**

A common mistake is to make assumptions about what a child and their family are experiencing or feeling. It is easy, for example, to assume that a child who has advanced AIDS or cancer is worried about dying. But he or she might have other very different concerns. An example is a little girl who was apparently frightened about dying. However, by allowing her to talk freely it emerged that she was neither scared of the dying process, nor scared of being dead, nor even of symptoms. What terrified her were worms! She knew she was going to be buried, and she couldn't bear the idea of worms eating her body. It was possible for a local funeral director to arrange for a lead-lined coffin, and after reassurance that she would get one of these, she was a great deal happier.

The important thing is to find out exactly what the child's fears are, before leaping in with solutions. Communication skills should be used to help us find out what the individual child and their family are concerned about. To do this we need to keep an open mind.

2.5.4.2 Distancing

Health workers in Africa often have personal experience of HIV or Cancer. Most have beloved children in their own lives, and the prospect of losing them is sometimes unthinkable. Many have family members who are living with HIV or who have died from AIDS or Cancer, and some may be HIV positive themselves. Caring for individuals who are a constant reminder of our own worst fears, or of family or friends with similar problems, can be very difficult. To cope, sometimes we may avoid caring for such patients. If we cannot avoid caring for them, we use avoidance in a subtly different way: by avoiding difficult conversations. As health workers, we need to develop self-awareness, recognize which kinds of patients 'push our buttons' and work out strategies for coping that don't block us from providing good care (see Chapter 19 – Caring for yourself).

2.5.4.3 Fear of doing harm

It is possible that you could give a child or parent some news that they are not ready to hear, and that could upset them. This happens rarely but in the event that you do say something a child is not ready for, in our experiences the psychological defences of children and their families tend to be subtle enough and strong enough to deal with any clumsy mistakes we have made. Remember that there is good evidence that children know much more than parents and health professionals think, but there is very little evidence that giving children too much information does any long-term harm[33]. Therefore, if in doubt, it is better to give the information than to withhold. If you use the 'WPC Chunk' method (see below), it is very unlikely that you will go wrong.

2.5.4.4 Fear of provoking strong emotions

Anger, crying, denial, depression, hatred and even laughter are some of the emotions and reactions that we associate with the death of a child. Most of us do not enjoy being on the receiving end of these emotions, and it is natural that we try to avoid them.

2.5.4.5 Perception of lack of skills

We all feel that we could use more skills, and never more so than in children's palliative care. We may have been on communication or counselling courses, but not felt that they fully deal with children's palliative care issues. If this is the case, be encouraged that it is very unlikely that you will do any harm by talking to children about difficult issues, and very likely that you will do a lot of good.

2.5.4.6 Sympathetic pain

Of course, we all fear illness and mortality, both for ourselves and for our loved ones. We may still have painful memories and experiences that our professional work can sometimes bring to the surface. We are taught to maintain a professional façade, so fear of losing control and expressing our own emotions can be an even bigger block to communication.

2.5.4.7 **Fear of 'having no solutions'**

This is something that is deeply rooted in health professionals, and we may not even realize that it is there. We feel that we ought to have a cure or a solution for our patients' problems, and we feel that we have failed if we don't. We may have been trained by humiliation, where admitting 'I don't know' to one of our senior's questions was almost a hanging offence. Therefore, in a children's palliative care situation, where we have no cure, where there is no hope of the child's survival, it is not surprising that we feel as if we have failed somehow.

However, the real myth is thinking that we have solutions to life and death in the first place. All of our patients will get sick, and they all will die eventually. If we think as health workers that we have all of the answers, this will make us feel useless and hopeless when we realize that we don't.

With the child, there are many ways that we can help them to feel better physically, emotionally and spiritually. With the parents and family, perhaps things seem a little less obvious, but there are always opportunities for health-workers to comfort, guide, reassure and, most important, create a presence or a rapport that enables healing before and after the death of a child. From the caregiver's point of view, such opportunities are tangible: one can teach parents how to cope, give advice on managing difficult behaviour, prepare the child's loved ones for grief, encourage the family to remain intact and provide a sense of safety and importance for surviving siblings[34,35]. Grieving families can benefit from communicating with their child about impending death[36]. Not communicating with the child about their impending death usually leaves a child feeling extremely isolated and fearful and can cause regrets later on for the parents.

2.6 **Difficult conversations: communicating with children and families in a children's palliative care setting**

It is important for the health worker to be able to connect with the child and family. If a good relationship and rapport has been established, this will help when later handling difficult questions. Some ways of connecting with the child and family include:

◆ *Remember the non-verbals:* Children are absolute experts in non-verbal communication. They have to be as they can't really express themselves any other way for the first few years. They are much better at it than you are, so take great care. They will be watching you, and the way you interact with their family, like hawks. As they get older, they will read as much into what you don't say as into what you do say. Just because you haven't spoken it, it doesn't mean you haven't said it. So, if you or the family is avoiding a thorny issue, remember that the child is likely to have picked up that there is something that is too bad or frightening to talk about. Imagine how that feels.

> Just because you haven't spoken it, it doesn't mean you haven't said it

◆ *Take time:* These conversations take time. If you are feeling rushed, take a deep breath and prepare yourself. It is counterproductive to rush it. Remember the old adage: 'more haste, less speed'.

◆ *Connect:* You will need to try and connect with the child and the parent/family. The child will look at how you communicate with their parent and how the parent responds to you and vice versa. So have an open and friendly manner, take time, shake hands and generally establish ease and rapport with both the child and the family.

- *Look at yourself:* You may have forgotten what the world looks like when you are two feet tall. Try sitting on the floor while the adult world buzzes around you. Believe me, to a child you probably look seriously scary, particularly if you are wearing a white coat, have a stethoscope round your neck or are carrying frightening instruments, boxes or other paraphernalia. So smile, make yourself smaller, get down to their level, crouch up and avoid big, fast, scary movements.

- *Respect space:* Respect the child's personal space. Wait until they come to you, or at least wait to be invited in. Don't be a cheek-pincher, an arm-puncher, a head-patter or a hair-ruffler.

- *Touch:* Once you are allowed closer, touch can be fine, or it can be deeply unwanted. The problem is that, sooner or later, you are going to have to touch if you want to examine, so you need to break the ice at some time. A very gentle touch on the hand, arm or possibly the cheek, can speak volumes to a child.

- *Make the environment child friendly:* Do you have pictures of nasty diseases on your walls? Take them down and replace them with something more soothing. It doesn't have to be Disney. Probably the best is to get the children you see to draw you some pictures or make you some models and stick that on the wall. Are there frightening instruments or equipment on display? Hide them. Do you have any toys or crayons in your room? If not, get some.

- *Ensure the child is comfortable:* It seems sensible, but make sure the child is comfortable (e.g. on mother's knee, on the floor playing with toys, on a bed, etc.). Does she need to be examined on the couch, or will mother's lap do? What is wrong with examining on the floor if the child is playing there happily anyway?

- *Offer regular support and praise:* At every opportunity make sure you say 'well done' or 'good girl', even if it is just for coming into your room without crying. The more you build a child's confidence, the more cooperative he will be.

- *Explain what you are doing:* If you need to undertake procedures that will be painful to the child, explain what you are doing and that it may hurt. Where possible, use distraction techniques or drugs to prevent and/or manage it. Whatever you do, don't be tempted to tell them that it will not hurt because if it does they will lose trust in you.

2.6.1 Understanding awareness

Before we can open the way for difficult discussions to happen, we need to understand that children with life-limiting illnesses can be more or less aware of what is happening and what everyone else knows or doesn't know. The same applies to the child's parents and other family members. These are called 'awareness contexts'[37] and there are four. If you have spent any time in palliative care you will recognize them immediately. Take, for example, the case of a child with HIV/AIDS. The family and health workers might be in one of the following four situations.

Box 2.2 Awareness contexts

1. Closed awareness: the child is not aware of HIV/AIDS and those who know conceal it.
2. Suspected awareness: the child is suspicious that something is wrong but is not certain.
3. Mutual pretence: the child, family and health workers all know but no one talks about it.
4. Open awareness: everyone knows and is open about it.

Very occasionally, children may indicate clearly that they do not want to know, but generally it is much easier for all concerned if children and families are in the 'open awareness' context as communication is much more open, which allows for fears and concerns to be aired and addressed, for better management plans to be negotiated and agreed, and for the child and family to feel more in control (which reduces fear).

Unfortunately, particularly in children's palliative care, a common finding is that child, family and health professionals are stuck in the mutual pretence[38] context. All collude with denial of the impending death, and all (to one extent or another) are 'rewarded' for this mutual pretence. Such rewards might include:

- The child avoids upsetting the parents and this eases the fear of rejection/isolation.
- The parents avoid 'role-conflict': this is the conflict between their role as the child's nurturer/protector with their potential role of bearers of bad news which will be upsetting for the child and other family members.
- The health professional avoids a role-conflict between the assumed role of 'the healer' and the actual role of 'the professional with no solution'.

Unfortunately, although the rewards of pretence and avoidance seem obvious, the problems with such approaches lie just below the surface. Mutual pretence leads to a major conflict between everyone's personal integrity (a wish to tell the truth) and the 'pretence roles' that they have become stuck in. Communication becomes a big problem, care suffers, and the child and family's quality of life is less than it could have been. Everyone loses.

That is not to say that avoidance, collusion and denial are entirely bad things. They are useful and valid coping mechanisms that we all use in many ways. They carry certain benefits for child and family[39]. They are usually done out of love, although sometimes they reflect control, which is arguably less healthy. They allow information to be managed and absorbed in stages. They provide a sense of protecting the child, although they may have the effect of isolating and patronizing the child. It is, superficially at least, easier for the family to cope with practical things if they are not being weighed down by difficult and emotional conversations.

However, there are real risks associated with ongoing denial and collusion. Blocked communication may increase a child's anxiety or depress her mood and can create a 'conspiracy of silence' and distrust. Rather than protecting the child, this may have the effect of isolating and patronizing the child. Just at a time where communication is crucial (to plan, prepare and adapt), communication is blocked. Health workers can feel alienated just when they need to feel connected, and they may even feel frustrated enough to push information when families are not receptive to it.

2.6.2 How to manage denial and collusion

This is an art, not a science, so there are no clear, one-size-fits-all answers. The art lies in being able to balance the risks and the benefits of allowing the denial to continue. In authors' experience, in most cases (particularly where the motivation is love rather than control) collusion and denial tend to melt away as events progress and as people adapt to the situation. Sometimes therefore, if you feel that there is no rush and that time will sort things out, 'masterly inactivity' might be the right option.

However, there are situations where you might need to push a bit. This is particularly the case where things are deteriorating fast and time is not a luxury you have, or where the child is clearly being isolated and upset by the collusion or denial.

In this case, the key message is that you need to do the following:

◆ *Investigate:* find out how much each person in the family wants to know by asking them.

◆ *Think:* is this the right moment, or would you be better off coming back? Do you know what forms of words you will use? If not practice. You wouldn't go into an exam without revision, or stand on stage without rehearsal.

◆ *Reflect back:* to all parties that you appreciate all the love and care that is being shown, and that you recognize that everyone is acting as they are, purely to prevent others being hurt. But also explain that, by not allowing communication, they may be inadvertently hurting their child. Use your own experiences or the evidence to back this up.

◆ *Explain the facts:*
  • In most cases, what parents think they are hiding, the child already knows.
  • By not communicating, parents are preventing their child from sharing their fears and concerns and are therefore preventing the child from being comforted.
  • That children are in fact very resilient and capable of dealing with bad news.
  • That, conversely, children do not deal well with feeling isolated or rejected.
  • That open communication tends to reduce anxiety all round, improve relationships and allows better communication, better planning and better care.
  • The evidence is that parents who sense that their child is aware of his or her imminent death later regret not having talked with their child (in fact in a study of 147 parents who had lost their children, not one regretted having talked about it)[40].

◆ *Balance up the pros and cons:* If you get stuck between a child who wants to know and parent(s) who refuse to allow him to be told, you need to learn the art of balancing several competing factors:
  • The risks of breaking the collusion versus the risks of holding it
  • The rights of the child versus the rights of the parents
  • The law of the land.

Box 2.3 Communication: Case Scenario 1

You are looking after Albert, a 10-year-old with advanced Burkitt's lymphoma which has failed to respond to treatment. His family cannot afford second line treatment. You and the parents both know he is going to die. The parents ask you not to tell him and forbid you from answering his questions about it. What do you do?

2.6.3 How to break bad news

This is an essential skill for anyone working in children's palliative care. It is at least as important as knowing which drugs to use for symptom control. It can be very hard, but it is crucial to enable preparation and planning for all concerned. Remember, it is our professional duty to inform children and their families about the benefits and risks of all of their treatments.

> To fail to try to obtain informed consent from parents and older children for our plans is to act negligently and unethically. Where the children are not able to give informed consent (e.g. when they are too young) informed assent should be obtained from them.

In resource-poor settings, where patients might be spending much needed money on pointless treatments and investigations, it is particularly important to make sure everyone is aware of what the real situation is.

> There may be good reasons why children and families don't want to hear the truth, but there are no good reasons why health professionals should be prepared to hide it.

Ideally, children and their families should not be chasing pointless investigations, taking useless medication, harbouring false hopes or sitting needlessly in a hospital bed when they could be at home.

It is *ok* to find it hard, we are only human. It is even *ok* to admit we are not up to it, but in this case it is our duty to ask for help from another health worker who is able to break difficult news.

2.6.3.1 The six-step approach for breaking bad news

There are six key steps to breaking bad news:

(1) setting the scene;

(2) finding out how much the child and family know;

(3) finding out how much the child and family want to know;

(4) sharing the information (use the WPC approach – see below);

(5) responding to the child's and family's feelings;

(6) planning and following through.

2.6.3.2 Setting the scene

Armies practise and train for battle, actors rehearse before they go on stage and we too should prepare ourselves in advance. To start with, work out how you are going to set about it. Make sure that you have fully grasped everything you can about the patient's condition and management to date, and that you have all the information you might need. Try to anticipate the kind of questions you might be asked (to do this, think about the kind of questions you would ask in their situation). Also, don't be embarrassed to practise speaking phrases and sentences in advance. Don't just think them, actually practise them. Get your mouth round them and see how it feels. You will feel more confident if you do. There are some useful phrases outlined in Section 2.8.

Work out in advance where the breaking of the news should happen and who should be there. Every situation will be different. Unlike with adult palliative care, where you may only be dealing with one person (the patient), in children's palliative care, there are normally many people who might need to be involved. If you suspect that the different people involved in the care of the child have different levels of knowledge or are approaching the situation very differently, it might be appropriate to see them separately. However, you need to make sure that you get to all the key decision makers in the same time frame, or you will risk causing tensions and conflict. It may or may not be appropriate for the child to be there. Often, and particularly with smaller children, parents tend to prefer having the news broken to them first, and then taking part in breaking the bad news to the child themselves.

2.6.3.3 Finding out how much the child and family knows

Try and find out how much each party to the conversation knows. Ask each one individually and try to prevent others blocking or interrupting. Take time, allow silence and space. When they speak, reflect back what they have said and be completely sure that you have understood exactly what they know before moving on to the next one.

2.6.3.4 Finding out how much the child and family want to know

This is the time to find out how much denial the child or family members wish (consciously or subconsciously) to use. If they signal that they are not ready, back off and review later on. Don't push information if they don't want it. To try and work this out, you can use questions such as *'Would you like me to tell you more about your child's condition?'*

2.6.3.5 Sharing the information

A good way is the 'WPC Chunk' method. WPC stands for *'warn'*, *'pause'* and *'check'*. It is simple and it works. Start off by mentally breaking the news into *chunks*. For example, if a child has a rapidly enlarging mediastinal lymphoma, there are actually several *chunks* of very bad news that need to be imparted:

- That he will die.
- That he will die soon.
- That he might suffer with unpleasant symptoms unless carefully managed (e.g. upper airway obstruction, dysphagia, haematemesis).
- That the family will need to learn what to do if any of these eventualities arise.

Very few people, if any, would be able to absorb all of these chunks of bad news in one go. People automatically cut out after a certain level of pain. Patients often describe hearing and remembering nothing after the first bit of bad news is broken. You might want to get it all over and done with, to get the bad news out in one go. That's understandable, but it won't work.

So, partly from compassion, and partly from pragmatism, we need to go very gently, and very slowly and at the pace that the person receiving the news wants to go. At the first sign of refusal, back off until he or she is ready to continue.

Box 2.4 The WPC chunk method of breaking bad news

1. Decide which *'chunk'* of bad news you are going to try to break.

2. **Warn:** This gives the person a chance to prepare and brace himself or herself. It probably also helps them to absorb the difficult information. *E.g. "I would like to talk to you about something that you will probably find difficult."*

3. **Pause:** This gives the person a chance to decide whether or not he/she still wants to go ahead, and also to react. If they assent (either verbally or non-verbally) go ahead and break the first chunk of bad news.

4. **Check back:** Ask what they have understood and correct or reinforce. This allows you to ensure that they have correctly understood you, and also acts to embed the news properly in the person's memory. This is important because, after traumatic events, people often forget what happened and what was said.

5. Decide whether they are ready to move on, and then break the next chunk of bad news using the same method.

2.6.3.6 Responding to the patient's feelings

Now just sit and wait. The child and family may react emotionally, calmly, rationally, irrationally, powerfully or numbly. Whatever the reaction, don't panic but stay calm and allow it to wash over you. However strong it is, it will fade and pass as long as you don't inflame it. Be gentle, use appropriate touch and show through your non-verbal communication that you have all the time in the world (even if you don't). Most importantly, whatever the response is, *validate it*. You might say something like 'it's OK to be angry/upset' or 'many people find it difficult to speak after hearing news like that', and so on.

Once the response settles, you should repeat the process until one of the following four things happen:

- There is no more bad news to break.
- They signal that they have had enough.
- You get the feeling that they have stopped hearing or absorbing.
- You feel that you personally cannot do anymore (which is fine, as long as you make sure that you arrange to come back).

2.6.3.7 Planning and following through

Once all the news is out, you have allowed time for individuals to react and express their emotions, and you have validated them, move from listening mode into a slightly more active mode. Begin to identify options, suggest sources of support and start negotiating management plans for the various problems and issues that you have identified. Whatever else you do, make sure that the family is able to make contact with you or a colleague over the next few days.

2.6.4 Disclosure of life-limiting illness (such as HIV/AIDS)

It is very hard to disclose to a child that he or she has a life-limiting disease. Disclosure of HIV status is a particular challenge due to the complex nature of the disease and the fact that the mother is likely to be the source of the infection. Disclosure of a positive HIV status can, and often does, lead to anxiety, guilt, anger, blame and stigma in the family.

There are many reasons why parents may not want their children to know that they are HIV positive. One of these is that the child is likely to want to know where they got the disease from and how their mother also got the disease, thus bringing up issues around sex that the family may not want to talk about. Parents might be worried about being seen as promiscuous or having to admit to the child that they had sex with someone who gave it to them. Some of the reasons given for not disclosing HIV status to a child include:

- to protect a child from social rejection,
- to protect him/her from fear or depression,
- parental sense of guilt or shame,
- parental fears of rejection by the child[41,42].

Studies have shown that children and adolescents who know what their diagnosis is are more likely to adhere to their treatment regimens and to be involved in discussions with regard to the management of their illness[43]. Benefits of disclosure also include:

- more open involvement in medical care decisions,
- increased opportunities for peer support,
- increased trust in health care providers and caregivers[44].

Nevertheless, informing children of their diagnosis and answering the questions that ensue are difficult tasks. Five stages of disclosing HIV diagnosis have been developed[45]:

Stage 1: Information gathering and trust building.

Stage 2: Education.

Stage 3: Determining when the time is right for disclosure.

Stage 4: The actual disclosure event.

Stage 5: Monitoring post-disclosure coping and managing disclosure-related bumps in the road.

Stage 1: Information gathering and trust building

Establishing a relationship with the health worker allows the family to begin to develop confidence and trust that the health worker has their child's best interest in mind. Prior to disclosure, the health worker should gather as much information about the child and the family as he or she can and in particular about their understanding of the child's disease. Comfort in sharing intimate details of beliefs and experiences may vary among family members and individuals comprising the team.

Stage 2: Education

The educational process involves an ongoing assessment of the knowledge and attitudes of the caregiver and child, as well as an ongoing sharing of facts and information. The goal here is to teach in small steps, continually assess readiness and always move towards the objective of full disclosure to the child.

Stage 3: Determining when the time is right for disclosure

A variety of factors may prompt the need to disclose a child's HIV status sooner than anticipated, including changes in the health status of the child or parent, who may be infected with HIV; a recent hospitalization; changes in medication that necessitate an increase in pill burden; or the need to begin a more difficult or risky medical regimen. Children frequently ask difficult questions when changes occur in their health, their medical regimen or their social situation (such as the illness of a parent). In addition, the death of parents or grandparents and other life-altering events may precipitate the need to disclose the child's HIV status.

A variety of factors can prompt caregivers to make the decision to disclose. These factors include questions asked by a child that suggest that he or she already knows; fear that a child will not be compliant with medication; changes in growth and development, such as reaching adolescence; wanting a child to be able to participate in specialized camping programmes for children with HIV and noticing a child's increasing interest in intimacy with opposite-sex peers.

Certainly, caregiver and patient autonomy and their right to confidentiality and privacy must be respected. Health care providers must take caregiver autonomy seriously and not merely endure it. Thus, lines of communication must be kept open and health care providers must perfect the art of listening well so that they can hear unspoken messages or discern 'hidden agendas' long before any points of crisis occur. This open communication also gives health care professionals a greater understanding of and (it is hoped) a greater respect for caregiver needs and caregiver ideas about what is best for a given child and his or her family.

Stage 4: The actual disclosure event

If stages 1 through 3 have been followed, the process of disclosure has been occurring in small steps for many months or years. In fact, each clinic visit can be viewed as an opportunity for movement towards diagnosis disclosure. Whenever possible, it is important to allow the caregiver/family to decide when and how to fully disclose to the child, but the health care provider can certainly offer suggestions about disclosure.

Some caregivers prefer to do the actual talking at the clinic, taking the primary role with the health care provider as backup/support, and some may elect to have the health care provider serve as the primary communicator. Others prefer to disclose the diagnosis to their child privately at home. Decisions regarding the general planning of disclosure (setting, timing, who will be there) can be delineated during one visit and, if desired by the caregivers, implemented at the next visit.

Because children's responses to the diagnosis vary considerably, it is important to prepare the caregiver for some of the possible responses that his or her child may have. It is common for the child's responses to occur at home after the clinic visit when the child's diagnosis was discussed. Some children will become very upset (angry or sad), whereas others will not want to discuss the issue. Some children show acceptance and understanding because they finally know why they must take so many medications and come for doctor visits so frequently, and why they have been so ill.

Stage 5: Monitoring post-disclosure coping and managing disclosure-related bumps in the road

It is important to monitor the impact of disclosure. Monitoring can occur in a variety of ways, for example by direct observation of a child, direct questioning regarding how a child feels about learning his or her diagnosis is also a valuable monitoring tool. Informal and casual checking with identified friends or other family members can serve as corroboration of clinic observations and the child's self-report. It is also common for children to have increased fears after learning their diagnosis. All children should be encouraged to discuss their fears and misconceptions so that they can be addressed in a sensitive manner.

Box 2.5 Communication: Case Scenario 2

Case study:

Jenny is a bright 13-year-old. She has presented with Kaposi's sarcoma and you have found her to be HIV positive. Both parents died of AIDS some time back and she has been living with her grandmother, who has not told Jenny how her parents died. Neither does Jenny know she might be HIV positive. You need to disclose all of this to her as you wish to start her on chemotherapy and she needs to be involved in giving consent. How would you go about breaking all of this bad news to her?

NB. If you can, role-play this study with a colleague or friend. It will be much more helpful to you. Allow your colleague to be the child.

2.6.5 How to manage anger

Anger is one of the hardest emotions to cope with and it can be quite frightening. However, it is quite normal for a child (particularly an adolescent) to feel angry about their situation. Expression of anger might also be helpful, so children should be encouraged to express their anger in a safe way such as stamping feet, tearing up paper, making mud balls and throwing them as far as possible or kicking a ball[46].

It is important, however, to remember that someone being angry *at* you isn't necessarily angry *with* you. They are probably just angry, sad and scared at the whole situation. If you find yourself in the midst of a major anger reaction, it is often helpful to remind yourself that nobody can maintain anger for any length of time if they are alone. Anger needs an audience. So, the best thing that you can do is to

◆ minimize yourself and your ego

◆ stay safe: keep a safe distance, close to an exit and leave at the first hint of impending violence

◆ appear open and non-threatening

◆ take a deep breath and allow the anger to wash over you – it will stop

◆ listen, listen, listen

◆ stay quiet

◆ don't interrupt or argue

◆ once the anger has dissipated, cautiously respond by reflecting back what you heard to be the main causes and focus for the anger

◆ legitimize it where possible

◆ ensure that everyone (including you) is safe. Don't put anyone in a risky situation, and get help if you think a risk is developing

◆ apologize as much as possible (even if you are apologizing for something that is outside your control)

◆ don't hold onto it after, but debrief as soon as possible.

2.7 **Dealing with difficult questions**

Of all the areas to do with communication in children's palliative care, being faced with difficult questions is one that health workers find most difficult and worrying. Children can and do use inopportune moments to ask their questions, and the idea of being floored by a difficult and painful one when we are neither ready nor prepared is not one that any of us cherishes.

Children don't always 'do' adult niceties. Questions from a child can be very blunt and to the point. Sometimes they can be frankly heart-rending. Chances are, they will ask when you least expect it and are least prepared for it.

However, the fact is, if you do manage to connect with a child, he or she will start asking you questions. Question-asking is a sign of trust, so we should be grateful for it. It means you are doing your job properly. If he or she is prepared to trust you with their concerns and fears, there is a very good chance that you can do something extremely helpful and worthwhile, which is to put their mind at rest and help them prepare for their death. After all, that is what children's palliative care is about.

2.7.1 **Answering difficult questions: useful tips**

Here are some tips that should get you through most situations.

◆ **Answer questions with questions** until you are sure that you are on the right wavelength. Remember, children and adults think differently and see the world differently. So, for example, if a dying child asks: 'What will happen with me?', don't launch immediately into death, God and heaven. They may well want to talk about that, but it might be something much more mundane. Answer their question with your own. For example ask: 'That's a good question. But, before I answer, what do you think might happen to you?' Once, I was answered with 'I think I might miss dinner because I have to wait for my medicines to arrive'. So, try and find out what is on the child's mind, otherwise you will probably end up answering the wrong question altogether! However, don't use your own questions to prevaricate once the child's question is clear. They will spot it and you will lose their trust.

- **Use clear language** appropriate to the child's age. Don't use jargon. Remember children may not even know some quite basic anatomical words (like 'chest' for example). Be very aware of the risks in using abstract language (e.g. 'eternal rest') or religious (e.g. 'gone to heaven'). Remember young children think concretely.

- **Talk clearly about what might happen after death:** Adults use a whole raft of euphemisms and abstract concepts to talk about death and after-death. These can be extremely confusing to children, and you may inadvertently cause significant distress if you do not watch what you say. A child who is asked if he wants to see his brother's body may wonder why he cannot see the head too. A child who has always been warned about the dangers of fire might be very scared at the idea of cremation. A child who has been told their mother is in heaven might worry that they do not visit or write. A child who has been told that their father can see them from heaven may be worried that the father will be cross if he sees them do something naughty in secret.

- **Give simple, clear and honest answers to questions:** If you do get into a conversation about death, be completely honest. Children tend not to ask adults until they have exhausted all other possible lines of enquiry (particularly other children, TV, books, overheard snippets of adult conversation and their own imaginations). The chances are that a child will only ask when one of two situations arises. One, they already know the answer and want you to confirm it. Two, they have a confused or worrying idea of what might happen and they need you to explain. Either way, you need to be honest, clear and straightforward. If you do not, you will either lose their trust or they will go away confused and worried. Neither option is good.

- **Don't go off on tangents, and don't use too many words**. More importantly, avoid rhetorical flourishes and metaphors. If you say his body will be buried and he will have a head-stone, don't blame him for thinking that after he dies you will separate his head from his body, turn his head into stone and bury the rest. If you describe death as eternal sleep, don't get mad when they won't go to bed. If you say she will go to heaven when she dies, don't blame her for thinking that she is going to be sent away from home, away from her family, away from her school to join a lot of dead strangers in a place she doesn't know. Use simple life imagery (e.g. when people die they do not breathe, eat, talk, think or feel any more; when dogs die they do not bark or run anymore; dead flowers do not grow or bloom any more).

- **Check back after explanations:** Once you have finished speaking, always get them to repeat their version of what you have just said. It is amazing how often children get the wrong end of the stick. Or perhaps, more accurately, it's amazing how often we give children the wrong end of the stick.

- **Be prepared to say you don't know:** Children live in a whole world that they don't know about. They are much more comfortable than adults about not knowing answers to things. Contrary to popular belief, they don't expect adults to know everything (even though they never seem to stop asking questions!). If you don't know, say so. You will gain trust. If you go on to help them find out the answer, you will also win a great deal of appreciation. Both will be very helpful as you get closer to the end and you need their cooperation and trust.

◆ **Don't be scared to show emotion**, but if you do, make sure that you explain it. On the whole, children are familiar with and comfortable with emotion, just as long as they understand where it is coming from and that it is not because of anything they have done wrong or might be punished for. If anyone (yourself included) gets upset during the consultation, make sure that you take time to explain that 'Mummy is upset because' or 'Daddy is feeling sad because'. Showing emotion can give permission for others to show emotion without risk that the child may wrongly interpret it as upset with, or because of, the child him/herself.

Box 2.6 Communication: Case Scenario 3

Case study:
William is a 6-year-old boy who has advanced HIV/AIDS and who has developed resistance to ARTs. His prognosis is very poor. One day, while playing, he asks you 'What will happen to me when I die'?
How do you answer?

NB. Role-play this scene if you can.

2.8 Useful phrases

Some useful phrases to help when communicating with children include:

◆ **To start a 2-way dialogue:**
'How are things going for you?'

◆ **Finding out how much the child knows:**
'Have you ever heard of XXX? Do you know what it means? Can you tell me what you know about it?'

◆ **Finding out how much the patient wants to know:**
'Some children like to know all there is to know, and some children prefer not to know. Which one are you?'

◆ **Warning that you are about to break bad news:**
'I need to talk to you about something. You might find it a bit difficult or sad. Can I talk to you about it? When can I talk to you about it?'

◆ **Checking back:**
'Most children would find it difficult to understand all of that in one go. It would be very helpful if you could tell me what you think I just said. That way I can make sure you have understood properly.'

◆ **Chunking:**
'I have said all I need to say about that now. I expect you are quite tired now? When you are ready, there is another thing I need to discuss. We don't have to talk about it now, but we can if you feel up to it. Shall we go on now or would you like to talk more later?'

◆ **Responding to patient/family feelings:**
'Could you tell me what you are feeling after hearing that?'

◆ **Planning and follow-through:**

'It's really important that you and I agree exactly what is going to happen next. Will you help me come up with a good plan?'

◆ **Dealing with denial:**

'You say you think that you will get better soon, but is there ever a time, even just for a few moments, when you are not so sure?'

◆ **Collusion:**

'I can see you would rather I didn't discuss that with XX. Can you share with me why you feel like that' or *'You must be finding it hard coping with all of that on your own?'*

◆ **Negotiating access to the child after collusion has been raised:**

'Perhaps we could work together to plan how much we can tell XX, and to discuss what effects this might have on him/her.'

◆ **Answering a difficult question and playing for time until you fully understand the question behind the question:**

'That's an interesting question. I wonder why do you ask that now?'

Or

'That's a tricky one. Let's talk about it. What do you think the answer might be?' or *'I wonder how it looks to you?'*

◆ **Admitting that you don't know:**

'I know you really want to know the answer, and if I knew it I promise I would tell you. But I am afraid I honestly don't know at the moment.'

Or

'I really wish I could answer that, but in all honesty I just do not know.'

◆ **Talking about death and the after-life:**

'Different people have all sorts of different beliefs about what happens after someone dies. We know that someone who has died cannot come back, call us or write to us. Being dead isn't like being in another village.'

Or

'These are some of the different things that people believe/I believe. I wonder what you believe? Shall we talk about it?'

Or

'Grown-ups use some strange words and sayings when they talk about death. That is because they find it hard to talk about. This can be very confusing for children, and children can often get the wrong idea or get upset because of what grown-ups say. Has anyone ever said anything to you about dying or what happens afterwards that you have found strange or upsetting?'

2.9 Involving siblings and other children

When a child is very sick and dying, and after their death, it is important that health workers are aware of other children who have been or are involved in their life. For example, it is important to support the siblings of children who are dying. Siblings will also experience the pain of seeing their brother or sister going through such an illness and dying and may well feel responsible or guilty for their death. They too will therefore need care and support during this time. Other groups of children who will be affected by the child's death are those in their community and school – time may need to be spent with these children allowing them to talk through some of their feelings about the death of the child. Much of what has been discussed in this chapter will also be relevant when communicating with siblings and friends of the child who is dying.

2.10 Young carers

As has been mentioned several times in this chapter, on some occasions the child who is sick and dying will be cared for by other young carers as the family unit may have broken down through illness or other reasons. These young people have therefore had to take on the responsibility of their parents and yet may not have the practical experience or emotional maturity to cope with all of this, so they will need special support in dealing with the situation. For many, they may feel guilty that they are not able to cope or to bring in money, food, etc. and care for their sibling. This may mean that they have little time for themselves, are unable to go to school and have little time for their friends, all of which may leave them lonely and isolated. Health workers will need to be sensitive in the way that they help and support them, and be aware that whilst they may be taking on the roles of adults, they are still children and so, the health worker needs to communicate with them in an age appropriate manner[47].

2.11 Communication: questions for you

(1) Reflect on your own practice and list the main barriers to communication with children that affect you.

(2) List those things you will do to make your communication and practice more child-friendly.

(3) Here are some common 'difficult' questions in children's palliative care. Think about them and work out what you would say. Don't just go through it in your head. Stand in front of a mirror and try getting the words out. Imagine the worst possible conversation and try speaking from both sides (child and health worker).

◆ Will it hurt when I die?

◆ Where will I go when I die?

◆ What will happen to my brother when I die?

◆ Will mummy be sad when I die?

Notes

1   Amery, J. & Lapwood, S. (2004). A study into the educational needs of children's hospice doctors: a descriptive quantitative and qualitative survey. *Palliative Medicine*, *18*(8), 727–33.

2   Amery, J., Rose, C. & Byarugaba, C. (2007). Implementation of a children's palliative care service at Hospice Africa Uganda. Abstract and oral presentation at Conference of The African Palliative Care Association. In *Proceedings of The Conference of The African Palliative Care Association Conference 2007 (to be published)*. 2nd African Palliative Care Conference Proceedings, Nairobi, September 2007. Available online at http://www.Apca.Co.Ug/Conferences&Workshops/Index.htm.

3   Amery, J., Rose, C. & Byarugaba, C. (2007). Children's palliative care educational needs assessment of health professionals at Hospice Africa Uganda. Abstract and poster presentation at Conference of The African Palliative Care Association. In *Proceedings of The Conference of The African Palliative Care Association Conference 2007* (to be published). 2nd African Palliative Care Conference Proceedings, Nairobi, September 2007. Available online at http://www.Apca.Co.Ug/Conferences&Workshops/Index.htm.

4   Amery, J., Rose, C. & Byarugaba, C. (2007). Development of a modular children's palliative care course for health professionals in Sub-Saharan Africa. Abstract and poster presentation at Conference of The African Palliative Care Association. In *Proceedings of The Conference of The African Palliative Care Association Conference 2007* (to be published). 2nd African Palliative Care Conference Proceedings, Nairobi. September 2007. Available online at http://www.Apca.Co.Ug/Conferences&Workshops/Index.htm.

5   Meryn, S. (1998). Improving doctor–patient communication: Not an option, but a necessity (Editorials). *BMJ*, *316*, 1922–30.

6 Faulkner, K. (1993). Children's understanding of death. In A. Armstrong-Dailey & S.Z. Goltzer (Eds.). *Hospice Care For Children*. (pp. 9–21). Oxford University Press, New York.

7 Bluebond-Langner, M. (1980). *The Private Worlds of Dying Children*. Princeton Paperbacks Series. Princeton University Press, Princeton.

8 Kreicbergs, Valdimarsdóttir, Onelöv, Henter & Steineck. (2004). Talking about death with children who have severe malignant disease. *New England Journal of Medicine, 351*, 1175–86.

9 Field, Marilyn, J. & Behrman, Richard E. (Eds.) (2001). Communication, goal setting, and care planning. *When Children Die: Improving Palliative and End-of-Life Care for Children and Their Families*. The National Academies Press, Washington.

10 Bikaako-Kajura, W., Luyirika, E., David W. Purcell et al. (2006). Disclosure of HIV status and adherence to daily drug regimens among HIV-infected children in Uganda. *AIDS And Behavior, 10*, 85–93.

11 Kai, J. (1996). Parents' difficulties and information needs in coping with acute illness in preschool children: A qualitative study. *BMJ, 313*(7063), 987–90.

12 Cole & Cole (2001). Prominent bio-social behavioural shifts in development. *Training Manual: Children And HIV/AIDS*. Mildmay International, London.

13 Erikson. (1993). Communicating with children: Helping children in distress. In Richman (Ed) *Save The Children Development Manual 2*. Save The Children, UK.

14 Freud. (1993). Communicating with children. Helping children in distress. In Richman (Ed) *Save The Children Development Manual 2*. Save The Children, UK.

15 Kohlberg. (2001). *Training Manual Children And HIV/AIDS*. Mildmay International, London.

16 Piaget. (1993). Communicating with Children. Helping children in distress. In Richman (Ed) *Save The Children Development Manual 2*. Save The Children, UK.

17 Bluebond Langer. (2006). Children's views on death. In Goldman, Hain & Liben (Eds.). *Oxford Textbook of Palliative Care for Children* (1st Edition). Oxford University Press, New York.

18 Adapted From: Maternal-Child HIV Training Course. AIDS Research & Family Care Clinic. Coast Province General Hospital, Mombasa, Kenya. August, 2001.

19 Moh Zimbabwe. In Tindyebwa, D., Kayita, J., Musoke, P., et al. (Eds.). *African Network for Care of Children Affected by HIVAIDS (ANECCA) Handbook on Paediatric AIDS in Africa*. (Revised Edition 2006). Available online at www.Anecca.org.

20 Joan Marston. (2006). Loss, grief, and bereavement in children. In Gwyther, Merriman, Mpanga, Sebuyira & Schietinger (Eds.). *A Clinical Guide to Supportive and Palliative Care for HIV/AIDS in Sub-Saharan Africa*. Foundation for Hospices in Sub-Saharan Africa. Available online at www.Fhssa.org.

21 Bluebond-Langner, M. (1980). *The Private Worlds of Dying Children*. Princeton Paperbacks Series. Princeton University Press, Princeton.

22 Bluebond-Langner, M. (1980). *The Private Worlds of Dying Children*. Princeton Paperbacks Series. Princeton University Press, Princeton.

23 Himelstein, B.P., Hilden, J.M., Boldt, A.M. & Weissman, D. (2004). Pediatric Palliative Care. *New England Journal of Medicine, 350*, 1752–62.

24 Zimbabwean Ministry of Health. (2006). *Palliative Care for Children: A Training Manual for Communities in Zimbabwe*.

25 Zimbabwean Ministry of Health. (2006). *Palliative Care for Children: A Training Manual for Communities in Zimbabwe*.

26 Zimbabwean Ministry of Health. (2006). *Palliative Care for Children: A Training Manual for Communities in Zimbabwe*.

27 Amery, J. & Lapwood, S. (2004). The Educational Needs of Children's Hospice Doctors in the UK. *Palliative Care*, September.

28 Amery, J., Rose, C., Byarugaba, C. & Agupio, G. (2008). *Educational Needs of Health Professionals in Uganda and Subsequent Children's Palliative Care Course Development and Evaluation*. Conference Proceedings – Children's Palliative Care Course Development and Evaluation. Speaking of Dying: What Are We Saying? 4th International Cardiff Conference on Paediatric palliative care.

29 CDC. 1999a. Achievements in public health. (1900–1999) Control of infectious diseases. *Morbidity and mortality weekly report,* July 30, 1999, 48(29);621–9. (also appeared in *Journal of the American Medical Association, 282*(11): 1029–32, 1999.) [Available online].

30 Ariès, Philippe. (1974). *Western Attitudes toward Death: From the Middle Ages to the Present.* (Trans. Patricia. M. Ranum). Johns Hopkins University Press, Baltimore

31 Malcolm A. Indepth section: American attitudes toward death. *The Journal of Popular Culture, 14*(Issue 4) 629–31.

32 Hayslip, B., Peveto, C.A. (2000). *Cultural Changes in Attitudes Toward Death, Dying, and Bereavement.* Springer Publishing Company.

33 Kreicbergs, Valdimarsdóttir, Onelöv, Henter & Steineck. (2004). Talking about death with children who have severe malignant disease. *New England Journal of Medicine,* Volume *351,* 1175–86.

34 Howell, D. (1993). The role of the primary physician. In A. Armstrong-Dailey & S.Z. Goltzer (Eds.) *Hospice Care for Children.* (pp. 172–88). Oxford University Press, New York.

35 Wolfe, L. (2004). Should parents speak with a dying child about impending death? *New England Journal of Medicine, 351,* 1175–86.

36 Faulkner, K. (1993). Children's understanding of death. In A. Armstrong-Dailey & S.Z. Goltzer (Eds.) *Hospice Care For Children.* (pp. 9–21). Oxford University Press, New York.

37 Glaser & Strauss. (1965). *Awareness And Dying.* Aldine, Chicago.

38 Bluebond-Langner, M. (1980). *The Private Worlds of Dying Children.* Princeton University Press, Princeton Paperbacks.

39 Regnard, C. (2004). *Helping The Patient With Advanced Disease: A Workbook In Current Learning In Palliative Care (CLIP)* No. 8: *Collusion And Denial.* Radcliffe Medical Press, Oxford. Available online at www.Radcliffe-Oxford.com.

40 Ulrika Kreicbergs, R.N., Valdimarsdóttir, U., Onelöv, E., Jan-Inge Henter & Steineck, G. (2004).Talking about death with children who have severe malignant disease. *New England Journal of Medicine, 351,* 1175–86.

41 Davis, J.K. & Shah, K. (1997). Bioethical aspects of HIV infection in children. *Clinical Pediatrics, 36*(10), 573–79.

42 Weiner, W.J. & Figueroa, C. (1998). *Personality and Social Psychology Bulletin, 24*(6), 563–74.

43 Bikaako-Kajura, W., Luyirika, E., Purcell, D. W., et al. (2006). Disclosure of HIV status and adherence to daily drug regimens among HIV-infected children in Uganda. *AIDS And Behavior, 10* **Suppl 1** (7), 85–93.

44 Davis, J.K. & Shah, K. (1997). Bioethical aspects of HIV infection in children. *Clinical Pediatrics, 36*(10), 573–79.

45 Doyle, D. and Woodruff, R. (2008). *Ethics Module: The IAHPC Manual of Palliative Care* (2nd Edition). IAHPC Press. Houston, USA.

46 Zimbabwean Ministry of Health. (2006). *Palliative Care for Children: A Training Manual for Communities in Zimbabwe.*

47 Zimbabwean Ministry of Health. (2006). *Palliative Care for Children: A Training Manual for Communities in Zimbabwe.*

Chapter 3

Play and development

Sue Boucher and Justin Amery

Key points

- Play is the single most important way that children learn about, grow confident with and manage the stresses of living in their world, providing developmental stimulation, distraction, exploration, socialisation and entertainment.

- As a result of their illness and circumstances, children with life-limiting illnesses are more vulnerable to developing learning disabilities and learning problems.

- Yet, because of their poor health and institutionalization, children with life-limiting illnesses are more likely than other children to miss out on play opportunities even though they need play to help them cope and come to terms with their illness.

- Despite having a limited life expectancy, children with a life-limiting illness have the right to develop to their full potential through a well-planned programme of focused stimulation.

- Even the sickest child can be helped to play.

- All children must therefore have the time and place to play, and painful procedures must not be carried out in play areas. Normal activities such as school, hobbies and visits by friends should be encouraged wherever possible.

3.1 Introduction

Anything that disrupts or restricts the normal social relationships in a family situation will critically endanger the development of a young child on all levels. Most of the children with whom you will come in contact with in children's palliative care will have suffered varying degrees of disruption and restriction to their normal family situations – either as a result of bereavement, their own life-limiting illness or that of a parent or sibling, poor nutrition or simple poverty, making them seriously at risk for developmental delays in a number of areas.

Health workers have an enormous responsibility (and a tremendous opportunity) to make a profound difference in the life and the development of children simply by playing and having fun. Isn't that a wonderful idea? Yet most health workers feel anxious about playing with children and lack confidence in how to go about it. This chapter aims to put that right, and enable readers to feel free and able to encourage and facilitate play even in the most resource poor settings.

3.2 **Child development and the importance of stimulation**

3.2.1 **Child development**

There is no scope in this book to deal fully with the theories of child development, but it is important for anyone working with children to understand that all of us – children and adults – develop as we get older. We also develop along different lines. Different theorists have described lines of physical, perceptual, cognitive, linguistic, social, emotional, moral and spiritual development.

For example, Piaget[1] describes various stages of cognitive development:

- Birth to six weeks: development of reflexes (e.g. sucking, eye tracking and palmar grasping), and then the development of these reflexes into voluntary actions (e.g. reflex grasping into intentional grasping).

- Six weeks to four months: development of habits (e.g. repeating passing their hand before their eyes).

- Four to nine months: development of coordination (e.g. intentional grasping) and repetition of the actions (e.g. hitting a mirror), a sense of object permanence (i.e. understanding that things still exist even if they cannot be seen).

- Nine to twelve months: development of logic, understanding of the link between means and ends of an action and the deliberate planning of steps to meet an objective.

- Twelve to eighteen months: discovery of new means to meet new goals and the beginning of insight, or true creativity.

- Toddler stage: The begining of the use of symbols (of which probably the most significant is language – words are actually symbols), which also enables memory and imagination. Thinking is egocentric, nonlogical and nonreversible. Self-control and autonomy begin to develop (the terrible twos), as do exploration, risk taking and experimentation.

- Pre-school stage: Broadened social horizons, greater engagement with others, development of fantasy and pretend play, eagerness for adventure and creativity and the development of responsibility.

- Childhood: Development of logic, systematic manipulation of symbols related to concrete objects, operational thinking (i.e. actions are reversible), the use of tools, ability to make things, use tools and acquisition of practical skills.

- Adolescence: Formation of personal and social identity[2], discovery of moral purpose, development of abstract concepts and formal reasoning.

More specific details of what happens at different stages can be found in Appendix 1. These charts can be very helpful as general indicators, but must not be understood in a fixed way. Development is an extremely fluid and dynamic thing. Tables and boxes cannot capture this fluidity, but they can be useful for illustrating the general direction and speed of flow.

However, for the purposes of this book, the important things to realize are as follows:

- We need to understand the principles of child development and what this means for our practise: Children are not simply 'mini-adults'. They see, feel and experience the world in a different way; use different thought processes to interpret it; and communicate and act differently to adults. If we don't understand this, we will find it very hard to understand children or be understood by them.

- Each child needs to be assessed and understood as an individual. Children can develop at different rates down different developmental lines; one child might develop quickly with physical and language skills, but not as quickly with intellectual skills. A child might be quite 'bright' cognitively, but have limited social skills. Therefore, we should not assume that an 'advanced' child is advanced in all areas, or that a 'slow' child is slow in all areas, nor should we ever label them as such.

◆ We must not pre-judge a child's development: Child development is not fixed but context dependent. A child with more stimulation in a particular area is likely to develop faster down that 'developmental line' than others. That is why children who have more experience of illness and death often have advanced understanding in that area. Therefore, we should not pre-judge a child's understanding on the basis of developmental charts.

◆ Tables often highlight what a child *cannot* do. Good health workers focus on what a child *can* do. Beware of focussing on tables and box checking. Focus on the child in front of you.

3.2.2 Critical learning periods

Children learn from the way they see and experience their world; from the way people treat them; from what they see, hear and experience from the moment they are born. Children are natural learners. Between birth and 5 years, and especially to 3 years, children grow and learn at the fastest rate of their lifetime, so it is easy to see the enormous opportunity parents and those who care for young children have in these early years, to help shape children's learning before they start school. The stimulating interaction between the child and its physical and social surroundings is extremely important. Any disturbance or major disruption of the structure of social relationships, such as the family, can significantly affect the development of young children on all levels.

> We learn more in the first five years of our life than in all the rest of our lives put together!

Kandel[3] describes the existence of critical learning periods in the preschool child's life. Very real chemical and physical changes take place in the brain during these critical learning periods. This is the time when a child learns a new skill (such as language or reading) with very little effort. During this period, the child's visual, mental and motor systems are ready to be used and, if triggered by the environment, they will be used together most effectively for the learning of the skill or task. In other words, the young child's brain is still 'plastic', and it can still grow, adapt and make new neuronal connections in response to stimuli. On the other hand, in the absence of relevant stimulation, parts of the brain become inactive, shrink down and eventually stop functioning altogether.

This phenomenon has been known for some time with eyesight. If a baby is born with correctable blindness, then he or she will regain sight if the problem (such as a squint or cataract) is corrected early in life[4]. However, if correction is delayed for a year or two, the child will not develop sight even if the problem is corrected because the part of the brain responsible for processing visual images has atrophied and/or been diverted to another function. It is not just eyesight that is affected in this way: motion, balance, hearing, speech and even the ability to form close and loving relationships can be permanently lost if a child is not properly stimulated in the crucial first few years.

The images of brain scans taken from healthy and understimulated children (see below) show what a profound impact understimulation can have on a child. You do not need to be a specialist to see the effects for yourself.

Brain stimulation for infants and young children is not that difficult to do. Touch, hearing, sight – all the infant's senses – can be stimulated by very simple methods such as talking, playing, holding and comforting the child, and by meeting his physical and psychological needs. Many of the children you will encounter in day-to-day practise will not have been exposed to the necessary conditions in their environment to make the most of these critical learning periods.

3.3 Play theory

Box 3.1 Excerpt from 'Readings from Childhood'[5]

Play has all the characteristics of a fine and complete educational process. It secures concentration for a great length of time. It develops initiative, imagination and intense interest. There is tremendous intellectual ferment, as well as complete emotional involvement. No other activity improves the personality so markedly. No other activity calls so fully on the resources of effort and energy which lie latent in the human being. Play is the most complete of all the educational processes for it influences the intellect, the emotions and the body of the child. It is the only activity in which the whole educational process is fully consummated, when experience induces learning and learning produces wisdom and character.

3.3.1 The importance of play – key theories

Play allows children to practise for later life[6], but it seems to be much more to it than that. Freud regarded play as cathartic. He believed that play could help children release negative feelings caused by traumatic events and substitute them with more positive ones; that it could help children come to understand painful situations and find ways to substitute pleasurable feelings for unpleasant ones; that it would help children to master their covert thoughts and overt actions; and lastly that it would help them to learn to interpret their experiences. Certainly, as children begin to realize their own vulnerability in their enormous world, play can help children reduce this sense of vulnerability. Perhaps that is why children like to play with miniature toys, reducing the overwhelming world of adults to a manageable size and one over which they have complete control.

Psychoanalytic theorists, such as Erik Erikson[7] suggested that play mirrors and supports a child's psychological and social development. In the first year of life, children use their sensory and motor skills to explore their own bodies. In the second year, they progress to manipulating objects in the environment. These play activities can help children develop their self-esteem and sense of empowerment by allowing them mastery of objects. Gradually, as they play, children go beyond control of objects to mastery of social interactions with their peers.

Piaget, a cognitive theorist, considered play to be a major tool for facilitating children's mental development and as a means of facilitating learning by exposing 'a child to new experiences and new possibilities of physical and mental activities for dealing with the world'. Piaget believed that people change their ways of thinking and behaving in order to adapt to their environments and that such adaptation is important for physical survival and psychological/intellectual growth. In Piaget's stage theory, the changes in play through each stage parallel different levels of cognitive and emotional development. They enable children to practise thoughts and behaviours that are acceptable to society so that they can act appropriately in different situations. Different kinds of play require different levels of cognitive sophistication, and that is why each different type of play is found at a specific stage of cognitive development.

Vygotsky, a socio-cultural theorist, believed that play serves as a tool of the mind to help children master their behaviours[8]. This theory suggests that the function of play is to help children develop self-regulation, expand the separation between their thoughts and actions and develop the skills needed to obtain a higher cognitive functioning. For example, when a child builds a car from wire or from blocks, he is learning to separate out the thought or image of the car (the toy) from the actual car he is trying to conceptualize or represent. This separation between actual and symbolic worlds, between thought and action, prepares children to develop abstract thinking. Thinking and acting are no longer simultaneous; behaviours are no longer driven by objects, but rather by children's symbolic thought. Play allows children to try out different thoughts and behaviours, mapping these to the real world, and therefore making children capable of using high-level mental functions (i.e. abstract thinking) to manipulate and monitor thoughts and ideas without direct and immediate reference to the real world. Therefore, play is an important educational strategy for facilitating children's development in cognitive, social/emotional, motor and language areas.

Caplan F. and Caplan T.[9], picking up Freud's themes, suggest that children deliberately create a make-believe play world for themselves in which they can experience a sense of freedom, control and mastery. In this world, they can manipulate reality and feel empowered. As they master their world, play helps children develop new competencies that lead to enhanced confidence and the resilience that they will need to face future challenges[10–12].

More recent theories have emphasized that the process is not one way[13–17]. In other words, it is not simply that play develops as the brain develops. It works the other way around as well. Play helps the brain to develop. A child's development is critically mediated by appropriate, affective relationships with loving and consistent caregivers as they relate to children through play[18]. Without play, children's brains and capacities will not develop healthily. This is of particular importance where children are already suffering with physical illnesses which themselves inhibit development.

3.3.2 The effects of play on a child's development

Play encourages physical development. It improves the child's physical and muscle development with activities such as throwing balls, lifting and carrying around objects, running around, climbing and building. While the child is playing, he is developing and improving his fine and large motor skills, gaining control over his body, refining his eye–hand co-ordination and developing his fitness levels. Play releases energy, provides challenges and allows the child to repeat and practise important skills.

Play encourages emotional development. Play helps the child to feel good about himself because there is no wrong or right way to play, so he does not experience failure. Through play the child learns to express and to understand his emotions, and it helps him to act out his inner fears and anxieties. Play encourages the child to take risks and to make decisions, to use his imagination and to look at things from new perspectives. Most importantly, it gives him an acceptable outlet for feelings of anger, hostility, frustration and joy.

Play encourages social development. It is through play that children at a very early age engage and interact in the world around them. Play can build children's self-confidence and empower their potential[19]. Play (particularly undirected free play) allows children to learn how to work in groups, to share, to negotiate, to resolve conflicts and to learn self-advocacy skills[20,21]. Playing with other children helps the child not to just think of himself. He develops consideration and empathy for others. Fantasy play allows him to take on a number of different social roles and helps him to become more aware of his own identity. He learns to share and to take turns, to be considerate, to lead and to follow and how to behave in order to be part of a group. Playing with others gives him the opportunity to forget his own worries and concerns and allows him to experience pure delight and happiness! When children play with adults the interactions that occur tell children that adults are fully paying attention to them and help to build trusting and enduring relationships[22–24].

Play encourages thinking and language development. Convincing evidence indicates that make-believe or dramatic play increases children's intellectual flexibility; such flexibility is considered a key element of the creative process[25]. Play also provides a base for building language[26]. When children pretend play, they are also involved in the communicative function of sharing objects with others. Hence, play is closely associated with language use and communication[27]. Less verbal children may be able to express their views, experiences and even frustrations through play, allowing others an opportunity to gain a fuller understanding of their perspective. Play has been shown to help children adjust to the school setting and to enhance children's learning readiness, learning behaviours and problem-solving skills[28,29].

Play promotes the young child's understanding of concepts. Through play he will learn what up and down means, hard and soft, big and small, etc. It provides him with opportunities to sort and classify, explore and solve problems and improves his ability to concentrate. Language development also takes place as the young child learns to communicate and share his ideas.

While the child is playing, he is unconsciously gathering information about his world. For example, when he builds with wooden blocks, he discovers that two squares put together make a rectangle or that two triangles can make a square. When he plays with sand and water, he learns about mass and volume, about floating and sinking and about how materials can be changed. Play encourages the child to think creatively and to be curious, to use his initiative and to plan. It improves his memory as well as his ability to reason.

Overall then, play is central to the life of the young child. It occupies most of his time between daily routines. It contributes to every single aspect of his development and lays the foundation for almost everything that he learns before he goes to school. Play is the means by which the child explores and masters his world and the non-verbal expression of his experience of reality. For children with life-limiting illnesses, or for children who have experienced trauma and stress, play is the most natural means by which he can get rid of aggression, come to terms with the trauma of illness and impending death and attempt to take control of his world. Through play the child expresses traumatic fixations, conflicts and hostilities. The child also uses play to disguise genuine conflicts and difficulties, or he may use play to relax tension and anxiety. Of greatest importance is the fact that he discharges aggression and seeks to overcome traumatic anxieties through play[30].

3.3.3 How children play

Children may play in different ways. These include the following, which can be used as indicators of stages reached in their social development:

- Solitary play, where the child plays by himself with his own toys, taking little notice of any other children nearby.

- Spectator play, where the child watches other children play, offering advice and asking questions but not becoming involved himself.

- Parallel play, where the child plays on his own near another child, sometimes with the same toys. They play next to each other but not with each other. Two-year-olds and young three-year-olds can often be seen playing in this manner.

- Associative play, where children play with one another, talking to each other and sharing toys but they do not have the same goal and each one is doing what he wants to do. Older three-year-olds and four-year-olds often play in this way.

♦ Co-operative play, where the children play together in a group with a shared goal, each taking on a specific role. This kind of play can become complex and have numerous rules and rituals attached and is common with five- and six-year-olds.

3.3.4 **Types of play**

There are different types of play and various ways of classifying them. For example[31,32]:

♦ Attunement play: When an infant makes eye contact with her mother, each experiences a spontaneous surge of emotions (joy). The baby responds with a radiant smile, the mother with her own smile and rhythmic vocalizations (baby talk). This is the grounding base of the state of play. It is known, through EEG and other imaging technologies, that the right cerebral cortex, which organizes emotional control, is 'attuned' in both infant and mother[33].

♦ Motor/physical play: Motor play provides critical opportunities for children to develop both individual gross and fine muscle strength and overall integration of muscles, nerves and brain functions. Learning about self-movement structures an individual's knowledge of the world – it is a way of *knowing*, and we actually, through movement and play, *think* in motion. For example, the play-driven movement of leaping upward is a lesson about gravity as well as one's body[34].

♦ Social play: By interacting with others in play settings, children learn social rules such as give and take, reciprocity, cooperation and sharing. Through a range of interactions with children at different social stages, children also learn to use moral reasoning to develop a mature sense of values.

  • Play and belonging[35]: The urge to play with others, in addition to being fun, is often driven by the desire to be accepted, to belong. This starts with 'parallel' play but later, as development proceeds, friendships begin to develop and empathy for others forms. Group loyalty and affection ensues, and with it the rudiments of a functioning community. In animals, affiliative play appears to be kindled by the release of certain hormones and neurotransmitters, but it requires the experience of play to make 'belonging' occur.

  • Rough and tumble play[36]: This seems to be necessary for the development and maintenance of social awareness, cooperation, fairness and altruism. Its nature and importance are generally unappreciated. However, it is important to realize that this is a state of play, not anarchy that must be controlled. This, and other games, sports and group activities, not only tolerate, but enjoy creative tension. Lack of experience with this pattern of play hampers the normal give and take necessary for social mastery and has been linked to poor control of violent impulses in later life.

♦ Language and narrative play[37]: Making sense of the world, its parts and one's particular place in it is a central aspect of early development. As we grow we are hear repeated stories, from our families, schools, friends, books and media. The security, meaning and enjoyment we get from hearing stories gives us permission to expand our own inner stream of consciousness and enrich our own personal narratives as our lives unfold.

♦ Constructive play: Constructive play is when children manipulate their environment to create things. This type of play occurs when children build towers and cities with blocks, play in the sand, construct contraptions on the woodworking bench and draw murals with chalk on the sidewalk. Constructive play allows children to experiment with objects; find out combinations that work and don't work; and learn basic knowledge about stacking, building, drawing, making music and constructing. Along with other special patterns of play, the curiosity about and playing with 'objects' is a pervasive innately fun pattern of play and creates its own 'states' of playfulness. Early on, toys take on highly personalized characteristics, and as skills in manipulating objects (i.e. banging on pans, skipping rocks, etc.) develop, the richer become the circuits in the brain. Hands playing with all types of objects help brains develop beyond strictly manipulative skills, with play as the driver of this development. The correlation of effective adult problem solving and earlier encouragement of and facility in manipulating objects has been established[38]. It also gives children a sense of accomplishment and empowers them with the control of their environment. Children who are comfortable in manipulating objects and materials also become good at manipulating words, ideas and concepts.

- Fantasy play[39,40]: Children learn to abstract, to try out new roles and possible situations, and to experiment with language and emotions with fantasy play. In addition, children develop flexible thinking; learn to create beyond the here and now; stretch their imaginations, use new words and word combinations in a risk-free environment, and use numbers and words to express ideas, concepts, dreams and histories.

- Games with rules: Developmentally, most children progress from an egocentric view of the world to an understanding of the importance of social contracts and rules. Part of this development occurs as they learn that games like Follow the Leader, Red Rover, Simon Says, soccer and other team sports cannot function without everyone adhering to the same set of rules. The 'games with rules' concept teaches children a critically important concept – the game of life has rules (laws) that we all must follow to function productively.

3.4 Facilitating and encouraging play with children

Children from some deprived settings, children who have been neglected or abused or children who have been sick for a long time may not be used to playing. It may be that a particular child has never seen a ball, or a crayon. In our experience, this is not uncommon, so you may need to show children initially what to do with some of the toys suggested below. However, take heart, most children need no more than a few seconds demonstration before they are trying to kick the ball or colour the paper with as much enthusiasm as the others.

Also, in many African children's palliative care settings, resources may not be available to buy expensive toys. But remember, children are able to make toys of pretty much anything. We have tried to suggest the toys below that can be easily made or are readily available as day-to-day household implements. Some things, such as books, may be harder to come by, but we have included them as they are very important. It is simple also to make picture books using drawings and cut-out pictures from magazines.

Remember that toys need to be safe and clean. In most children's palliative care settings, there is a cross-infection risk, so toys should be kept clean and well maintained and thrown out if they become unsafe (e.g. with splinters, loose parts, parts that can be swallowed or pushed into noses and ears). Strings on toys should be less than 30 cm and should ideally detach if much pressure is applied. Try to avoid toys that shoot things like darts, arrows, plastic bullets or pellets. You might also think that it is not ideal for children to be encouraged to play with pretend guns or weapons as these can encourage violent play.

3.4.1 Playing with children from 0 to 18 months

Suitable toys:

- Mobiles – hung over the crib about a foot from the baby's eye level
- Pictures (drawn or painted by adults, other children or cut from magazines) stuck on walls and on the ceiling

- Music toys, rattles (e.g. plastic bottles containing pebbles, bottles filled to different levels with water)
- Stacking toys and nested boxes or cups
- Pots and pans, plastic containers, spoon in a plastic cup
- Large puzzles, books with rhymes and picture books
- Materials of different textures to squeeze and chew
- Toys that float
- Toys to pull on a string (e.g. painted plastic bottles) or to bang together (e.g. spoons and pots)
- Large dolls.

Play ideas for caregivers of 0- to 18-month-old children:

- Respond to baby's sounds
- Make eye contact
- Concentrate on social and gross motor play
- Smile at the baby. Let the baby play with your fingers
- Talk and sing to the baby
- Say rhymes with hand actions
- Play 'peek-a-boo,' 'bye-bye,' and hiding games
- Look and make faces in a mirror
- Play at 'losing' and 'finding' things
- Name objects as you give them to the baby
- Speak to baby while dressing him
- Let baby lie on tummy while playing
- Shake a rattle
- Focus on an interesting and colourful toy
- Get baby to touch different textures
- Encourage him to crawl to toys out of his reach
- Put him outside with other children.

3.4.2 Playing with children from 18 months to 3 years

Suitable toys:

- Outdoor play equipment (ropes, swings, tyres)
- Things to ride on
- Push-pull toys (such as wire cars)
- Sandpit and sandpit toys (such as spoons, funnels, plastic bottles and tins with lids)
- Weaving and beading materials
- Large crayons, paints and pencils
- Blackboard and chalk
- Wooden blocks of different shapes and sizes

- Large packing boxes for climbing in and out
- Dress-up clothes
- Stuffed animals
- Dolls
- Kitchen implements
- Picture books
- Music and story CDs
- Simple musical instruments
- Play dough (see appendix for recipe).

Play ideas for caregivers of 1- to 2-year-olds:

- Encourage child to crawl and move around – focus on gross motor development
- Hide things, 'lose' things, and let children hide things from you
- Play catching and chasing games
- Build something with blocks
- Play follow-the-leader
- Play guessing games
- Act out stories
- Let children copy your activities (such as cleaning the house)
- Read and sing to the children
- Help children to classify objects (sort them into groups)
- Tell stories and let children supply missing words
- Singing, clapping and dancing
- Show the children how the toys work and encourage them to do it themselves
- Use books, sensory toys, reactive toys, building blocks and balls.

Play ideas for 2- to 3-year-olds:

- Concentrate on activities to develop social, gross and fine motor skills
- Show the children different animals
- Teach them the names of the animals and the sounds they make
- Let the children walk and move like different animals
- Play on the musical instruments
- Blow bubbles high and low and encourage children to catch them
- Pack and unpack the box of balls to teach children the concept of 'in and out'
- Roll, throw and kick the balls
- Count the balls
- Draw pictures using large pieces of paper and crayons.

3.4.3 Playing with children from 3 to 6 years

Suitable toys:

- Things to play with and climb on such as skipping ropes, swings, tyres, earth mounds and so on

- Balls and bats
- Empty cardboard boxes
- Dolls for dressing and undressing
- Large puzzles or board games
- Toy vehicles (bought or made with wire)
- Rhythm instruments like drums
- Beads, blocks, buttons
- Peg boards
- Dress-up outfits
- Toy phones
- Doll houses
- Housekeeping toys
- Toy animals
- Construction sets
- Crayons, paints, pencils
- Play dough, drawing paper, glue
- Sand play
- Story books, books on CD, radio, TV
- Puppets made from socks and buttons.

Play ideas for caregivers of 3- to 6-year-olds:

- Concentrate on educational, fine and gross motor play
- Hold make-believe telephone conversations
- Play hide-and-seek
- Singing and dancing
- Practise motor skills with card games and board games
- Play 'counting' and 'number' games
- Pretend to be animals and different people
- Use hand puppets with different voices
- Read to the children and act out the stories
- Talk about the pictures and different colours in the book
- Play 'matching' games and 'counting' games
- Encourage children to create stories while looking through books and magazines
- Let the children name body parts
- Ask the children, what we do with our eyes, ears, nose and mouth
- Teach the children their full name and age
- Let them draw the outlines of their hands and count their fingers
- Clay or play dough: Roll small balls, make small snakes, press snakes flat on table, mould into geometric shapes and various objects
- Ask them the colours of the clay and other toys
- Play dress up with the clothes.

- Let the children 'pretend play' with tea sets and shop toys
- Let the children sing songs with movements
- Encourage sand and water play
- Provide them with crayons, paint and paper
- Play with balls
- Discuss different colours and shapes.

3.4.4 Playing with children from 6 to 9 years

Suitable toys:

- Scooters, skateboards, carts
- Ball sports and games
- Kites
- Board games
- Dolls
- Toy vehicles
- Materials for construction such as wood, wire, paper and glue, clay
- Puzzles
- Toys or disused computers and keyboards
- Dress-up outfits
- Doll houses
- Miniature people and vehicles
- Art materials – crayons, pastels, paints, play dough paper for drawing
- Books and CD's.

Play ideas for caregivers of 6- to 9-year-olds:

- Be observant of children's play
- Provide opportunities for children to play make-believe games
- Encourage children to create and build things
- Help children to organize and classify things
- Allow children to play competitively at games and play situations
- Use puppets to tell stories
- Play language games, e.g. ask children to find 'rhyming' words or synonyms
- Encourage creative writing and poetry
- Play singing and dancing games, and encourage children to make up their own songs and chants
- Attach written names to objects to encourage reading ability
- Play team sports
- Tell jokes and riddles
- Read to the children
- Let the children read to you
- Take children on outings to interesting places and encourage them to explore their world.

3.4.5 **Compiling a play programme for an individual child**

In practise it may be difficult for health workers to have time to assess the needs of individual children and then compile a specific play programme based upon their needs. If so, don't worry. In the section below, we have suggested generic play programmes for different age groups. However, in the ideal word, each child should be assessed against the 'normal' developmental milestones. There are different groups of developmental milestones: physical, perceptual, linguistic, social and moral. These can be found in the appendices of this chapter. As with all developmental models, these need to be handled with care. Different children will progress at different speeds and not always in the order suggested. However, they are useful for picking up areas where children may require extra stimulation.

You should not attempt to assess a child immediately or in one sitting. Ideally, you should ask other colleagues who know the children to help. However, over a period you should be able to identify which areas (if any) the child is lagging behind in, and then try and plan activities which help stimulate that area. For example, children lagging in gross motor skills will benefit from games to encourage sitting, reaching, crawling, standing, walking and running. Children struggling with social development will benefit from play involving touch and contact, including peek-a-boo games, mutual water play, singing together, reading together and so on.

Once an individual programme has been planned, it should be noted clearly so that everyone involved with the child is aware which types of play are to be encouraged. This might be on the front of the child's notes, by the bed or in a folder kept for the individual child. Ideally, these notes should be in simple language such as:

'Talk to me often, sing to me, encourage me to reach for objects and congratulate me if I manage, encourage me to play with my hands and feet'. These kinds of instructions are clear and easy for everyone to use.

3.4.6 **Planning the day**

A good day care programme will take into consideration the unique and specific needs and requirements of every group such as their age, their state of health and their abilities. It should provide the children with the correct balance of activities and be stimulating but not too demanding or tiring. There needs to be time for the children to run about freely and explore the outdoor equipment; time for them to be calm; time for them to express themselves creatively through art and musical activities; time for them to talk and time for them to listen and learn; time for them to think and solve problems and time for them to rest and eat and renew their energy levels. Caregivers need to plan their days carefully but also be flexible and willing to change or do something out of routine if it will benefit and stimulate the children.

Adapt and change the times of the following programmes to suit your specific needs. However, a good programme must have the following important elements:

- Regular times for routines such as nappy changing, toileting, washing hands, eating, resting or sleeping. Try to keep these at the same time every day so the children know what to expect.
- A variety of activities that stimulate children – change the toys they play with, the books they look at and the music they listen to.
- A balance of energetic, physical activities and calmer activities.
- Plenty of time for the quality individual interaction between caregivers and each child.
- The purpose of day care is to develop the whole child, so their cognitive, physical, social, emotional, spiritual, normative and creative needs are met.

3.4.6.1 **Example of a day programme for babies (0–1 year)**

7:00 – 8:30	Children arrive. Give individual attention to each one. Attend to any physical needs, e.g. nappy change. Breakfast, if necessary. Put the younger babies down to sleep.
8:30 – 9:30	Spend time with those who are awake – playing with toys, looking at pictures in books, singing and doing finger rhymes. Play music for them to listen to.
9:30 – 10:00	Change nappies and clothing if needed. Give bottle or appropriate finger snack.
10:00 – 11:00	If the weather is suitable, take the babies outdoors. Stay in the shade if it is hot or find a warm sunny spot in the winter. Give them individual attention, lots of cuddles and talk to them.
11:00 – 12:30	Change nappies. Give a bottle or feed them lunch.
12:30 – 14:20	Nap time. Play with and talk to babies who are awake. Calm time. Play calming music.
14:30 – 15:00	Change nappies. Give bottles or snack.
15:00 – 16:30	Take outdoors to play if the weather permits. Play, talk and give individual attention.
16:30 – 17:00	Change nappies. Prepare for them to go home. Dress in appropriate clothing.

POINTS TO REMEMBER

- Babies need lots of physical contact and cuddles.
- Babies must not be left in wet or soiled nappies. Change these as soon as possible.
- Babies should never be left to cry unattended.
- Talk to them, sing to them, play music to them and play with them.

3.4.6.2 **Example of a day programme for toddlers (1–3 years)**

7:00 – 8:30	Children arrive. Greet each child individually with a smile and a hug. Change nappies and clothing if necessary. Feed breakfast if this is needed.
8:30 – 9:15	Indoor activities such as playing with construction toys, blocks, puzzles, dolls, etc. Provide paper and crayons for drawing, and pictures for cutting and pasting. Provide play dough and toys to go with the play dough. Talk to the children and play with them.
9:15 – 9:30	Toilet routine and hand washing. Change nappies if necessary.
9:30 – 10:00	A healthy snack with something to drink afterwards.
10:00 – 10:30	Play music and let them sing, dance and move or involve them in a creative activity where they can draw and paint, cut and stick.
10:30 – 11:45	Play calming music. Let them rest and take a nap if they need to. Those who are awake can play in the garden. Watch them!
11:45 – 12:00	Wash hands and toilet routine. Change nappies if needed.
12:00 – 12:30	Lunch and something to drink afterwards.
12:30 – 12:45	Story time – tell or read them a short story. Use dolls, puppets or books with bright pictures
12:45 – 14:00	Resting time. Calm, restful activities for children who are awake.

14:00 – 14:45	Outdoor play if the weather permits.
14:45 – 15:00	Change nappies. Toilet routine and wash hands.
15:00 – 15:15	Feed them a healthy snack with something to drink afterwards.
15:15 16:15	Quiet indoor activities. You can read another story. Play dough and drawing/painting activities, etc.
16:15 – 16:45	Toilet routine. Prepare for going home. Quieter activities.
16:45 – 17:00	Pay individual attention to each child as they leave.

POINTS TO REMEMBER

- ◆ Giving a toddler loving attention is even more important than any activity you can do with him or her.
- ◆ Language development is vital: talk, sing and listen to them.

3.4.6.3 **A day programme for children (3–6 years)**

7:00 – 8:00	Children arrive. Welcome each child with a smile. Have quiet activities available. Feed breakfast if this is needed.
8:00 – 8:15	Informal discussion time. Encourage children to tell you any news they have. Talk about the weather, the day ahead and any activities that you have planned.
8:15 – 8:45	Planned activities to develop skills and understanding of concepts. School readiness activities for children going into Grade 1.
8:45 – 9:30	Free play time. If there is more than one caregiver, let children choose whether to play inside the play room or outdoors. Caregivers must be observant while the children play, making sure that they play safely. Rotate the toys regularly for stimulation.
9:30 – 9:45	Toilet routine and hand washing.
9:45 – 10:00	Feed them a healthy snack with something to drink afterwards.
10:00 – 10:30	Play music and let them sing, dance and move to music or involve them all in a craft activity. Discuss things of interest to them.
10:30 – 11:45	Free play time (as above).
11:45 – 12:00	Wash hands and toilet routine.
12:00 – 12:30	Lunch and something to drink afterwards.
12:30 – 12:45	Story time – tell or read them a short story. Use dolls, puppets or books with bright pictures.
12:45 – 14:00	Resting time. Calm, restful activities for children who are awake.
14:00 – 14:45	Outdoor play if the weather permits.
14:45 – 15:00	Toilet routine and wash hands.
15:00 – 15:15	Feed them a healthy snack with something to drink afterwards.
15:15 – 16:15	Quiet indoor activities. You can read another story. Offer play dough and drawing activities.
16:15 – 16:45	Toilet routine. Prepare for going home. Quieter activities.
16:45 – 17:00	Pay individual attention to each child as they leave.

POINTS TO REMEMBER

- Children of this age still need a lot of individual attention.
- Encourage independence but always offer support.

3.5 Setting up the children's play area

It may be that you have very little space in which to operate. However, in case you do, we have suggested below some ideas for how you might want to set up an area for the children in your care.

In general terms it is good to have

- a cognitive (thinking) area: for children to think and learn
- a book area: for children to read and be read to
- a fantasy area: for dressing up and puppet plays
- a creative area: for painting, drawing, creative play and crafts
- an outdoor area: for energetic play
- a sleeping area: for sleep and rest.

3.5.1 The thinking area

This is an area where the children are able to use their minds constructively. They might engage in building with blocks or construction toys; build puzzles and play games which require them to think and problem solve. This section of the playroom needs shelving in order to display a selection of these toys and games. These toys should be rotated on a weekly basis so the children do not get bored with them.

If you possibly can, get some different shaped and sized wooden blocks as these are one of the most wonderful educational toys that you can provide for young children. They should be stored neatly in a cupboard as packing them away correctly is every bit as valuable a learning opportunity for the children as playing with them. Ideally, try to make at least 10–20 of each size block so there are enough for children to create interesting structures. Blocks can be made out of any wood, as long as it is sanded and smooth. It is important that blocks are made to specific measurements: two square blocks put together must be of the same length as one of the rectangular blocks. This helps children learn about shape and size and fractions, balance and structures, symmetry and asymmetry, doubling and halving. The lessons are endless. Keep toys clean by washing them thoroughly every few weeks. Add disinfectant to the water. Other toys you might include are:

- construction toys (e.g. wooden blocks, duplo, etc.)
- puzzles
- board games like bingo, matching games and counting games
- stacking and nesting toys
- threading beads and cotton reels
- shape sorting toys.

3.5.2 The book corner

Choose a quiet corner of the playroom for the book corner. Offer a selection of books, displayed on shelving, with soft cushions for the children to sit on and enjoy looking at the books. Change the books at regular intervals so the children constantly have something new to look at. You should include:

- books that are sturdy and appropriate for the age groups
- books with pictures that relate to the child's life world and culture
- books with pictures of nature and animals
- books with stories that educate and make the child feel secure
- carefully selected books about death and dying and the cycles of life where this is appropriate.

3.5.3 The fantasy area

This part of the room will have old clothes, dress-up clothes, old shoes and hats for the children to use for dressing up for fantasy play, play furniture, dolls and toy (or real, but safe) kitchen utensils. This area should have sufficient storage space for the dress-up clothing and after playing in this area the children need to be reminded to pack the things away in the drawers or boxes provided for storage. You might include:

- play furniture like chairs, table, household equipment
- toy pots and pans, plates, cups and utensils
- dress-up clothes including old adult shirts, skirts, shorts, shoes, hats, etc
- old or toy telephones and computers with keyboards
- dolls, dolls clothing, a doll's house, doll's furniture
- a long mirror securely attached to a wall to look at themselves when they dress up.

3.5.4 The creative area

This could be in a sheltered fringe area outside, or inside. There should be a table with chairs for children to sit at while they are busy with the creative activities, another table for play dough and an easel for painting activities. Every day children need to be given the opportunity to express their creativity through painting, drawing, colouring, pasting or modelling with play dough.

A plastic sheet or newspapers on the floor can also be used for box construction's activities. Supply children with all kinds of empty food containers such as boxes, cartons, egg trays, plastic bottles and polystyrene trays. Provide glue and paper to stick the boxes and cartons together to make things. Allow them to paint and decorate their box constructions if they want to. You may provide:

- a sturdy easel or easels, paint pots and strong paint brushes
- paints, crayons, felt tip pens, coloured chalk
- scrap paper
- blunt nosed scissors and glue (make up wallpaper glue or a paste made with flour and water)
- play dough
- toys to use with the play dough
- a plastic mat or an endless supply of newspaper.

3.5.5 **The sheltered outdoor area (fringe area)**

It is useful to have an area attached to the building where the children can play outdoors but under shelter. It is desirable to use this area for the placing of senso-pathic trays. These are large plastic basins or fibre-glass trays used to hold water, sand and other interesting sensory materials such as sawdust and dry maize meal. Ideally, these trays should be raised to the waist height of the child. Anything with water in must be raised and carefully supervised to prevent small children from falling in and drowning. Large, shallow plastic bowls placed on a table at the child's waist height can also be used. The creative/art area could be situated in the fringe area if there is not enough space in the play room. You may provide:

- trays or large bowls, ideally at the child's waist height, for putting substances in (e.g. water, sawdust, sand, dry maize meal; bird seed; mud; finger paint; cornflour with a little water; pebbles, etc.)
- a selection of toys and equipment for putting with the above substances, e.g. toys, cars and figures (animals or people), floating toys, tubing, things to pour from and into
- different sizes of plastic containers and spoons.

3.5.6 **The outdoor area**

When planning the outdoor area, it is important to take safety into account. Make sure that all areas can be watched at all times, and fence or block off areas where the children can play without being seen. Ideally, try to provide a sand pit; a level area for running games and ball games; and a climbing area. Sand pits should be covered at the end of every day to prevent animals soiling in them and once a month sterilized either by emptying 4 x 250 g packets of coarse salt into the sand and spraying with water or sprinkling one cup of swimming pool chlorine into the sand and spraying with water until diluted. If you have climbing structures such as poles or swings, ensure that they are not on paved ground and that they are kept in good condition. Regularly check for frayed ropes, loose bolts, raised nails, worn chains and hinges, loose wooden planks or bars on any climbing equipment and repair immediately. Prevent the children from playing on the broken equipment until it has been repaired. Apart from the jungle gyms, children need plenty of opportunities to develop their balancing skills. Old tyres make wonderful balancing equipment.

Plant them firmly in the ground so only the top half can be seen. Use a variety of sizes and plant them next to one another to form a bridge for the children to walk over. You might provide:

- wheeled toys
- bats and balls
- areas for climbing and rolling
- stilts
- hula hoops
- balancing beams
- old tyres half buried (never use tyres with steel belts inside)
- skipping ropes (must always be supervised as ropes can be dangerous)
- sand pit and toys.

As far as possible, there should be washable flooring, a covered or sheltered outdoor area and a safe, contained outdoor area. You will need plenty of shelving and lockable storage (unfortunately items tend to go missing). If you are providing food you will need a safe kitchen and eating area. You will of course also need toilets.

3.5.7 The sleeping area

If possible it is best to have a separate area for children to sleep, as children with life-limiting illnesses will get tired very quickly and need to sleep frequently. This room needs to have plenty of mats or mattresses for the children, ideally with pictures and mobiles for them to look at as they go to sleep and when they wake up. Children must never be left to cry unattended in this room. You may wish to play soothing music for the children while they rest.

3.5.8 Storage

You can never have enough shelving or enough cupboard space! The kitchen and bathroom should have some cupboards that are out of the children's reach and are able to be locked for the storage of medications, household cleaning substances, etc.

Some storage tips:

- If games, puzzles, books and toys are not stored in a systematic manner, very soon you will find yourself with boxes of toys all mixed up together. Children do not play constructively, nor can they gain much stimulation from playing with such a jumble of unrelated toys.

- Keep each toy or set of toys in a separate container. Collect ice cream containers for the smaller toys and bigger boxes or containers for the larger ones. Write on each container with permanent markers so it is easy to see where things belong. Train the children to tidy up after themselves when they have finished playing by putting the toys in the correct container and back on the shelf. Sing a 'Tidy up' song to make it fun. Do not offer the children all the toys to play with every day. Alternate the toys you put into the sand pit and the senso-pathic trays every day. Others should be rotated on a weekly basis. This provides stimulation and encourages constructive and productive play.

- If you have puzzles with broken boxes, store the pieces in containers or cheap plastic boxes with lids. Number each container and write that number on the back of each puzzle piece that belongs in it. This makes it easy to find where stray puzzle pieces belong. Cut out the picture and put the number on it before throwing the broken box away. Store the boxes and pictures in number order.

- It would be an advantage to have an outdoor storage area for storing the wheeled toys, sand pit toys and other outdoor toys and equipment such as balls and bats, etc.

3.6 Specific activities

3.6.1 Painting

You can use the following:

- Paints or nursery dyes – powder paint can be mixed with wallpaper glue and water to make it go further.
- Paint pots with lids and plugs: seal at the end of every day.
- Paint brushes: wash every day – do not leave in the paint overnight.
- Scrap paper: ask the community to collect scrap paper for drawing and painting on.
- Lots of newspaper to save table tops and floors from the mess!

3.6.2 Drawing

Drawing in some form or another is probably the first form of creative expression for children, and it provides traumatized children and children in distress a means of expressing their pain and anxiety. That is why it is important that the children are given an opportunity to draw every day. Provide different media for them depending on their age and their fine motor control.

You can use:

- paper of all shapes, colours and sizes
- crayons
- coloured chalk (quickly dip the chalk in water before use)
- pastels
- charcoal
- pencils and pens
- white boards and white board markers.

3.6.3 Cutting and pasting activities

Children should only be allowed to cut out under adult supervision as scissors can be dangerous. Only use blunt nosed scissors, but make sure that they are fairly sharp otherwise the children get frustrated.

You need:

- a few pairs of blunt-nosed safety scissors
- pictures for cutting out (collect old cards, pictures from magazines, adverts, pamphlets, etc.)
- glue – make a jug of wallpaper glue which can be used to thicken powder paint and as glue for paper: you can make glue by mixing flour and water to a paste
- paper of all sizes and colours.

3.6.4 Box construction

This is a wonderful, creative activity which encourages children to create machines, houses and structures using waste materials. Get the community to save all their packaging from food (cardboard boxes, plastic tubs, etc.) and the insides of toilet rolls, wax paper rolls and paper towel rolls, etc.

You will need:

- old boxes, cartons, lids, etc.
- paper or sheets of cardboard
- stickers – printers who print stickers and labels often have overruns which they are willing to donate
- craft glue or flour and water paste
- paint – once the child has made something, he may want to paint it.

3.6.5 Musical activities

Music should be a part of every day for the young child. Let the children sing songs while they play, while they tidy up the play room, while they wash their hands and before they eat their food, they can sing a prayer of thanks. Teach them songs and simple rhymes with hand actions and songs and rhymes with actions that involve their whole body. Teach the children songs that will help them learn and remember important things like the names of body parts, hygiene and values. Songs are also a good way to help children to remember the order of the alphabet or the order of numbers. Number songs and rhymes can teach children how to count, add and subtract.

3.6.6 Dancing and moving to music

If you have a CD player, a radio or even just a drum or tambourine, encourage children to listen to the music or the beat, to dance and move to the beat and to clap in time to music. Train the children to listen to:

- the pulse and the rhythm of the song
- to hear when the music gets louder and when it gets softer
- when the song has high and low pitched notes
- what instruments are being played in the song
- whether the song is fast or slow or somewhere in-between.

3.6.7 Making and playing musical (percussion) instruments

Make simple musical instruments for the children to play in time to music:

- Shakers can be made with plastic yoghurt cartons – put some maize rice, stones or plain rice inside and cover with a large sticker or paper and elastic band. Shake in time to the music.
- Make rhythm sticks by cutting pieces of thick dowel rods, old broom sticks or plastic tubing about 20 cm in length. They can bang these together.
- Make kitchen drums by hitting a plastic cup with a teaspoon, a metal pot with a metal spoon, banging pot lids together, etc.
- Saw dry coconut shells in half. Bang together in time to music.

3.6.8 Making play dough

Ingredients: 3 cups white cake or bread flour, 1 cup salt, 1 small 12 g packet of cream of tartar, 3 tablespoons oil, 3 cups of water, food colouring, a few drops of essence (e.g. lemon, vanilla, strawberry, etc.)

- Mix flour, salt and cream of tartar in a heavy metal pot.
- Mix water, oil and food colouring and slowly add to the flour mixture, stirring with a wooden spoon. Add the essence (optional).
- Cook over a low heat, stirring all the time.
- Just before the play dough is completely cooked, remove it from the stove and allow it to finish cooking in its own heat.
- Knead and store in an airtight container. It can be kept for two to three weeks.

3.6.9 Outdoor activities

Specific activities to develop the children's large motor skills should take place regularly – at least once a week. Let them crawl through things, balance on things and jump over things. Take the time to teach the children how to hop, jump with two feet together, skip, gallop, jump and turn their bodies while they are in the air and how to play hopscotch. You can draw a hopscotch on concrete or tar with chalk. Let them catch and throw bean bags, large balls, tennis balls. Get them to hit the balls with a bat, bounce the balls and kick the balls. Balance bean bags on their heads and other parts of their bodies. Teach them how to use the hula hoop or place the hula hoops on the ground and play games where they jump from one to the other. Play musical statues and musical bumps – play music or bang a drum and when you stop they must stand like a statue or sit down. Play games where they must run and stop and quickly change direction.

You need:

- bean bags – make your own from strong material and fill with maize rice or plastic beads
- balls – big balls and small balls
- skipping ropes – only use these under adult supervision
- hula hoops
- bats – plastic or wooden cricket bats: you can make your own by rolling newspaper into a long tube shape and securing with thick packaging tape.

3.7 **Record keeping**

Record keeping is a vital part of running a Day Care and records must be comprehensive, clear and kept up-to-date. Each child should have a file that contains all the important information relating to him/her. Ensure that any confidential information is kept in a locked cabinet or cupboard and is made accessible only to those who have the right to see that. It is essential to record the following information for each child:

- surname, full name, gender and date of birth
- the child's home language
- home address and contact numbers of parents/guardians
- details of who has permission to fetch the child
- medical history of the child
- admission and discharge register
- attendance register
- written permission for guardians for any planned excursions outside of the facility.

In addition to the above records, it is vital that a record is kept of the child's developmental progress. You can use the Milestones charts and the Checklist charts as a guide to help you devise a system to record the child's progress. Caregivers should make a written note of any progress and/or any regression they may observe in the child's development, behaviour or emotional state. These notes can be used to develop individualized stimulation and care programmes for children, especially those with special needs.

3.8 **Questions for you**

1. Think of some of the children you have seen recently. Can you think of any who would benefit from play activities?
2. Think of a child you know who is 2–3, and another who is 4–6. Try and think of a play programme for them which will help stimulate them in ways that they need and would enjoy
3. How could you improve the play and stimulation facilities at your place of work?

Notes

1 Piaget, J. (1977). The essential Piaget. Gruber Howard E. & J. Jacques Voneche (Eds.). Basic Books, New York.

2 Erikson. (1956). *Journal of the American Psychoanalytic Association*, 4, 56–121.

3 Kandel, E.R., Schwartz, J.H. & Jessell, T.M. (1991). *Principles of Neural Science* (3rd Edition). Elsevier, New York.

4 Kellman, P. & Arterberry, M. (1998). *The Cradle of Knowledge*. MIT Press, Cambridge, MA, USA.

5 Scarfe, N.V. (1966). Readings from Childhood Education: Articles of Lasting Value. *Association for Childhood Education International*. Maryland, US.

6 Saracho, O.N. & Spodek, B. (1995). Children's play and early childhood education: Insights from history and theory. *Journal of Education*, *177*(3), 129–49.

7 Hughes, F.P. (1999). *Children, Play and Development* (3rd Edition). Allyn & Bacon, Boston.

8 Cited in Bodrova, E. & Leong, D. (1996). *Tools of the Mind: The Vygotskian Approach to Early Childhood Education*. Merrill, Columbus, OH.

9 Caplan, F. & Caplan, T. (1973). *The Power of Play*. Doubleday, New York.

10 Hurwitz, S.C. (2002/2003). To be successful: Let them play! *Child Education*, *79*,101–2.

11 Erickson, R.J. (1985). Play contributes to the full emotional development of the child. *Education*, *105*, 261–63.

12 Band, E.B. & Weisz, J.R. (1988). How to feel better when it feels bad: Children's perspectives on coping with everyday stress. *Developmental Psychology*, *24*, 247–53.

13 Caplan, F. & Caplan, T. (1973). *The Power of Play*. Doubleday, New York.

14 Pepler, D. J. (1982). Play and divergent thinking. In D.J. Pepler & K.H. Rubin (Eds.), *The Play of Children: Current Theory and Research* (Vol. 6, pp. 64–78). Karger, New York.

15 Shonkoff, J.P. & Phillips, D.A. (Eds.). (2000). *From Neurons to Neighborhoods: The Science of Early Childhood Development*. National Academy Press, Washington, DC.

16 Frost, J.L. (1998). *Neuroscience, Play and Brain Development*. Paper presented at: IPA/USA Triennial National Conference. Longmont, CO. June 18–21. Available online at www.eric.ed.gov/ERICDocs/data/ ericdocs2/content storage 01/0000000b/80/11/ 56/d6.pdf. Accessed June 22, 2006

17 Tamis-LeMonda, C.S., Shannon, J.D., Cabrera, N.J. & Lamb, M.E. (2004). Fathers and mothers at play with their 2- and 3-year-olds: Contributions to language and cognitive development. *Child Development,75*, 1806–20.

18 Shonkoff, J.P. & Phillips, D.A. (Eds.). (2000). *From Neurons to Neighborhoods: The Science of Early Childhood Development*. National Academy Press, Washington, DC.

19 Trawick-Smith, J. (1994). *Interactions in the Classroom: Facilitating Play in the Early Years*. Macmillan, New York.

20 Pellegrini, A.D. & Smith, P.K. (1998). The development of play during childhood: Forms and possible functions. *Child Psychology and Psychiatry Review*, *3*, 51–7.

21 McElwain, E.L. & Volling, B.L. (2005). Preschool children's interactions with friends and older siblings: Relationship specificity and joint contributions to problem behaviors. *Journal of Family Psychology*, *19*, 486–96.

22 Tamis-LeMonda, C.S., Shannon, J.D., Cabrera, N.J. & Lamb, M.E. (2004). Fathers and mothers at play with their 2- and 3-year-olds: Contributions to language and cognitive development. *Child Development*, *75*, 1806–20.

23 Smith, D. (2002). How play influences children's development at home and school. *Journal of Physical Education, Recreation Dance*, *66*, 19–23.

24 Tsao, L. (2002). How much do we know about the importance of play in child development? *Child Education*, *78*, 230–33.

25 Hughes, F. P. (1999). *Children, Play, and Development* (3rd Edition). Allyn and Bacon, Boston.

26 Saltz, E. & Brodie, J. (1982). Pretend-play training in childhood: A review and critique. In D. J. Pepler & K. H. Rubin (Eds.) *The Play of Children: Current Theory and Research*. (Vol. 6, pp. 97–113). Karger, New York.

27 McCune-Nicolich, L. & Bruskin, C. (1982). Combinatorial competency in symbolic play and language. In D. J. Pepler & K. H. Rubin (Eds.) *The Play of Children: Current Theory and Research* (Vol. 6, pp. 30–45). Karger, New York.

28 Pellegrini, A.D. & Boyd, B. (1993). The role of play in early childhood development and education: Issues in definition and function. In B. Spodek (Ed). *Handbook of Research on the Education of Young Children*. (pp. 105–21) MacMillan, New York.

29 Fisher, E.P. (1992). The impact of play on development: A meta-analysis. *Play Cult, 5*, 159.

30 Hartley, Frank & Goldenson. (1999). *Understanding Children's Play*. Routledge, London.

31 'National Institute for Play': www.nifplay.org

32 Child development Insititute: www.childdevelopmentinfo.com

33 Schore, A.N. The seventh annual John Bowlby memorial lecture. Minds in the making: Attachment, the self-organizing brain, and developmentally-oriented psychoanalytic psychotherapy. *British Journal of Psychotherapy, 17*, 299–328.

34 Sheets-Johnstone, Maxine (1999). The Primacy of Movement, Johns-Benjamin, *Advances in Consciousness Research*. Vol. 14.

35 Opie. I. (1993). *The People in the Playground*. Oxford University Press, New York.

36 Pelligrini, A.D. (1988). Rough-and-Tumble play from childhood through adolescence. In D. Fromberg & D. Bergen (Eds.) *Play from Birth to Twelve and Beyond: Contexts, Perspectives, and Meanings*. (pp. 401–8). Garland, New York.

37 Paley, V.G. (1992). *You Can't Say You Can't Play*. Harvard University Press, Cambridge MA.

38 Frank Wilson (1999). *The Hand: How Its Use Shapes the Brain, Language, and Human Culture* (Vintage).

39 Singer, Dorothy, G. & Singer, Jerome, L. (1990). *The House of Make-Believe: Children's Play and the Developing Imagination*.

40 Winnicott, D. W. (1999). *Playing and Reality*. Routledge, London.

Appendix 1: Developmental milestones

Table 3.1 Physical and motor developmental milestones

Age	Large motor milestones	Fine motor milestones
6 months	Lifts head when on stomach Controls head and arm movements Rolls over Makes movements of excitement with body	Grasps things Transfers objects from one hand to the other
1 year	Has control of legs and feet Stands holding on to things Moves around obstacles by side-stepping Waves goodbye	Picks up things using thumb and fore-finger Can hold a cup to drink from Begins to eat without help Uncontrolled scribbling on paper
18 months	Crawls up stairs Walks on his own Enjoys pushing or pulling toys Throws a large ball underhand	Drinks from a cup with both hands Can feed himself with a spoon Makes lines on paper with a crayon Passes object from one hand to the other
2 years	Runs but falls when turning a corner Can walk backwards Kicks and throws a large ball Climbs steps with both feet on every step Uses feet to propel a riding/wheeled toy Capable of bowel and bladder control Climbs up on chair, turns and sits down	Turns pages in a book one at a time Builds a tower of six blocks Puts small items into a container and takes them out again Can put objects together and take them apart Holds crayons in fist and scribbles on the paper
3 years	Stands on one leg Goes up stairs with one foot on each step Can catch and throw a large ball	Builds a tower of 10 cubes Begins to show hand dominance Can do large buttons and zips
4 years	Jumps up and down Goes down stairs one foot at a time Can pedal a tricycle Dresses and undresses with help Climbs trees and ladders	Holds a crayon using a tripod grip (thumb + 2 fingers) Draws a circle and a cross Cuts paper in half with scissors Threads small wooden beads on a string
5 years	Skips Walks backwards Dresses and undresses alone Can run fast in a circle	Copies a square and a triangle Catches a ball thrown from 1 metre away Can use a pencil to trace simple pictures Cuts on a line with scissors
6 years	Very active Can turn a somersault Jumps and hops forwards without falling Balances on either foot for 10 seconds	Copies a diamond Can use a pencil to trace letters and numbers Cuts along a curved or angular line with scissors

Table 3.2 Perceptual developmental milestones

Age	Perceptual milestones
1 month	Reacts to light by closing his eyes Prefers to watch moving objects
4 months	Turns his eyes in the direction of an object Reacts to different colours and shows preference for some
6 months	Follows a dangling toy from side to side Eyes move together Turns head towards sounds and familiar voices Pays attention to music Shows likes and dislikes for certain foods
1 year	Drops toys and watches where they go Watches people and activities Points to objects 1–2 metres away
2 years	Recognizes and expresses pain and its location Fits shapes into correctly shaped holes
3 years	Eye–hand movements are better coordinated
4 years	Can match colours that are the same and name a few of them
5 years	Identifies and names most colours

Table 3.3 Language developmental milestones

Age	Language milestones
6 months	Makes sounds to draw attention Double syllable sounds such as 'mumum' and 'dada' Withdraws from an angry voice and smiles and coos at a friendly voice Cannot understand 'No!' or 'danger'
1 year	Imitates sounds that are heard Babbles two or three words repeatedly Recognizes own name Follows simple instructions, e.g. 'Come here'.
18 months	Uses many understandable words (up to 50 words) Uses one word to convey a whole thought, e.g. 'me' for 'give it to me' Can locate and point to familiar objects when asked to do so Enjoys songs and rhymes and tries to join in
2 years	Uses 50 to 300 words and learns new ones every day Refers to self as 'me' or 'I', e.g. 'Me want that.' Joins two to three words in sentences (known as telegraphic speech, i.e. uses only words that have meaning, e.g. 'Me go out') Understands far more than they are able to express
3 years	Has a vocabulary of approximately 900 words and speaks in sentences Constantly asks questions and often talks to himself Can remember and sing simple rhymes and songs

Table 3.3 (continued) Language developmental milestones

Age	Language milestones
4 years	Has a vocabulary of approximately 1500 words Uses the pronouns *I, you* and *me* correctly Will often talk aloud and explain what they are doing Asks even more questions than before Many babyish substitutions in speech, e.g. 'wif' for 'with' or 'dat' for 'that' Can answer questions like 'Whose?' 'How many?' 'Where?' 'Why?' Begins to correctly use the past tense of verbs, e.g. 'Mommy *went* to work'.
5 years	Has a vocabulary of approximately 2000 words Fluent speech with few babyish substitutions Enjoys word play and making up *silly* words Can tell a familiar story while looking at a picture book Understands humour and enjoys hearing and telling jokes
6 years	Has a vocabulary of approximately 2500 words, has fluent speech and talks a lot Remembers and sings short poems, rhymes and songs Enjoys jokes and riddles with humour that is not very subtle Can listen to stories for extended length of time and sing short songs, and rhymes

Table 3.4 Cognitive developmental milestones

Age	Cognitive milestones
6 months	Drops things intentionally and repeatedly and watches where they go Imitates activities like playing a drum Is aware of own body and starts putting things offered in mouth Concentration develops and he examines objects more closely
1 year	Enjoys games where objects are hidden Begins to understand that a toy dog, a picture of a dog and a real dog are all 'dogs'
18 months	Discovers cause and effect, e.g. If I hit the pot with the spoon it makes a loud noise Keen to explore and get to know about the things around him Carries out requests that use memory, e.g. 'Go to your room and fetch your teddy'.
2 years	Begins to understand what different things are for and what belongs together Will use an object for other than what it is intended, e.g. will make car noises and push a block on the floor Does simple classification based on one attribute, e.g. separates toy cars from blocks Names objects in picture books and enjoys being read to
3 years	Likes to look at books and pretends to read Listens attentively to age-appropriate stories Can rote count to 10 but does not fully understand the *values* of the numbers Has a good memory Knows if he/she is a boy or a girl Begins imaginative play
4 years	Understands and names the sequence of daily events Learns to build simple puzzles (12–20 pieces) Can recognize missing parts from a picture or puzzle Understands what 'most' means and begins to understand number values Plays complex fantasy games

(continued)

Table 3.4 (continued) Cognitive developmental milestones

Age	Cognitive milestones
5 years	Understands concept of same, e.g. same shape, or same size Understands what money is for Eager to learn new things Understands 'more' and 'less' Understands 'first', 'second' and 'last' Can order objects, e.g. from tallest to shortest Arrives at some understanding about death and dying Can recognize his own written name and some familiar words and letters
6 years	Can count objects correctly to 20 and recognizes numerals 1–10 Loves listening to stories and looking at picture books Knows letters of the alphabet and understands that they are used to form words

Table 3.5 Emotional and social developmental milestones

Age	Emotional milestones	Social milestones
6 months	Shows delight and distress Smiles at a face Enjoys being cuddled	Recognizes mother Distinguishes between familiar people and strangers
1 year	Has developed emotional attachment to mother and protests separation from her Displays anger Gives affection Often shy with strangers	Plays 'peek-a-boo' games Waves good-bye Gives and takes objects Interested in his own image in the mirror
18 months	Very dependent behaviour Very upset when separated from mother May develop a fear of bathing	Often does the opposite of what he is told to do
2 years	Has temper tantrums Shows resentment towards a new baby May have blanket or stuffed toy for comfort Defiant and says 'No!' a lot	Likes people but still very egocentric Has difficulty in sharing Plays alongside other children, not with them
3 years	Has developed a sense of humour and enjoys playing tricks Affectionate towards parents/caregivers Temper tantrums may continue	Begins to share and be less selfish May show interest in specific friends Starts to project his own experiences on dolls and other fantasy toys
4 years	Fear of dark may surface Begins to gain some self-control and use language rather than tantrums to express anger Likes to make people laugh	Intense curiosity and interest in other children's bodies Can play in a group Begins to take turns Begins to identify with same-sex parent and imitates him/her

Table 3.5 (continued) Emotional and social developmental milestones

Age	Emotional milestones	Social milestones
5 years	Understands responsibility and guilt Feels pride in things he has done Failure makes him frustrated	Prefers to play with other children May tease other children and use name-calling May have a 'best' friend Becomes competitive and fights occur Prefers gender-appropriate activities
6 years	Continues to gain self-control	Plays in a group where there is a division of roles and sharing of common goals Prefers some children over others and groups can become exclusive Can be very generous and caring

Table 3.6 Moral developmental milestones

Age	Moral and normative milestones
Birth – 2 years	Lack of moral judgement and control The child learns right and wrong mostly from the result of pain or pleasure The child accepts norms without questioning
2–3 years	Punishment and reward begin to play an important role in the development of norms The child trusts parents/caregivers fully for moral judgement and the setting of norms
3–5 years	The child is controlled morally by rules set by adults Moral behaviour is aimed mainly at avoiding punishment He understands that his behaviour can please or displease adults and begins to behave accordingly He reasons that he can misbehave as long as the adult can't see him! He begins to form a better idea of what is 'right' and 'wrong' from the example set by his parents and caregivers His conduct is less impulsive
5–7 years	He begins to differentiate between 'good' and 'bad' He becomes aware of guilt and learns to apologize for bad behaviour He develops a reasonable sense of responsibility, independence and manners

Table 3.7 Spiritual developmental milestones

Age	Spiritual milestones
Birth –2 years	Pre-religious Bible stories and church services are of little value to the child
2–3 years	Cannot respond to the message of any religion, but responds to the love that he experiences from those who tell him about God

(continued)

Table 3.7 (continued) Spiritual developmental milestones

Age	Spiritual milestones
3–5 years	The child defines God in human terms (e.g. like his dad, only stronger and more powerful) Begins to listen to stories from scriptures but does not relate them to real life Begins to pray – prayers are egocentric and concrete, e.g. prays about personal situation, family members, his toys, food, etc.
5–7 years	Responds to Bible stories with less emotion and more thinking Prayers become less about himself and his own needs and start to include others

Developmental checklists

Use the following checklists to help you determine any delays in normal development for specific children and to chart their progress over a number of months. If you have access to a photocopier, make copies of the appropriate checklists for each child and keep them in a file for easy reference. As the child grows and matures, add the next suitable checklist to the file.

Assess each child according to their age to see if and where the delays are. Use the checklist *closest in age* to the child you are testing.

If the child has reached less than half of the milestones on that checklist, use the previous checklist for that child. In this way you can use the results to find out how severe the delays are and as a guide in the planning of your daily and weekly programmes. You can also use them to decide whether you need to call in the help and services of a professional such as a psychologist, a speech therapist or an occupational therapist.

The checklists will direct you to the areas that need to be worked on and stimulated for each child or for groups of children. Repeat the tests every 2–3 months to see if there has been any improvement. In some instances, you may find that milestones mentioned are not within the particular child's realm of experience, for example he or she may never have been exposed to a puzzle. In this case, either cross that milestone off the checklist or substitute it with another similar activity with which the child *will* be familiar.

To make the assessment more accurate and informative you may wish to use these marks as a code

Does it well	Can do it but not well	Almost able to do it	Cannot not do it at all
☺	✓	●	✗

Checklist for a child aged Birth–2 Months

CHILD'S NAME: _____ D.O.B. _____

*Important background information that could affect results:*_____

_____

_____

	Action	Date	Date	Date
Birth	Sucking reflex: sucks on anything placed in mouth			
	Rooting reflex: opens mouth and turns head towards the side his cheek is stroked			
	Startle reflex: splays arms and hands in response to loud noises or unexpected movements then brings them in to chest			
	Step reflex: when baby is held upright with feet touching a firm surface, he will make little stepping movements forward			
	Grasp reflex: grasps anything placed in his hand, clenches it briefly, then just lets go			
	Responds positively to comforting actions and cries loudly during painful activity			
	Makes eye contact or stares at object for 5–10 seconds			
One month	Lifts head when lying on tummy			
	Moves head from side to side			
	Brings hands to face			
	Stares at faces			
	Blinks at bright lights			
	Responds to sounds			
Two months	Vocalizes: gurgles and coos			
	Reflexes fade and are replaced by voluntary movements			
	Holds head up for short periods			
	Follows objects with eyes across field of vision			
	Turns head and eyes towards an interesting sound			
	Stares at own image in a mirror			
	Tries to push at a dangling toy			
	Notices own hands			

Checklist for a child aged approximately 3 Months

CHILD'S NAME: _____ D.O.B._____

*Important background information that could affect results:*_____

_____

_____

	Action	Date	Date	Date
Large motor	Raises head and chest when lying on tummy and can support upper body with arms			
	Kicks legs and moves arms about when lying on back			
	Pushes down with legs when placed on a hard surface			
	Can sit with support			
Fine motor	Opens and shuts hands and can shake a rattle			
	Can bring hands together			
Perceptual	Can follow a moving object with eyes			
	Recognizes familiar faces and objects at a distance			
	Beginning to use hands and eyes in a co-ordinated manner			
	Turns head towards the direction of a sound			
	Recognizes familiar voices			
Language	Coos and gurgles with vowel sounds 'ah, eh, oh' in response to what he sees, hears and feels			
	Likes to babble and make up sounds			
	May be able to imitate some vowel sounds			
Cognitive	Shows anticipation of regular activity like bathing and feeding			
	Knows the difference between parents/caregivers and strangers			
	Explores objects with mouth			
Social and Emotional	Beginning to develop a social smile			
	Enjoys playing with people and may cry when playing stops			
	Imitates movements and facial expressions			
	Will laugh when tickled			

Checklist for a child aged approximately 6 Months

CHILD'S NAME: _____ D.O.B. _____

*Important background information that could affect results:*_____

_____

_____

	Action	Date	Date	Date
Large motor	Lifts head when on stomach and wriggles forward			
	Controls head and arm movements			
	Sits			
Fine motor	Grasps things			
	Transfers objects from one hand to the other			
Perceptual	Follows dangling toy from side to side			
	Eyes move together when following a moving object			
	Turns head towards sounds and familiar voices			
	Pays attention to music			
Language	Makes sounds to draw attention			
	Makes double syllable sounds such as 'mumum' and 'dada'			
	Smiles and coos at a friendly voice			
Cognitive	Watches where dropped items go			
	Imitates simple activities			
	Puts things offered in mouth			
	Examines objects closely			
Social and Emotional	Shows delight and distress			
	Smiles at a face			
	Enjoys being cuddled			
	Recognizes mother or caregivers			
	Distinguishes between familiar people and strangers			

Checklist for a child aged approximately 9 Months

CHILD'S NAME: _____ D.O.B. _____

Important background information that could affect results: _____

_____

_____

	Action	Date	Date	Date
Large motor	Starting to crawl/can crawl			
	Can sit upright without support			
	Gets up on hands and feet and rocks or lunges forwards			
	Can stand while holding on to something			
Fine motor	Passes objects from hand to hand			
	Manipulates objects with hands, e.g. bangs cups			
	Can pick up small objects using finger and thumb			
Perceptual	Looks for dropped objects			
	Close inspection of smaller objects			
	Is good at imitating sounds heard and begins to imitate words			
Language	Begins to show an understanding of common words			
	Makes two syllable sounds and may use words like 'mama'			
	Responds to own name and familiar words			
Cognitive	Shows an understanding of language, e.g. will wave goodbye when asked, if this has been taught			
	Turns head away when finished eating			
	Can work out how to get something that is out of reach			
	Eagerly explores his world using his hands and his mouth			
Social and Emotional	Wary or afraid of strangers			
	Emergence of self – distinct personality traits become obvious			
	Cries when caregiver leaves him			
	Shows affection to parents and/or caregivers			

Checklist for a child aged approximately 1 Year

CHILD'S NAME: _____ D.O.B. _____

*Important background information that could affect results:*_____

	Action	Date	Date	Date
Large motor	Has control over legs and feet			
	Can stand holding on to something			
	Moves around obstacles by side-stepping			
	Waves goodbye			
Fine motor	Picks up things using thumb and fore-finger			
	Can hold a cup to drink from			
	Starts to eat without help			
	Makes uncontrolled scribbles on paper			
Perceptual	Drops toys and watches where they go			
	Watches people and activities			
	Sees and points to objects 1–2 metres away			
	Shows preferences and dislikes for certain foods			
Language	Babbles repeatedly and imitates sounds that are heard			
	Recognizes and says his/her own name and animal sounds			
	Follows simple instructions like 'Come here'			
Cognitive	Looks to see where you hide an object			
	Can recognize pictures of known objects in books			
	Understands simple questions, e.g. 'Where's your nose?'			
	Shakes his/her head for 'No!'			
Social and Emotional	Cries when separated from mother/prime caregiver			
	Displays anger			
	Is loving and affectionate			
	Gives away and accepts objects			
	Interested in his/her own image in a mirror			

Checklist for a child aged approximately 18 Months

CHILD'S NAME: _____ D.O.B. _____

Important background information that could affect results: _____

_____

_____

	Action	Date	Date	Date
Large motor	Walks on his/her own			
	Can push and pull wheeled toys			
	Throws a large ball underhand			
	Crawls up stairs			
Fine motor	Drinks from a cup with both hands			
	Can feed himself/herself with a spoon			
	Makes lines on paper with a crayon			
	Passes object from one hand to the other when offered a second object			
	Can turn the pages of a book			
Perceptual	Enjoys looking at pictures in books			
	Responds to music and singing			
Language	Uses many understandable words (up to 50 words)			
	Enjoys songs and rhymes and tries to join in			
	Can locate and point to familiar objects when asked to do so			
Cognitive	Keen to explore and know about the things around him/her			
	Can carry out a request that uses memory, e.g. 'Go to the kitchen and fetch a spoon'.			
	Understands cause and effect: to test this you can ask him/her to make a loud noise with a toy or his body			
Social and Emotional	Very dependent behaviour			
	Gets upset when separated from mother or prime caregiver			
	Likes to do the opposite of what he/she is told to do			

Checklist for a child aged approximately 2 Years

CHILD'S NAME: _____ D.O.B. _____

*Important background information that could affect results:*_____

_____

_____

	Action	Date	Date	Date
Large motor	Runs			
	Jumps with both feet together			
	Can walk backwards			
	Can kick and throw a large ball			
	Can climb up and down steps with both feet on every step			
	Can use feet to ride on and move a wheeled toy			
	Has control over his/her bowel and bladder			
	Can climb up on a chair, turn and sit down			
Fine motor	Can build a tower of 6 blocks			
	Holds crayon or paintbrush and makes controlled movements			
	Can put small objects in a container and take them out again			
	Can feed himself/herself			
Perceptual	Fits a shape into the same shaped hole			
	Responds to and can locate pain			
Language	Uses 50 to 300 words and learns new ones every day			
	Understands far more than he/she is able to express			
	Joins 2–3 words in sentences, e.g. 'Me go outside'.			
Cognitive	Understands what things are for and what belongs together			
	Does simple classification based on one attribute, e.g. separates toy cars from blocks			
	Names objects in picture books and enjoys being read to			
Social and Emotional	Has temper tantrums			
	Likes to be around people			
	Plays *alongside* other children			

Checklist for a child aged approximately 3 Years

CHILD'S NAME: _____ D.O.B. _____

*Important background information that could affect results:*_____

_____

_____

	Action	Date	Date	Date
Large motor	Stands on one leg for about 6 seconds			
	Goes *up* stairs with one foot on each step			
	Stands up from a kneeling position without using his/her hands			
	Can catch and throw a large ball without losing balance			
Fine motor	Builds a tower of 10 blocks			
	Can do up buttons and thread 6 large beads onto a string			
	Can copy straight lines and a cross			
	Holds crayons between his/her thumb and fingers			
Perceptual	Can distinguish between and match various shapes			
	Can distinguish between and match different colours			
Language	Speaks in complete sentences			
	Can remember and sing simple songs and rhymes			
	Listens attentively to stories appropriate to his/her age			
Cognitive	Can count to 10			
	Has a good memory			
	Likes to look at books			
	Knows if he/she is a boy or a girl			
	Participates in imaginative/fantasy play			
Social and Emotional	Has a sense of humour and enjoys playing tricks			
	Affectionate towards parents/caregivers			
	Beginning to share and be less selfish			
	Fantasy play reflects his/her own experiences			

Checklist for a child aged approximately 4 Years

CHILD'S NAME: _____ D.O.B. _____

Important background information that could affect results: _____

_____

_____

	Action	Date	Date	Date
Large motor	Jumps up and down			
	Dresses and undresses with help			
	Goes *down* stairs one foot at a time			
	Climbs trees and ladders			
	Can pedal a tricycle			
Fine motor	Holds a crayon using a tripod grip (thumb + 2 fingers)			
	Cuts paper in half with scissors			
	Threads 12 small beads on a string			
	Can model with playdough and clay			
	Can draw a recognizable figure of a man			
Perceptual	Can build a 12–24 piece puzzle			
	Can name four or more colours			
Language	Uses the pronouns *I, you* and *me* correctly			
	Can answer questions like 'Whose?', 'Where?', 'Why?'			
	Uses the past tense of verbs, e.g. 'Mommy *went* to work'.			
Cognitive	Understands and names the sequence of daily events			
	Understands the value of the lower numbers, e.g. $3 = \blacklozenge\ \blacklozenge\ \blacklozenge$			
	Can name parts missing from a picture or a puzzle			
	Understands what 'most' means			
Social and Emotional	Plays complex fantasy games			
	Can play co-operatively in a group			
	Is willing to take turns with toys			

Checklist for a child aged approximately 5 Years

CHILD'S NAME: _____ D.O.B. _____

*Important background information that could affect results:*_____

_____

_____

	Action	Date	Date	Date
Large motor	Can run fast in a circle			
	Walks backwards			
	Dresses and undresses without adult assistance			
Fine motor	Copies a square and a triangle			
	Can use a pencil to trace simple pictures			
	Catches a ball thrown from 1 metre away			
	Cuts on a line with scissors			
Perceptual	Can build a puzzle with 24–36 pieces			
	Can name most of the more common colours			
Language	Uses fluent speech			
	Can tell a familiar story while looking at a picture book			
	Understands humour and enjoys hearing and telling jokes			
Cognitive	Is eager to learn new things			
	Understands concept of same, e.g. same shape, or same size			
	Understands 'first', 'second' and 'last'			
	Reads his own name and some familiar words/letters			
	Understands what money is for			
	Understands 'more' and 'less'			
	Can order objects, e.g. from tallest to shortest			
Social and Emotional	Has a 'best' friend			
	Is competitive – i.e. likes to do well in a contest situation			
	Shows pride in his/her accomplishments			
	Prefers to play gender-related games (e.g. boys play with cars)			

Checklist for a child aged approximately 6 Years

CHILD'S NAME: _____ D.O.B. _____

*Important background information that could affect results:*_____

_____

_____

	Action	Date	Date	Date
Large motor	Can skip and gallop			
	Can turn a somersault			
	Jumps and hops forward without falling			
	Can balance on either foot for 10 seconds			
Fine motor	Copies a diamond			
	Cuts on an angular or curved line with scissors			
	Can use a pencil to trace and copy letters and numbers			
Perceptual	Can distinguish small differences in shapes			
	Can distinguish differences in the orientation of a letter, e.g. between p, b, q and d or f and t			
Language	Speech is fluent and he/she has a large vocabulary			
	Understands and enjoys simple jokes and riddles			
	Remembers short rhymes and can sing familiar songs			
	Can listen to age appropriate stories for 20–30 minutes			
Cognitive	Rote counts to 20			
	Knows numerals and number values from 1–10			
	Recognizes letters of the alphabet (especially in his/her name)			
	Shows an interest in learning to read			
Social and Emotional	Takes a role in group play and co-operates within the group			
	Knows how to be generous and caring			
	Can feel some empathy for other children			

Chapter 4

Assessment and management planning

Caroline Rose and Justin Amery

Key points

- You might feel fairly confident about this subject, and so perhaps think this chapter will not be very useful to you.
- If so, we beg to differ – this chapter is probably the most important in the whole book.
- As Derek Doyle once said, the heart and soul of good palliative care is 'immaculate assessment'.
- Children have a very broad range of needs, all of which need to be assessed and factored in to a good children's palliative care assessment and management plan.
- To understand these needs, keep interviewing the child and family until you can picture in your mind what it is like to be the child from the moment they wake up to the moment they sleep – a 'typical day'.
- From this picture of a 'typical day' distil all of the child's and family's main concerns into a clear and holistic problem list.
- Develop a SMART* management plan for each of these problems which hopes for the best but plans for the worst.
- If the child and family do not have easy access to your services 24 hours per day, never leave them until you have prepared them and equipped them for all eventualities.

*Specific, measurable, acceptable, realistic and time-framed.

4.1 Introduction

This chapter describes the heart and soul of good children's palliative care. It tells you how to get from knowing nothing about a child and family to having a full, comprehensive and holistic management plan for every problem the child and family are facing as part of their battle with HIV/AIDS, cancer or other life-limiting conditions. It is no exaggeration to say, if you get this bit right, the rest is straightforward. On the other hand, if you get it wrong, the care you provide will be suboptimal at best and poor at worst.

In principle, the steps are straightforward.

Table 4.1 Five steps to excellent children's palliative care

1. Assess the child and family holistically.
2. Develop a problem list covering physical, psychosocial and spiritual needs.
3. Design a management plan for each of these problems.
4. Carry out the management plan.
5. Review and adapt the problem list and management plan as things progress.

In practise, there are plenty of ways you can trip up.

If you don't know where you are on the map, there is no way of working out how to get to your destination. If you don't know what a child's problems are, you have no hope addressing those problems. Without good assessment of children and families, it is impossible to develop a good and holistic management plan, so you will not be able to provide good children's palliative care. This is self-evident. Unfortunately, learning resources for health professionals tend to focus much more on symptom-control skills than assessment skills[1]. Perhaps it is therefore not surprising that, in the authors' experience, health workers often run into difficulties because of failure to assess children and families thoroughly.

No matter what is the reason though, there is no doubt that assessment in children's palliative care is something that is crucial, yet something which tends to be done very badly. We hope that readers will avoid the temptation of skipping this chapter in a rush to get to the chapters on symptom control and instead take time to read and reflect on their assessment skills and practise.

4.2 **Background**

While the authors have not found any published literature on the assessment of children and young people with palliative care needs in Africa, there is some literature relating to the subject in the United Kingdom. Some of the principles and practise of this literature can be applied in the African setting.

In 1991, the Department of Health in the United Kingdom published a report 'Welfare of Children & Young People in Hospital'[2,3] which was concerned not only with hospital care but also with holistic care in the community. The key theme of this report was that there should be a comprehensive assessment process for chronically ill children and that all health areas should have clear policies for this. In 2000, the UK Department of Health published a second report[4] which stated that:

> Assessments should have a clear objective to reach understanding of the specific needs of the child and other members of the family; and to agree a realistic and achievable plan for the provision of support and services to meet those needs. *It should be recognised that assessment is not a single event but a continuing process,* which allows flexibility and choice as the child and family's circumstances change.

In 2003, the UK Association for children's palliative care (ACT)[5] produced a document detailing the specific needs of assessing children with life-limiting illnesses. It states:

> It may be tempting for groups of professionals to make assessments based on their own observations and experience and to decide what would be best for a particular family. The child and family must be at the centre of the process and a non-judgmental approach by professionals with the time and ability to listen will form the basis of assessment. The family's home, culture and wider community network

will be important considerations . . . Partnership is the theme throughout this guidance, not only with the family but also with other professionals, services and organizations.

4.3 Aims of assessment

The aims of assessment[6] should be to

(1) provide **factual information** on the child and family members;

(2) **explore ideas, concerns and expectations** of child and family members;

(3) develop a **clear problem list;**

(4) discuss and agree a **clear management plan**.

4.4 Principles of assessment

There are some basic principles of assessment which will serve you well if you keep to them. These are as follows:

◆ **Keep the child in the centre of your focus**: Trust him, respect her autonomy and address issues of confidentiality and consent. The rights of children to have their views heard have been enshrined in law in the UN Convention on the Rights of the Child[7].

◆ **Trust the child and family**: They are the primary carers and are experts in the care of the child.

◆ **Home should be the centre of care and the model for caring**[8]: Wherever possible, keep the child at home. When this is not possible, model the care and the environment on the home as much as possible.

◆ **Listen, listen, listen**: The child and family will tell you what their ideas, fears and needs are. If you do not know all of them by the end of the assessment process, you are not finished.

◆ **Be open, clear and honest**: Use simple, non-jargon language. Talking about death and dying is hard, but most children and families prefer to know so that they can prepare themselves and others. Many parents have said that receiving timely and accurate information is one of the most important areas for them[9].

◆ **Be holistic**: A child and family can be distressed by physical, psychological, social, financial or spiritual needs. Only by assessing them all can you develop a good management plan. No two families will be the same. What seems minor to one family may be the most pressing need causing great anxiety to another[10].

◆ **Think partnership**: The importance of partnership has been further reinforced by a substantial number of research findings[11-13]. Your main partnership is with the child and family. However, you need to form partnerships with other community and professional carers and health workers. Partnership working ensures that parents or caregivers feel respected and informed, that staff are being open and honest with them and that they in turn are confident about providing vital information about their child, themselves and their circumstances[14].

◆ **Key-working**: If more than one health worker is involved, it is sensible to negotiate and agree one key-worker that child, family, carers and professionals recognize. This will help ensure consistency and good communication.

◆ **The assessment should be a process not a single event**: For a start, the whole assessment is often too much to do all in one go, so keep going back until it is finished. Secondly, in

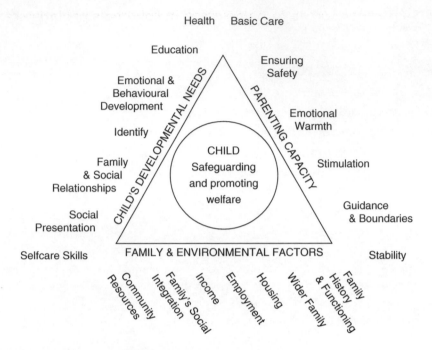

Fig. 4.1 The assessment framework[15].

children's palliative care, things change, often quite rapidly. As problems come and go, your assessment will need to be constantly revisited and updated.

◆ **Review**: The needs of a dying child and his/her family can change rapidly and dramatically. This week's assessment may be very different to last week's.

4.5 **Dimensions of a child's needs**

The chances are that if you are reading this then you come from a medical or nursing background. If that is the case, particularly if you are a doctor, you will have been firmly taught the bio-medical model of assessment (history, examination, special investigations, diagnosis and treatment). Unfortunately, although this framework has its place with some of the physical causes of symptoms, in most areas of children's palliative care it is woefully inadequate. A child can suffer for many different reasons. A child has many different needs, any of which, if blocked or adversely affected, will cause the child to suffer in one way or another. Now the reality is that, in most African health care settings, we will not have the resources to meet all of the child's needs, but that doesn't mean we should not know what they are.

The following framework is one of many theoretical models. It has been outlined below as an illustration of all the areas you need to think about when assessing a child's palliative care needs. When you read it, try and imagine you are a 12-year-old child with end-stage AIDS or cancer, feeling very unwell, as well as being disabled, disfigured and unable to self-care. Try and think which of the needs on the right hand column might be unfulfilled, and reflect on how that would make you feel.

4.5.1 **Summary of areas to be assessed in children's palliative care**

Table 4.2 Summary of areas to be assessed

Health	Includes
Growth and development Physical and mental wellbeing	◆ Freedom from pain and disease ◆ Adequate and nutritious diet ◆ Appropriate health care ◆ Exercise ◆ Immunizations ◆ Developmental checks, dental and optical care ◆ Sex education ◆ Substance misuse education
Education	Includes
All areas of a child's cognitive development from birth to maturity	◆ Opportunities for play and interaction with other children ◆ Access to learning ◆ Acquisition of skills and interests ◆ To experience success and achievement
Emotional and behavioural development Concerns the appropriateness of response demonstrated in feelings and actions by a child, initially to parents and caregivers and, as the child grows older, to others beyond the family.	Includes ◆ Nature and quality of early attachments ◆ Characteristics of temperament ◆ Adaptation to change ◆ Response to stress ◆ Degree of appropriate self control.
Identity Concerns the child's growing sense of self as a separate and valued person.	Includes ◆ Child's view of self and abilities ◆ Self-image and self-esteem ◆ Having a positive sense of individuality. ◆ Feelings of belonging and acceptance (by family, peer group and wider society, including other cultural groups) (Race, religion, age, gender and disability may all contribute to this)
Family and social relationships Concerns development of empathy and the capacity to place self in someone else's shoes.	Includes ◆ Stable and affectionate relationship with parents or caregivers ◆ Good relationships with siblings ◆ Age appropriate friendships with peers and other significant persons in the child's life ◆ Response of family to these relationships.
Social presentation Concerns child's growing understanding of the way in which appearance, behaviour and any impairment are perceived by the outside world and the impression being given.	Includes ◆ Appropriateness of dress for age, gender, culture and religion ◆ Cleanliness and personal hygiene ◆ Availability of advice from parents or caregivers about presentation created in different settings

(Continued)

Table 4.2 (continued) Summary of areas to be assessed

Family history and functioning	Includes ◆ Genetic and psychosocial factors ◆ Who is living in the household and how they are related to the child? ◆ Significant changes in family/household composition ◆ Chronology of significant life events and their meaning to family members ◆ Nature of family functioning, including wider family roles and responsibilities, decision-making processes, family hierarchies and sibling relationships ◆ Who are considered to be members of the extended family and what is their role?
Housing	Includes ◆ What basic amenities and facilities are there? ◆ Is housing accessible and suitable to the needs of the sick child?
Employment and income	Includes ◆ Who is working in the household, their pattern of work and any changes? ◆ How is work or the absence of work viewed by family members? ◆ How does it affect their relationship with the child? ◆ Income available over a sustained period of time ◆ Sufficiency of income to meet the family's needs
Family's social integration	Includes ◆ The wider context of the local neighbourhood and community and its impact on the child and parents ◆ Degree of the family's integration or isolation, their family groups, peer groups, friendship and social networks and the importance attached to them.
Community resources	Includes ◆ Description of all facilities and services in a neighbourhood, including health care services, schools, places of worship, transport, shops and leisure.

4.6 **The process of assessment**

4.6.1 **Step 1: Make a good impression**

First impression matters. It is very important that the child and family recognize you as someone who wants to help, who is able to help and who is prepared to be honest and open with them. Therefore, make a point of explaining what you wish to do early on.

4.6.2 **Step 2: Explain the process**

You need to explain to the child and family that they should try to be honest and open with you, even about difficult issues. The explanation should cover the following:

◆ What the process will involve?

◆ How the assessment will lead to a problem list and management plan?

◆ Who else might be involved (health workers, community volunteers, other professionals, etc.)?

◆ What will happen afterwards?

Ideally, you should have some written and pictorial information about your service, the assessment process and what services you might be able to offer.

4.6.3 Step 3: Involve the child

From even a very young age, children will be able to give information about their functional abilities and, provided with an atmosphere in which their views are respected and given validity, they will be able to describe feelings and needs[16]. Try and think how you might involve the child in the assessment process taking into account their age, development, disability and culture. It will be necessary to build a rapport that will help the child to feel understood, establishing the most appropriate method of communication (see Chapter 2 – Communicating with children and their families).

4.6.4 Step 4: Identifying family situation, structures and dynamics

It is very important early on to get a clear feel for how each family 'works', its culture and its environment. Every family has a different way of dealing with issues, problems and decisions (see Chapter 13: Psychosocial and family care). Each family's financial and social circumstances are different. These variations mean that similar problems will have very different effects on different families. If you can understand all of this early, you will have a much better chance of developing a management plan that is realistic and tailored to the particular needs of the family.

While we have not found any research on the effects of culture and ethnic background on children's palliative care services in Africa, it is (anecdotally) clear to those with knowledge of Africa and the West that family structures, decision-making processes and hierarchies can be quite different to the Western nuclear family model. It may be that the parents are not the ultimate decision-makers and that other family members need to be involved. It may be that some families are very private and not keen to seek help outside the family. It may be that the main carer for the child is another child. There may be many children in the family, who may or may not be first-degree siblings to the child, but who nevertheless are very close. All of the family structures, dynamics and decision-making processes need to be clarified and documented before a proper assessment and management plan can be developed.

4.6.5 Step 5: Establish the 'typical day'

A very good way to get a feel for what the main problems are is to ask the child and family to describe their typical day. This has two benefits. Firstly, it will give you a wealth of information that you won't get simply by completing pro-forma record sheets. Secondly, because it is familiar, it is a good way of helping the child and family build confidence, overcome shyness and develop trust in you.

The description should be in great detail. Try and get them to tell you everything from the moment they wake up to the moment they go to sleep. Get them to include small details about what they eat and when, when they go to the toilet, what jobs they do and when, when they play and with whom, what they do at school and so on.

Box 4.1 Exercise: Your own typical day

Think about your own typical day. Better still, find a child you know well and ask them about theirs. Start from the moment they wake up and don't finish listening and writing until the moment they go to bed at night. As you listen, begin to realize and note down that they are giving very rich information about their physical, psychological, social, family, community and educational functioning.

4.6.6 **Step 6: Establishing functional abilities**

From this discussion, and from your observations, try and make sure that you have a good idea of what are called the child's functional abilities. These are all the things a child needs to be able to do to live a full and healthy life. This is called a 'functional assessment'. An example of what you should assess is included below. We have included a column for scoring on the right as an example, but many people are suspicious of scoring systems because they are very subjective in these kinds of circumstances. If you have this concern, a better way is to avoid scoring and simply add descriptions of what the child can do or cannot do.

So, for example, a child might only be able to walk with support from a parent. You can either score this '1/2 (partly dependent)' or simply say 'can walk only with the aid of parent'. You decide which way you would prefer.

Table 4.3 Form for establishing functional abilities of a chilld

Item	Score (or decsription)
	0 = fully independent, 1= partly dependent, 2 = fully dependent
Breathing	
Cardiovascular	
Maintaining comfort	
Maintaining body temperature	
Vision	
Hearing	
Mobility/co-ordination	
Personal care: feeding, bathing, dressing, toileting, taking medication	
Bladder management	
Bowel management	
Language, communication	
Sleep	
Play, development, social interaction	
Problem solving, memory	
Safety	

Where the child is older, you should also consider:

♦ transition to independent living
♦ further education
♦ employment issues
♦ sexual needs

4.6.7 Step 7: Clinical assessment

You may be surprised to find that the clinical assessment comes so far down the list of tasks in the assessment process. However, if you think about it, it makes sense that the assessment of what is abnormal should only come after assessment of what is normal (i.e. the background, routines, family structures and abilities of the child). So, before starting on the clinical assessment, you should have a very clear idea of what it is like to be the child.

In children's palliative care, the aim of the clinical assessment is to identify and clarify particular causes of distress. Before you start, remember the concept of total pain. Pain and distress come from a variety of causes: physical, psychological, social, financial, spiritual and cultural. Although we may come from medical backgrounds, and be happier dealing with physical problems and treatments, it is vital that we do not forget all of the possible aspects of suffering in order that we give ourselves the best chance of coming up with a management plan that addresses all of the child's and family's needs.

The issues to be addressed in the clinical assessment should include:

+ physical symptoms
+ relevant past medical history
+ drug history
+ allergies
+ psychological and emotional concerns
+ spiritual concerns.

For each symptom, you should ask enough supplementary questions to enable you to come up with a differential diagnosis. These act as medical 'sieves' to help you narrow down the likely causes. Specific questions for specific symptoms can be found in the relevant section in this handbook. It is beyond the scope of this handbook to detail generic clinical skills, but obviously all health workers involved in children's palliative care need to have a good understanding of medical history-taking and examination skills. Readers should refer to other learning resources if necessary.

4.6.8 Step 8: Examining the child

At some point during the assessment process you will need to examine the child. The big difference between examining children and adults is that children may not cooperate and, if they do, they may stop cooperating at any time. That means you have to forget your hopes of a smooth 15 minute systematic, textbook examination. You need to be a bit more creative.

> Try to avoid starting the examination unless you have whittled your differential diagnoses down to 3 or fewer possibilities, and you know exactly what clinical signs you are looking for to help you confirm or rule out the differentials.

4.6.8.1 Some tips for examining children

+ Remember that the examination starts as soon as a child walks through the door. If he walks in normally, smiles at you, says hello, notices a small crayon and starts colouring, you have established that he has no major lateralizing signs and that gross motor, fine motor, speech, vision and sensation functions are probably all normal. In other words, you have pretty much done a fairly comprehensive gross neurological exam, at least for the kind of pathology you are likely to see in children's palliative care.

- During the history, keep whittling away at your differential diagnoses. Don't examine unless you have whittled your differential down to 3 or fewer possibilities.

- Use simple words. For example, most children understand 'please show me your tummy' but not 'I am going to examine your chest'.

- Once you have got down to three differentials, ask yourself: 'If I could examine only one thing for each diagnosis, what would it be?' and then examine those immediately. So, for example, if you suspect a chest infection, chest auscultation is likely to be the most discriminatory exam. If you suspect abdominal lymphadenopathy, abdominal palpation is the most useful. You can always go back and do a systematic examination later (if the child allows you).

- Break it up: you can check glands at the same time as stroking a cheek, or a pulse when holding a hand.

- Leave intrusive examinations (e.g. throat and ears) until last.

4.6.9 **Step 9: Special investigations**

In a resource-poor setting, you may well have access only to a limited number of investigations, and even these might prove too costly. In many situations in children's palliative care, special investigations are not required. Nevertheless, there are some times when they are helpful, particularly when you are trying to rule out reversible causes of symptoms (e.g. infective causes of pain or fever, radiosensitive tumours causing local symptoms, raised calcium and so on). The key thing is to be discriminating. This is particularly the case where a family has to pay much needed money. If a test will be very helpful and may affect the management plan, it is worth doing. If it is for curiosity, or will not significantly affect the management plan, you should refrain from ordering it.

Do I really need this test?
When ordering tests, be discriminating.
Ask yourself: 'What might I do differently when I get this result back?'
If the answer is: 'Not much', then don't do it!

4.7 **Management planning in children's palliative care**

Working together with child, family and colleagues to achieve an agreed, achievable and realistic management plan is possibly one of the greatest challenges to children's palliative care in the African context. Yet, without it, it is next to impossible to provide good children's palliative care.

Good children's palliative care management planning means hoping for the best and planning for the worst.

Management planning means hoping for the best and planning for the worst. Planning for the worst means discussing the worst with the child and family, and that can be a painful and difficult task in children's palliative care. If this is true for you, you are not alone. Many studies have shown how health workers delay difficult discussions and care planning until it is too late, leaving the child and family to suffer needlessly[17–19]. However, think about how you would feel about a health worker who avoided telling you the truth and left you to face difficult and tragic consequences unforeseen and unprepared.

> To withhold important information from our patients is immoral, unethical and negligent.

You might also find it challenging to have to discuss difficult and painful issues. You might find it frustrating to have to put a great deal of time and energy into what might be considered to be managerial and administrative work. Trying to set up collaborative working systems with families and co-workers can be frustrating, time-consuming and energy-sapping in the initial stages, particularly to busy health workers already overwhelmed by a large number of longer-surviving HIV-infected children and adults. Nevertheless, if we are to be effective as care providers for patients and families affected by HIV/AIDS and cancers, it is fundamentally important to work within this collaborative, comprehensive framework.

So, it is absolutely essential that you do brace yourself, prepare yourself and spare no effort in arranging and facilitating all necessary discussions to ensure that a holistic, realistic, all-encompassing and collaborative management plan is written, reviewed and updated. Ultimately, once the plan and systems are up and running, you will find that you provide better care and achieve greater job satisfaction and support as a result.

4.7.1 The challenges of management planning

This is the true art of children's palliative care. At its simplest, management planning is straightforward. You work out a problem list at the end of the assessment stage, and then you attach a management plan for each problem. In practise however, things can get be a bit more complicated.

◆ Holistic children's palliative care implies identification and management of physical, psychological, social and spiritual problems. Hence problem lists are often long and complex, requiring well-organized, clear and updated management plans.

◆ Decision-making in children's palliative care is often difficult – involving discussions about prognosis, the risks and benefits of different therapies, the effects of complex family dynamics and the effect of ethical and legal issues.

◆ The question of how 'quality of life' is best served is complex and often not easy to achieve consensus on.

◆ Problems with child, family and health worker guilt, fear, denial, avoidance and collusion can make the development of genuine problem lists and management plans very difficult.

◆ Needs of individual children are constantly changing with time and with progress of the disease. These changing needs often require the input of many different professional and voluntary carers (particularly with HIV/AIDS) so the potential for confusion and miscommunication is enormous.

◆ The need for continuity of care dictates that comprehensive clinical records be kept and made available to all health workers involved in an individual case. This poses significant challenges for over-stretched and under-resourced health management systems and services[20]. Concerns about stigmatization of children with HIV and cancer limit the acceptability of patient-held record cards.

- Continuity in care providers is much more challenging, given the high levels of attrition, transfers and mobility of health care workers in the African setting.

4.7.2 Management planning: When?

- Planning should start the moment you meet the child and family.
- Planning should be ongoing and re-visited frequently as needed.
- Planning should be 'normalized' by incorporating it into routine care.
- Don't wait until a crisis happens in order to address it: if you are on the ball and preparing for the worst, unanticipated crises should not happen.
- Do not defer these discussions until it is too late for meaningful discussion.

4.7.3 Management planning: Who?

- You
- The child
- The immediate family.
- Other family members who have a decision-making function about the child.
- Health workers who have an active involvement in the child's care.
- Other community or voluntary carers who might be involved.

4.7.4 Management planning: How?

- Be positive, respectful and focused on the values, concerns, cultural beliefs and care preferences of the patient and family.
- Be aware of the fears, concerns and expectations of the child and family members.
- Discuss and agree a problem list including all relevant physical, social, psychological and spiritual problems.
- For each problem lay out clearly the possible scenarios, from best to worst, so that the child and family are aware (but use the breaking bad news approach if you are to share any new and difficult information – see Chapter 2 – Communicating with children and their families).
- For each problem and scenario, detail a plan.
- For each plan be clear:
  - Who will be involved
  - What will be done
  - When it will be done
- Record the plan in a clear health record, ideally with a copy going with the child and family to ensure continuity and adherence.
- Access to essential drugs and supplies.
- Community-level support structures.

4.7.5 Management planning: What? – the problem list

The problem list and action plan are at the heart of good children's palliative care. If you create a good, holistic problem list with an associated action plan, the chances are you will perform as well as you can perform. If you don't, you won't. It's as simple as that.

So, spend time on creating the problem list. As you go through the assessment process, keep a separate sheet of paper on which you can jot down problems as they arise. Otherwise you will forget them at the end.

You can create a problem list anyway you like. Some people prefer to use a blank sheet of paper and create it as they go, others prefer to have a pro-forma tick list, others a half-way house between the two. However, as a general rule it is sensible to have a problem list with an action plan included. Children's palliative care problem lists can be very long, so it is easy to get confused about which actions treatments are associated with which problems. If you associate an action plan with each problem on the list, you and your colleagues will be clear about the plans and stick to them.

As an aide memoir, you should have thought about all of the following areas when you write a problem list. It is adapted from the Gold Standards Framework 'PEPSI-COLA' sheet[21]. You do not need to use this format, but it should prompt you to think broadly and give you ideas for how you want to develop your own problem list and management plan.

Table 4.4 The PEPSI-COLA assessment framework

Problem	Action plan
P – Physical	
Functional problems Physical symptoms Medication – regular & PRN Compliance/stopping non-essentials Complementary therapies	
E – Emotional	
Understanding expectations Fears/Security Relationships	
P – Personal (for child and family members)	
Family dynamics and relationships Play Isolation Education Spiritual/religious needs	
S – Social Support	
Nutrition Financial issues Housing issues Care for the carers Practical support	
I – Information/communication	

Problems that might arise because of some key things not known/understood by:
   ◆ the child,
   ◆ family members,
   ◆ fellow health workers,
   ◆ others
(for example, factors that might affect drug adherence, place of care or fears about death and dying).	

(Continued)

Table 4.4 (continued) The PEPSI-COLA assessment framework

Problem	Action plan
C – Control	
Has the child and family had a chance to choose where possible? Is their dignity protected as much as possible? Have they been involved in treatment options/management plan ? Have they specified what they want to happen after death? Place of death.	
O – Out of Hours/Emergency	
What will happen if you are not around? Has cover been planned? If not, do the family know what to do? Have they got enough drugs? Do they have enough info?	
L – Late	
End-of-life/terminal management plan. Has non-palliative treatment been stopped? Are the child and family aware that this is the final stage? Has spiritual care been addressed? How often will you review? Have late stage symptoms been controlled?	
A – Afterwards	
Bereavement support. Assessment/audit of your performance. Does the team have opportunities for debrief and support?	

Permission 1: Adapted with permission from the Gold Standards Framework, Keri Thomas 2002.

4.8 **Reviewing**

It can be very hard in a resource-poor context to provide regular follow-up and review. You may only see a child and family once or twice before they move off up country or find they can no longer afford transport to get to you. They may have no easy phone contact. However, that does not excuse poor planning and preparation. If you know you will not be able to review for a longer period than you would ideally wish, you need to make sure that:

◆ the child and family are absolutely clear about the management plan for each problem

◆ you have anticipated the worst case scenarios (even the ones that are very hard to discuss like choking, heavy bleeding or fitting)

◆ you have talked through these scenarios with the family and made sure that they are absolutely clear what to do if any of them actually happen

◆ you have given written or pictorial information to back this up

◆ you have calculated how much of each of their drugs they will need (worst case) and left more than enough to cover it

◆ you have made sure that they have sufficient food, money and equipment to manage

◆ you have helped them draft in additional help from family and friends if needed

◆ you have given them a contact number (if possible) so that at least they can talk through concerns that might arise over the phone.

Box 4.2 Assessment case scenario

Case study:

Abigail is a 9-year-old girl with Burkitt's Lymphoma. She presented to the ward with Spinal cord compression, causing paralysis of the lower limbs and urinary incontinence. Despite chemotherapy and steroids these have not resolved. She is still unable to control her bowels but is often constipated; her mother has been manually evacuating some hard stool this week.

She is not able to walk and currently needs her mother with her to do everything; her mother carries her to places such as the toilet and the shop. She spends a lot of time lying on her bed and has got a pressure sore on each of her hips. Her mother is 8 months pregnant and carrying her is getting increasingly difficult.

She is unable to get to school and is missing playing football with her friends which used to be her favourite thing to do.

She has a good appetite but complains she is often hungry as when she is at the hospital her mother doesn't have enough money to buy food. She is able to feed herself.

She is able to communicate well, she hears well but is only able to see out of one eye as she had a tumour in the other one and the sight has not returned.

- What is the problem list?
- Write actions for each problem.
- Who else would you like to involve?
- What other information would you like to find out?

4.9 Questions for you

(1) Find a child you know and sit with him/her: write out a description of their own 'typical day' from the moment they wake up through until the next morning. Reflect on how well you do this with your patients.

(2) Reflect on your own practise in children's palliative care assessment. List what you think you do well and then list what you think you do not do so well?

(3) For those areas you think you do not do so well, write a plan for how you might change your practise?

(4) Reflect on the clinical record sheet you use for children's palliative care. Does it capture the essential elements discussed in this chapter? If not, how would you improve it?

Notes

1 Amery, J. & Lapwood, S. (2004). A study into the educational needs of children's hospice doctors: a descriptive quantitative and qualitative survey. *Palliative Medicine, 18*(8), 727–33.

2 Department of Health. (1991). *Welfare of Children and Young People in Hospital.* NHS Executive HMSO, London.

3 Department of Health. (1996). *Child Health in the Community: A Guide to Good Practice.* NHS Executive, HMSO, London.

4 Department of Health, Department for Education & Employment and The Home Office. (2000). *Framework for the Assessment of Children in Need and their Families.* HMSO, London.

5 The Association for Children's Palliative Care (ACT). (2003). *Assessment of Children with Life-Limiting Conditions and Their Families: A Guide to Effective Care Planning.* Available online at www.Act.org.

6 The Association for Children's Palliative Care (ACT). (2003). *Assessment of Children with Life-Limiting Conditions and Their Families: A Guide to Effective Care Planning.* Available online at www.Act.org.

7 UN Convention on The Rights of The Child. Available online at http://www.Unhchr.Ch/Html/Menu2/6/Crc/Treaties/Crc.Htm. 1991

8 The Association for Children's Palliative Care (ACT). (1993). *ACT Charter for Children with Life-Threatening Conditions and their Families.* ACT, Bristol. Available online at www.Act.org. Revised in 1998.

9 Kirk, S. & Glendenning, C. (2000). *Supporting Families Caring for A Technology-Dependent Child in The Community.* National Primary Care Research and Development Centre, Manchester.

10 Association for Children's Palliative Care (ACT)/Royal College of Paediatrics & Child Health. (1997). *Guide to The Development of Children's Palliative Care Services.* ACT, Bristol and Children's Palliative Care, London.

11 Butt, J. & Box, C. (1998). *Family Centred. A Study of the Use of Family Centres by Black Families.* REU, London.

12 Aldgate, J. & Bradley, M. (1999). *Supporting Families Through Short-Term Fostering.* The Stationery Office, London.

13 Tunstill, J. & Aldgate, J. (2000). *From Policy to Practice: Services for Children in Need.* The Stationery Office, London.

14 Department of Health. (2000). *Framework for the Assessment of Children in Need and their Families.* The Stationery Office, London.

15 Department of Health. (2000). *Framework for the Assessment of Children in Need and their Families.* The Stationery Office, London.

16 Marchant, R. (2001). *The Assessment of Children with Complex Needs, Child's World: Assessing Children in Need.* Jessica Kingsley Publishers, London.

17 Wenger, N.S., Kanouse, D.E., Collins, R.L., et al. (2001). End-of-Life discussions and preferences among persons with HIV. *JAMA, 285,* 2880–7.

18 Mouton, C., Teno, J.M., Mor, V. & Piette, J. (1997). Communications of preferences for care among human immunodeficiency virus-infected patients. Barriers to informed decisions. *Archives of Family Medicine, 6,* 342–7.

19 Curtis, J.R. & Patrick, D.L. (1997). Barriers to communication about end-of-life care in AIDS patients. *Journal of General Internal Medicine, 12,* 736–41.

20 Tindyebwa, D., Kayita, J., Musoke, P., et al. (Eds.). (2006). *African Network for Care of Children Affected by HIV/AIDS (ANECCA). Handbook on Paediatric AIDS in Africa.* (Revised Edition). Available online at www.Anecca.org.

21 Keri, Thomas & Department of Health. (2005). *PEPSI COLA Aide Memoire – Gold Standards Framework.* Government Stationary Office. London.

Section 2

Symptom control in children's palliative care

This section covers the management of the physical symptoms that you are likely to come across in the African children's palliative care context. It also covers HIV/AIDS. This might seem odd. HIV/AIDS is, after all, a disease not a symptom. We do not, for example, have a section on cancer. The reasons for this are that, in Africa, HIV/AIDS presents an enormous problem; the clusters of symptoms are unique; and the use of anti-retroviral therapy creates some particular challenges when it comes to prescribing palliative care drugs.

Apart from the chapter on HIV/AIDS (Chapter 12), the other chapter cover pain management and then symptoms related to particular systems (e.g. respiratory, gastrointestinal, neurological and so on).

Finally, in Section 4 we bring it all together with the chapter on end of life care. This chapter does repeat and reinforce some of the symptom control advice given in previous chapters and incorporates advice on psychosocial issues and bereavement from later chapters. The authors believe some repetition is warranted as end-of-life care is unique: it is often a more intense phase of management in which many of the strands of care come together, hopefully in a smooth and systematic way, in order to help the child and family achieve a death which is comfortable and dignified.

2.1 Four rules of symptom control in children's palliative care

Before moving on to the individual chapters, we thought you might like to read our simple rules for symptom control in children's palliative care. Remember them well. They have helped the authors out of many a tricky situation!

2.1.1 Rule one – Don't panic!

Symptom control can be very frightening, particularly in children. Fortunately, they are also usually very straightforward and quick to treat. Of course you must treat quickly – leaving a child to suffer is wrong. But you have time to take a deep breath and a quick think. Remember the adage: more haste, less speed. Have you really assessed properly? What is the child telling you? Is there something that is causing/worsening the symptoms that can be quickly relieved? What about non-pharmacological treatments? What would the right drug, dose and route be?

2.1.2 Rule two – Immaculate assessment

If you perform a thorough assessment of all of the child's and family's needs: physical, psychological, familial, social, spiritual, financial and the community; you will almost certainly develop a thorough problem list. With a good problem list, you will be able to draw up an effective and achievable management plan. Without one, you won't. Immaculate assessments lead to immaculate children's palliative care. Poor assessments lead to poor children's palliative care, as simple as that.

2.1.3 **Rule three – Hope for the best, prepare for the worst**

Fortunately, most symptoms are treatable, and many can be almost entirely removed. However, always keep in the back of your mind those symptoms that can be difficult to treat – neuropathic pains or dystonia or stridor, for example. Think also of other reasons why your symptom management may not work. Perhaps the patient will not understand and dose himself wrongly, perhaps you will miscalculate and give insufficient doses or quantities, perhaps you have missed that the grandmother is very fearful of drugs such as morphine and will block the mother using them when they get home. Think, think, think – and then prepare your strategy.

2.1.4 **Rule four – Treat what you can treat**

Sometimes, perhaps more often than not, it will not be clear to you what is causing the child's symptoms. But if you work your way through the chapters below, pick out individual symptoms and treat them accordingly, you will almost certainly make the child feel much better. Hopefully, when you have done that you can think and assess a bit more, and the truth about underlying pathology will emerge.

Chapter 5

Pain

Justin Amery, Michelle Meiring, Renee Albertyn
and Sat Jassal

Key points

- Take time to assess properly.
- Always use non-pharmacological methods – it's amazing how effective these are in children.
- Always start with paracetamol and an NSAID.
- If that's not enough, go for morphine (codeine doesn't seem to add much).
- If anxiety is a major factor, add a benzodiazepine.
- If the pain is shooting, burning or in a dermatome add amitriptyline, or carbamazepine.
- If the pain is related to seizures or spasm, add an anticonvulsant and/or benzodiazepine.
- If the pain is intractable and you suspect thalamic involvement, try ketamine or nitrous oxide (if it is available).

5.1 Cracking some myths about pain relief in children's palliative care

Unfortunately, children's palliative care is beset by professional myths which may seriously undermine your ability to make the child and family feel better. Here are the main ones. Arm yourself with the evidence so you can stand up for your patient when the time comes.

Box 5.1 Case study – Sarah

Sarah is a 10- year-old total orphan alone on the oncology ward. She has disseminated lymphoma in her brain, spine, neck and abdomen. Last time you met her you found that she had grade 5/5 pain in her head and abdomen. You decided to start her on morphine and (because she had no carer) you taught her how to give herself the correct dose at the correct time. Fortunately she responded very well and was soon able to get out of bed and start playing with other children in the ward. However, when you visit her today, you find her back in bed, moaning and obviously in severe pain. She says the nurse took her morphine away. You find the nurse in charge who tells you that Sarah is just making a fuss, her pain is not that bad, that she cannot be trusted to take her own morphine and (in any event) morphine is addictive and dangerous in children. What do you do?

5.1.1 The myth: Children and infants don't really feel much pain

The facts

◆ If anything, children are more sensitive to some pain than adults.

◆ By 26 weeks gestation, pain pathways and the cortical and sub cortical pain centres are well developed[1].

◆ Behavioural[2,3] and physiological[4] studies have shown that even very young infants respond to painful stimuli.

◆ Premature infants undergoing surgery with minimal anesthesia have significantly higher stress responses and significantly higher rates of complications and mortality than those given deeper anesthesia.[5,6]

5.1.2 The myth: Even if young children experience pain, they have no memory and it has no lasting effect

The facts

◆ Pain and distress can endure in even the tiny child's memory, resulting in disturbances of feeding, sleeping and the stability of the state of arousal[7].

◆ Preliminary data even suggest that early experiences of pain may produce permanent structural and functional reorganization of developing nociceptive neural pathways, which in turn may affect future experiences of pain[8].

◆ Prolonged untreated pain increases length of hospital stays and in addition could have a negative impact on healing.

5.1.3 The myth: Exposing children to opioid medications will run the risk of drug addiction

The facts

◆ Thirty-nine per cent of physicians are concerned about the risk of addiction resulting from the use of opioid analgesics in young patients[9].

◆ Children are at no more risk of becoming addicted to opioids than adults[10,11].

◆ Addiction is a psychological dependence – not experienced in patients with true pain on therapeutic doses and so very rare in the palliative care setting.

5.1.4 The myth: Children cannot be relied upon to decide their own level of analgesia

The facts

◆ Patient-controlled analgesia has been used successfully and safely in children as young as 6 years, with a high degree of satisfaction reported by the children and their parents[12,13]. Patient-controlled analgesic pumps (PCA pumps) are very unlikely to be available to you. However, what we can take from this is that children can be allowed to indicate how much of their morphine they think they need, and (in the author's experience in Africa) older children are able to manage it by themselves.

5.1.5 The myth: If children are in pain, they'll tell you and probably over exaggerate

The facts

- In day-to-day life, children can exaggerate their pain experiences, often to seek attention. However, the children's palliative care setting is far from being day-to-day.

- Children are better able to hide their pain than to fake it[14]. In other words, children often *mask* the presence of pain, possibly because they have come to fear injections or other procedures[15].

- Some children may be in some level of pain much of the time, and think nothing can be done – so they don't complain.

- Some children equate feeling pain with being taken to the hospital – a place they don't want to go.

- Some children may not complain of pain because they don't want their parents to be upset or unhappy.

- Some children, especially very young ones, may not have the ability to really communicate what they are feeling about pain.

5.1.6 The myth: We medical professionals are good at assessing childhood pain

The facts

- Medical professionals consistently and significantly under-rate children's pain[16].

- The tendency toward under-medication for pain is even more pronounced in children than in adults[17].

- Medical professionals (and other adults) often have a concern that children may feign or exaggerate suffering to obtain some secondary gain which causes them to discount children's reports of pain[18].

- Because pain is sometimes difficult to treat, medical professionals may diminish the seriousness of children's suffering and alleviate their own frustration by blaming children for protesting too much[19].

5.1.7 The myth: FACES scales are not reliable with African children and they are not able to use them

The facts

- While it is true that they have not specifically been tested in Africa, the Wong-Baker FACES scale has been tested across many cultures, in developed and developing world, and is valid and reliable, and can be used with confidence to assess pain/distress.

- It is also worth noting that evidence suggests that children have a subculture of their own regardless of their parents' cultural orientation[20–22].

- The authors of this chapter have varying experiences of uses of the FACES scales. In Uganda, we have found them very helpful, but less so in South Africa. What we can agree on is that:
  - FACES scales probably indicate 'distress' rather than pain specifically. However, in practise, this is a fine distinction and probably makes little difference to management.
  - FACES scales, like any other tools, cannot be relied upon in isolation. They need to be taken in the context of a holistic history and examination (see below).

5.1.8 **The myth: Play therapy won't work for African children as the concept of play for African children is different**

The facts

◆ Children respond extremely well to touch, distraction, relaxation techniques, music, art and play to help relieve distressing symptoms.

◆ There are a number of successful projects in Africa using play and art therapy to relieve distressing problems in children with AIDS (see Chapter 3, Play and development)[23,24].

◆ These therapies should be mainstream in any palliative care service for children (ACT Charter, UK)[25].

5.2 **Pain assessment**

Like any other symptom, you cannot properly manage pain unless you properly assess it. Like any other assessment, it is much easier if you start by developing a trusted and open relationship with the family and by doing your homework. So read the medical folders/medical notes and letters if there are any, and make sure that you ask the child and family.

Before moving on to pain assessment, a word of warning: pain assessments are important, but need to be combined with a careful evaluation of the presenting symptoms and diagnosis. Look for symptoms that are known to be painful (e.g. meningitis, gastro-oesophageal reflux) or that can cause anxiety and pain (e.g. pneumonia, vomiting). It is important to treat the pain if it is there and not wait.

There are three main ways you can assess a child's pain. These are as follows:

(1) Ask the child: the quickest and most accurate, provided that the child is able to tell you.

(2) Ask the family (or known carer). This is the next best way, and important as a cross-check even when the child has already told you. It is extremely important to include the mother/caregiver in the assessment process. Nobody knows the child better than the mother. Check for previous exposure to pain, verbal pain indicators, premorbid personality.

(3) Try to assess it yourself: This is the least accurate option, but better than nothing if you are stuck. Think of your own body changes when you are in pain: you may feel pale, you are probably tensed or hunched up and your heart probably races; your face may be tight or even crying. All of these can be the same in children. But again, remember the evidence that shows that health professionals consistently underestimate children's pain when they don't double check with the child and mother/guardian. Take care however, especially of babies and very young children. With this group, do not trust your own judgement too much. Very young children are often too ill, or too tired to respond to pain stimuli. The absence of verbal or non-verbal pain indicators does not necessarily mean that the child is pain-free.

5.2.1 **Asking the child**

Just as in adult palliative care, the aim of the pain assessment is to determine what is causing the pain in order to be able to work out which management is most likely to work. The object of pain assessment is to capture the various dimensions of the pain, including the following:

◆ Intensity: You can use a variety of rating scales that can be helpful here, but the Wong-Baker FACES scales are probably the best tested in practise, at least in the West. The child is asked to identify their own pain intensity from the faces offered. They are suitable for children of around five upwards. Older children might find a straightforward Numerical Rating Scale (NRS) easier.

- Location and radiation: body charts work very well with children.
- Radiation: children find this one trickier to answer.
- Duration and changes with time: children may have difficulty pinning down time frames, as most children do not fully understand concepts of time until 7 or 8 years old.
- Description: children can usually answer this one with help.
- Any associations, exacerbating and relieving factors: this one is a bit hit and miss, but still worth asking.

Children, just like adults, might need a bit of prompting to help them to help you. Beware of asking leading questions – children often want to please the adult and might tell you what they think you want to hear. You might find the following suggestions helpful. Note the use of parochial language (such as 'hurt' instead of 'pain'). Obviously the exact words you use will vary on the child's native language, but just try to imagine yourself as the child in order to think of which words will make most sense. If you are stuck ask either the family or use a slightly older child to 'translate' for you (this tip is often amazingly successful). Remember however that children may not realize how much they are hurting because of constant pain[26].

Use prompting questions such as:

- Do you have a hurt/pain?
- Can you show me where it hurts?
- Does it hurt anywhere else?
- When did the hurt start?
- Do you know what might have started the hurt?
- How much does it hurt? (You can use a pain scale at this point.)
- Can you tell me any words that might describe the hurt?
- What helps to take away the hurt? What made it worse?

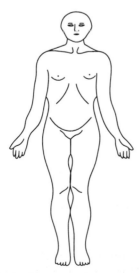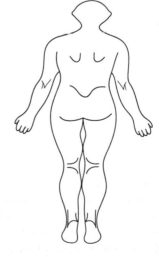

Fig. 5.1 Body chart.

5.2.1.1 The Wong-Baker FACES scale

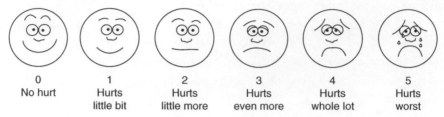

0	1	2	3	4	5
No hurt	Hurts little bit	Hurts little more	Hurts even more	Hurts whole lot	Hurts worst

Fig. 5.2 Wong-Baker FACES Scale[27].
Permission 1: Printed with permission of Elsevier Ltd. Oxford.
Source: Hockenberry, M.J., Wilson, D., Winkelstein, M.L.(2005) *Wong's Essentials of Pediatric Nursing*, 7 Edn. St. Louis, p. 1259. Used With Permission. Copyright, Mosby.

Original instructions: Explain to the person that each face is for a person who feels happy because he has no pain (hurt) or sad because he has some or a lot of pain. **Face 0** is very happy because he doesn't hurt at all. **Face 1** hurts just a little bit. **Face 2** hurts a little more. **Face 3** hurts even more. **Face 4** hurts a whole lot. **Face 5** hurts as much as you can imagine, although you don't have to be crying to feel this bad. Ask the person to choose the face that best describes how he is feeling.

Brief word instructions: Point to each face using the words to describe the pain intensity. Ask the child to choose the face that best describes own pain and record the appropriate number.

5.2.1.2 The Faces pain scale

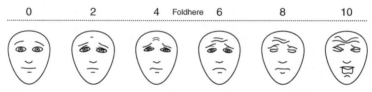

Fig. 5.3 The Faces pain scale.

The *Faces* pain scale has been revised so that the scale is from zero to ten rather than zero to five as in the Wong-Baker measure. The affective qualities including the smile and tears have been removed. When using the Faces Pain Scale Revised, you no longer have to include a statement such as 'You can experience the worst pain and not be crying'.

Original instructions: Explain to the person that each face is for a person who feels happy because he has no pain (hurt) or sad because he has some or a lot of pain. **Face 0** is very happy because he doesn't hurt at all. **Face 1** hurts just a little bit. **Face 2** hurts a little more. **Face 3** hurts even more. **Face 4** hurts a whole lot. **Face 5** hurts as much as you can imagine, although you don't have to be crying to feel this bad. Ask the person to choose the face that best describes how he is feeling.

Brief word instructions: Point to each face using the words to describe the pain intensity. Ask the child to choose the face that best describes own pain and record the appropriate number.

As mentioned above, be careful when using a pain measurement tool. You need to understand the parameters in the tool as well as how to interpret the score. Most importantly, no tool is perfect. Many told are far from perfect (including the ones described above). Read Chapter 4 (Assessment and management planning) to remind yourself of the importance of holistic history-taking from the child and mother/guardian, and proper physical examination.

The numerical rating scale is from 0 to 5
0 being the lowest score = No Pain
5 is the highest score = Worst pain possible

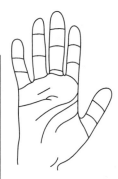

Use of the five fingers of the hand to grade severity
of patient's pain, starting with the little finger
upwards:
- Little finger – Mild Pain
- Up to Ring finger – Moderate pain
- Middle finger – Moderately severe pain
- Index finger – Severe pain
- Thumb – Overwhelming pain

Fig. 5.4 Numerical rating scale

5.2.2 **Asking the family or carer**

Ideally, the best person to ask is the parent or main caregiver. If they are not around, ask anyone who knows the child better than you do. It may be a nurse, volunteer on the ward or an older child in a nearby bed. Remember from the myths outlined above, hard as it is for our pride to accept, we health professionals are not very good at assessing pain in children. The important thing is that we are looking for verification of our own assessment.

- Try to discover additional concerns and/or meanings that the family or carers are attributing to changes in the child's behaviour.
- Ask the family or carer the same questions you asked the child.
- Use the same rating scales and charts.
- Ask the family or carers if they have noticed any signs of pain (particularly facial expression, body movements, quality of cry, stillness or withdrawal, change in favourite activities or sleeping, etc.).

Ultimately, you may well find that the accounts you receive vary, but no one said that the assessment of pain is a science! In fact it is an art, and this is where your own intuition and judgement comes in. Pain is an individual experience – no two people will experience pain in exactly the same way. Each child needs an individual plan.

5.2.3 **Your own 'objective' pain assessment**

A warning: take care here. Remember, on the whole, we health professionals are likely to underestimate the pain. Also, as children get older, facial expression and cry become less useful as indicators of pain, probably because older children develop a much wider repertoire of behaviour learnt from those around them (including language). In other words, how pain is expressed varies with age and with culture, which is probably one of the reasons why it is hard for health professionals to be accurate.

However, our assessment can still be valid, particularly if we use a framework to help us assess. Remember that pain generates a sympathetic nervous response, and therefore we can expect to see some of the following in a child who is in pain.

5.2.3.1 **The touch visual pain scale**

One of the authors (Renee Albertyn) has developed a scale particularly for use in the African context. This is the TVP (touch visual pain) scale. It was specifically designed to measure pain, anxiety and discomfort in infants less than one year of age. This involves the observation of sympathetic nervous system responses such as heart rate. Look for:

- Flexed and tensed body and limb postures
- Increases in the heart and breathing rate: but remember these can be drug induced or drug inhibited.
- Pallor
- Sweating
- Overly quiet or crying
- Withdrawn or clingy
- Wincing
- Moaning
- Restlessness.

(N.B. All of the above changes become less pronounced in chronic pain)

5.2.3.1.1 Instructions for the TVP

(1) Fill in background characteristics on the other side.

(2) Gently take away the sheets to observe the whole body of the child.

(3) Observe the child, using your eyes and hands starting from the feet.

(4) Fill in the tactile and visual score, score a 1 for each behaviour you observe.

(5) Add the 'ones' and score may range from 0 to 10.

(6) Place a mark on both numeric scales (below the tactile and visual score) which represent, in your expert opinion, the extent of pain and discomfort the child experiences at that specific time.

Scores:

- 0–3: observe patient, no real pain or anxiety present;
- 4–6: possible pain and anxiety/discomfort;
- 6–10: definite intervention required.

For possible anxiety, eliminate aspects such as hunger, thirst, uncomfortable position, separation anxiety (mother just left), need for a diaper change, etc.

For possible pain, consider aspects such as the time that the last dose of analgesia was given, whether analgesia was correctly given (dose and route), any painful procedures that could cause pain reaction, type of drugs and drug combinations.

Patient initials	Ward
Folder number:	Date:
Date of birth:	Time:
Gender:	Diagnosis:
Analgesic treatment (dosage and time):	
Tactile and visual score	**Present?**
Additional information:	
Observer:_____	
	Total score:

Do not react to the first assessment, always work with a baseline assessment obtained on admission. If in doubt, do three assessments, 30 minutes apart after repositioning the patient in a more comfortable position.

5.2.3.2 Clinical signs of neonates in pain

Neonates are particularly hard to assess for pain. Generally a baby who is pain free will be relaxed and soft to the touch. A baby in pain will be tense, watchful and agitated.

5.2.3.3 The FLACC scale

The FLACC scale[28] (see below) has been developed to help quantify clinical signs of childhood pain changes and is particularly useful to help improve consistency of assessment where different health professionals are involved. Again, use with care. It can lend a misleading air of objectivity to something which remains subjective.

Table 5.1 The FLACC scale

	SUGGESTED AGE GROUP: 2 months to 7 years		
	SCORING		
CATEGORIES	**0**	**1**	**2**
Face	No particular expression or smile	Occasional grimace or frown, withdrawn, disinterested	Frequent to constant quivering chin, clenched jaw
Legs	Normal position or relaxed	Uneasy, restless, tense	Kicking or legs drawn up
Activity	Lying quietly, normal position, moves easily	Squirming, shifting, back and forth, tense	Arched, rigid or jerking
Cry	No cry (awake or asleep)	Moans or whimpers, occasional complaint	Crying steadily, screams or sobs, frequent complaints
Consolability	Content, relaxed	Reassured by occasional touching, hugging or being talked to, distractible	Difficult to console or comfort

Each of the five categories: (**F**) Face; (**L**) Legs; (**A**) Activity; (**C**) Cry; (**C**) Consolability, is scored from 0–2 which results in a total score between 0 and 10 (*Merkel et al. 1997*)
Permission 2: Reproduced with permission from the Regents of the University of Michigan, © 2002

5.3 Pain diaries and flow sheets

Another way of assessing pain is to monitor it over time. In many ways this is much more useful in practise than the 'snapshot' tools suggested above, particularly where the pain is chronic. After all, when we are treating pain, we need to know how the pain improves (or does not improve) over time. Children and families can make up their own diary, which should include at least the time, the duration, the context in which pain has occurred and some sort of pain intensity assessment. A really helpful example was developed at Derian House Hospice in the UK, and this is shown below, with the chart filled out by a fictional family. We have used it successfully at Hospice Africa Uganda.

Table 5.2 The derian house pain diary

Time	Monday	Tuesday	Wednesday	Thursday	Friday	Saturday	Sunday
06:00							
07:00							
08:00							
09:00							
10:00							
11:00							
12:00							
13:00							
14:00							
15:00							
16:00							
17:00							
18:00							
19:00							
20:00							
21:00							
22:00							
23:00							
00:00							
01:00							
02:00							
03:00							
04:00							
05:00							

Permission 3: Reprinted with permission of Derian House Hospice

Key

Asleep		Awake & content		Uncomfortable	
Distressed		Severe distress			

5.4 The extent of the children's palliative care pain problem in Africa

In the African palliative care setting pain is very, very common. It is likely that most of the children you will see will be suffering with pain. In cancer, around 75% of patients suffer with pain[29]. While estimates vary, estimates of the frequency of pain in patients with AIDS generally range from 40% to 80%. Furthermore, the intensity of pain in AIDS appears to be comparable with, or even exceed, pain experienced by cancer patients. Worse still, the evidence suggests that pain is dramatically undertreated in patients with AIDS and that opioid analgesics in particular are underutilized[30].

These global findings are reproduced in Africa. The WHO estimates that there are 9 million new cases of cancer in the world, half of which are in the developing world (WHO 1996). In patients with AIDS reporting severe pain, 85% receive less than adequate treatment[31].

5.5 Causes of pain in children with cancer or HIV/AIDS

5.5.1 Classification of pain

There are three broad types of pain. The types of pain and their characteristics are outlined below.

Nociceptive pain

- So called because it results from stimulation of 'nociceptors' (pain receptors).
- Two subtypes: somatic (e.g. skin, connective tissue, muscle and bone) and visceral pain (e.g. internal organs and other hollow viscera).
- Somatic pain is usually well localized and often sharp and acute.
- Visceral pain less well localized and often described as deep, dull, aching, gnawing or spasmodic.
- Nociceptive pain tends to respond to non-opioids and opioids.

Neuropathic pain

- Due to damage to nerve tissue.
- Tends to be described as burning, tingling, stabbing, shooting, electric or allodynic.
- May respond to paracetamol, NSAIDs and opioids, but may need additional adjuvants (see below); Neuropathic pain usually needs the pain adjuvant therapy.

Thalamic pain

- Due to damage to the thalamus or spinothalamic pathway (e.g. CVA, infections, neurodegenerative conditions).
- Incompletely understood.
- In children often associated with conditions which interfere with communication, so often very difficult to identify and assess.
- Responds poorly to traditional analgesics or adjuvants.
- Reports and anecdotal experience suggest that the use of anaesthetics (e.g. nitrous oxide or ketamine) or possibly methadone is most likely to be effective.

(Sympathetic pain and psychogenic pain are considered in Chapter 13: Psychosocial and family care)

Box 5.2 Case study – Different types of pain

Isaac is a 12-year old boy with HIV/AIDS. He is on ARTs. He has now mainly recovered from severe viral encephalitis, but has been left with a slight weakness down his right side. Recently, he developed myositis in his left thigh. He complains of various pains. Firstly, he is getting intense, throbbing, localized pain in his left thigh. He says this pain is 5/5, always present and worse when the leg is moved or touched. It is associated with a fever. Secondly, he has started getting tingling, burning and shooting pains in his feet since starting his ARTs. Thirdly, he just feels as if the whole right side of his body is uncomfortable. He hates anything touching it, and likes to remain undressed as clothes irritate it. Occasionally, he gets burning or tearing like pains down the whole of his right side.

Isaac has three different types of pain, caused by three different triggers. Having read the section above, try and work out what these pains types are.

5.5.2 **Common causes of pain in children's palliative care in Africa**

In studies of adults with HIV/AIDS, the most common causes of pain are[32]:

- ◆ Pain-related to HIV/AIDS (45%)
  - HIV neuropathy
  - HIV myelopathy
  - Kaposi's sarcoma
  - Secondary infections (intestines, skin)
  - Organomegaly
  - Arthritis/Vasculitis
  - Myopathy/Myositis.
- ◆ Pain related to HIV/AIDS therapy (15–30%)
  - Antiretrovirals, anti-virals
  - Anti-mycobacterials, PCP prophylaxis
  - Chemotherapy (vincristine)
  - Radiation
  - Surgery
  - Procedures (bronchoscopy, biopsies).
- ◆ Pain unrelated to AIDS (25–40%)
  - Disc disease
  - Diabetic neuropathy.

HIV-related conditions that are observed to cause pain particularly in children include[33]:

- ◆ Meningitis and sinusitis (headaches)
- ◆ Otitis media
- ◆ Shingles
- ◆ Cellulitis and abscesses
- ◆ Severe candida dermatitis
- ◆ Dental caries
- ◆ Intestinal infections, such as mycobacterium avium intracellulare (MAI) and
- ◆ Cryptosporidium
- ◆ Hepatosplenomegaly
- ◆ Oral and esophageal candidiasis and
- ◆ Spasticity associated with encephalopathy that causes painful muscle spasms.

In cancer pain is usually due to direct invasion of pain-sensitive structures by the neoplasm[35,36]. The structures most often involved are bone and neural tissue, but pain also can occur when there is an obstruction of a hollow viscus, distention of organ capsules, distortion or occlusion of blood vessels and infiltration of soft tissues. In about one-quarter of patients, the cause relates to an anti-cancer treatment, and fewer than 10% have pain unrelated to the cancer or its treatment. Many patients, particularly those with advanced illness, have multiple causes and several sources of pain.

Other contributing factors are as follows:

◆ The intensity with which a child experiences pain is influenced by emotional factors (e.g. anxiety, fear, isolation) and cognitive factors (e.g. meaning ascribed to the pain, memory of similar experiences).

◆ Therefore, two children with virtually identical tissue damage may experience pain with different degrees of intensity. Specific factors influencing pain include:

  • fear and anxiety, e.g. being in strange surroundings

  • separation from family

  • painful procedures

  • social stigma

  • spiritual distress can all contribute to children's experience of pain.

Box 5.3 AIDS pain syndromes and most common diagnoses in AIDS[34]

Pain type	N	%
Somatic pain	107	71
Neuropathic pain	69	46
Visceral pain	44	29
Headache	69	46
Pain diagnosis		
Joint pains	47	31
Polyneuropathy	42	28
Muscle	40	27
Skin	23	15
Bone	31	20
Abdominal	25	17
Chest	19	13
Radiculopathy	18	12

5.6 Principles of pain management in children

5.6.1 The concept of total pain

The principles of pain management in children are the same as in adults. Just as in adults, pain can come from a variety of sources: physical, psychological, social and spiritual. The concept of total pain, first used by Cicely Saunders, is useful here.

She said that 'Total pain is a crisis at every level':

◆ Physical, uncontrolled pain

◆ Emotional pain due to (for example) anxiety, sadness, anger or fear

◆ Social pain due to carer strain, loss of confidence, fear and distress

◆ Spiritual pain due to anguish, suffering, hopelessness and meaninglessness.

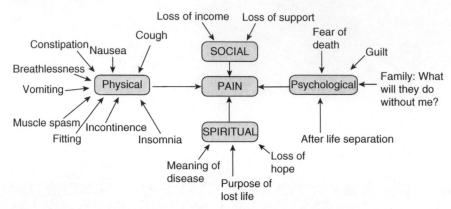

Fig. 5.5 Total pain.

5.7 **Non-pharmacological approaches to pain treatment in children[37]**

Non-pharmacological approaches can be highly effective. Recently, the international research review body, the Cochrane Collaboration[38], reviewed all literature on the subject and that non-pharmacological techniques are highly effective (see box below). They are not commonly used in Africa but arguably, in view of the problems getting hold of strong analgesics in many areas, they should be core learning for medical professionals caring for children. They are easy to learn and should be used when possible to give the child some control in the management of pain. One needs also to be culturally and religiously sensitive as some non-pharmacological approaches may not be acceptable to all patients.

Results of the Cochrane Review on psychological interventions for procedural pain and distress in children and adolescents

The largest effect sizes for treatment improvement over control conditions exist for distraction, hypnosis, self-reported distress, behavioural measures of distress and combined cognitive-behavioural interventions. Promising but limited evidence exists for the efficacy of numerous other psychological interventions including: information/preparation, nurse coaching plus distraction, parent positioning plus distraction and distraction plus suggestion.

5.7.1 **Distraction**

Distraction is used to focus the child's attention away from the pain. For children, simple distraction techniques can be very effective in decreasing the pain. Simple measures such as looking at books, blowing bubbles and counting are favourite distraction techniques for children. Touch can be an important distraction technique by stroking, patting and rocking infants as well as children who are in distress.

Deep breathing is the easiest technique to use with young children. The child is instructed to take a deep breath through the nose and blow it out through the mouth. Making a conscious effort to count the child's respirations focuses attention on the breathing. For school-age children, asking them to hold their breath during a painful procedure transfers their focus to their breathing and not on the procedure. Asking children to 'blow away their pain' has also been discussed as an effective distraction tool[39]. Parents should be taught distraction techniques and encouraged to hold their children for comfort as much as possible. Parent coaching gives them a way to participate in decreasing their child's pain and also may provide some benefit in decreasing parent anxiety and worry.

Table 5.3 Distraction techniques in children

Age	Methods
0–2 years	Touching, stroking, patting, rocking, playing music, using mobiles over the crib
2–4 years	Puppet play, storytelling, reading books, breathing, blowing bubbles
4–6 years	Breathing, storytelling, puppet play, talking about favourite places, TV shows, activities
6–11 years	Music, breathing, counting, eye fixation, thumb squeezing, talking about favourite places, activities on TV shows, humour

5.7.2 Muscle relaxation

Muscle relaxation is used to decrease mental and physical tension. It is used most effectively in older children and adolescents because it involves the relaxation of voluntary skeletal muscles. Slowly each muscle is tensed and then relaxed in a systematic way. Attention is placed on breathing which causes the individual to be aware of the feelings of tension and relaxation. Once breathing is under control, attention is focused on the muscles to promote progressive relaxation. This technique is useful prior to an anxiety producing procedure. Conscious awareness of the tension creates a more relaxed state, enabling the procedure to be completed more easily. A muscle relaxation exercise can be used with most children over 5 years of age.

Box 5.4 Muscle relaxation exercise

- Make yourself as comfortable as possible.
- Move around in your chair or bed until you feel good.
- Close your eyes when you are ready.
- Take a deep breath through your nose and breathe out slowly.
- Breathe again in and out slowly.
- Now focus on your hand, make a tight fist and hold it, hold it, now let it relax.
- Focus your attention on the muscles of your arm, push down your elbow against the arm of the chair or onto the bed, hold it, hold it and now relax your arm.
- Let's begin relaxing the muscles of our head and neck. Lift your eyebrows up as high as possible, hold those muscles tight, hold them, now relax and let them go.
- Squint your eyes and wrinkle your nose, hold those muscles tight, hold them, now relax and let them go.

Box 5.4 Muscle relaxation exercise *(continued)*

- Bite your teeth together and make a smile, hold those muscles tight, hold them, now relax and let them go.
- Pull your chin down toward your chest, hold it tight, hold it, now relax and let it go.
- Take a deep breath, hold it, hold it, pull your shoulders back, now relax and let it go.
- Pull your stomach in and try to hold it, hold it tight, now relax those muscles and let them go.
- Lift your leg and hold it out straight, hold it, hold it, now relax and let it rest again on the floor or bed.
- Point your toes towards the ceiling, hold them tight, keep them pointed, now relax them and let them go.
- Take another deep breath through your nose and let it out slowly through your mouth, breathe in again slowly and let it out through your mouth.
- Notice how relaxed your muscles feel?

5.7.3 Hypnosis

Hypnosis involves enabling the child to focus very closely on something with a consequent reduction in peripheral awareness (and so a reduction in pain awareness where pain is present). Most of us know that a kick on the shin hurts less when we are really concentrating on playing in a football match than a similar kick when we are feeling cold, miserable and tired and doing nothing in particular. In this state it is possible to enhance control, especially over unwanted sensations, such as pain, which can be placed at the periphery of awareness, altered or even eliminated[40]. Talking a child through guided imagery is in itself a form of hypnosis (see next section). Hypnosis does require a motivated child, and it may take a few practises for a child to get good at it; but parents can be taught to hypnotize their children and children can also be taught to hypnotize themselves. Therefore, it is less useful for one-off procedures, but good for regular procedures (such as lumbar punctures or bone marrow biopsies).

5.7.4 Guided imagery

Guided imagery engages the child by focusing on a pleasant activity, providing distraction from the pain or changing the perception of the painful experience. Guided imagery is used to give the child the opportunity to imagine being in a more pleasant situation. The effective use of imagery involves all of the child's senses. When imagining a favourite place the child is asked to feel the warmth all around, see the colours, smell the odours and hear the sounds. This helps the child create a clear scene in their mind. It is important to stress that every child needs a favourite place to go that is safe. This safe place provides a means of escape. A guided imagery exercise can be used with school age children and adolescents. The child needs to be able to trust you and ideally you need to be able to speak the same language.

Both hypnosis and guided imagery are excellent options – provided that there are no language barriers that could prevent insight into and understanding of the process involved.

5.7.4.1 Favourite imagery scenes for children

Visual imagery

- Favourite places
- Animals

- Flowers
- TV
- Favourite room
- Favourite sport.

Auditory imagery

- Conversations with significant others
- Favourite song
- Playing a musical instrument
- Listening to music
- Environmental sounds (waves, birdsong etc.).

Movement imagery

- Flying
- Swimming
- Any activity.

Box 5.5 Guided imagery exercise

Say the following in a slow, gentle voice . . .

- Make yourself as comfortable as possible.
- Move around in your chair or bed.
- Take a deep breath through your nose and breathe out slowly.
- I am going to count and with each number you will notice yourself becoming more comfortable.
- 12, breathing softly.
- 11-10-9-8, you can close your eyes if you wish.
- You may want to imagine in your mind a place that is special to you.
- It may be at the seashore, by a river, in the mountains.
- There may be other people there with you, or you might want to be by yourself.
- 7-6-5-4, you can enjoy this special place and know that your mind will remember it when you need to return.
- 3-2-1, your breathing is now slow and easy.
- The muscles of your face are relaxed.
- Let yourself see, feel and hear the surroundings of that special place.
- It is yours.
- (Pause a few minutes and let them enjoy that special place)
- When you are ready to return from that special place all your own, you will become more aware of my voice, aware of the light in the room.
- You may want to stretch your muscles, take a deep breath.
- You can open your eyes when you are ready.

5.7.5 Reinforcement of coping behaviour

Once pain has settled or been successfully treated, it is very important to remind and congratulate the child about how well they have coped (even if they have not coped brilliantly). This instills a sense of achievement procedure that allows the child time to recover, focuses the child's attention on successful coping and instills a sense of achievement. That does not mean however you should ignore problems that happened. These should be mentioned and talked through[41] but then looked at from a more positive light in order to try and reduce fear of them next time.

5.8 Principles of pharmacological pain management in children's palliative care

5.8.1 How the drugs work

It is not really necessary to understand the full theory of how drugs work to be able to perform good children's palliative care. However, at least we should all understand that pain is a complex phenomenon involving several different parts of the nervous system. As the table below describes, different drugs work in different ways. If we understand that, we will understand how to attack pain from different directions and on different fronts, thereby improving our chances of success.

Table 5.4 How analgesics work

Site of action	Drug
CNS prostaglandins	Paracetamol
Central pain receptors	Opioids
Visceral pain receptors	Opioids
Peripheral cyclo-oxygenase receptors	NSAID
Peripheral nerves	Local anaesthetics
Dorsal horn of the spinal cord	Opioids
Enhanced 'descending inhibition' (the same principle as rubbing your leg when you have banged it)	Opioids Antidepressants and methadone
GABA inhibitory system (pain seems less when you are relaxed than when you are anxious and tense)	Benzodiazepines Anticonvulsants
Inhibition of the glutamate excitatory system (an apparently perverse system which makes chronic pain feel worse the longer you have it – probably evolutionarily useful)	Anticonvulsants, methadone

5.8.2 The WHO pain ladder

Just as in adults, we use the WHO pain ladder to address children's pain pharmacologically. A common mistake is to drop the lower drug when moving to the next step, but in fact children who are taking paracetamol, a NSAID and morphine will get better relief than childen on morphine alone (as can be understood by reading Table 5.4).

Table 5.5 The WHO pain ladder

Step 3 - Moderate to severe pain	Strong opioid plus paracetamol, non-steroidal anti-inflammatory drugs (NSAIDs) +/– adjuvant
Step 2 - Moderate pain	Weaker opioid plus paracetamol, non-steroidal anti-inflammatory drugs (NSAIDs) +/– adjuvant
Step 1 - Mild pain	Paracetamol and/or non-steroidal anti-inflammatory drugs (NSAIDs) +/– adjuvant

Medication is prescribed based on the pain severity, moving up the steps of the ladder from non-opioid medications to weak opioids to stronger opioids as the pain increases in intensity. The ladder represents a model that begins with mild analgesics and progresses to stronger analgesics for persistent or increasing pain.

The choice of drugs should be based on the severity of the pain, i.e. if children report very severe pain, they should be started on a strong opioid such as morphine. If treatment at one step does not work, then do not try other drugs of the same level, but go up the ladder.

Use adjuvant therapy at any level of the ladder, where available, nerve blocks and epidural injections/infusions are a further option for uncontrolled pain.

Step 1 – Non-opioids
Non-opioids are the first line medication for mild pain and include paracetamol and non-steroidal anti-inflammatory drugs (NSAIDs). Paracetamol is cheap and available as tablets, suspension or as a suppository. It also acts as an anti-pyretic. It is a safe and effective medication. NSAIDs (e.g. ibuprofen and diclofenac) are very useful in the management of pain, especially bone, joint and inflammatory pains. They should be avoided if the platelet count is less than 20, unless the child is imminently dying and should be used with caution in renal disease. Avoid in children with peptic ulcer disease or aspirin sensitive asthma. Ibuprofen is cheap and widely available. It comes in tablet and suspension form. Diclofenac is also a very useful NSAID and comes as both a tablet and in suppository form. Aspirin should be avoided in children below 12 years if there is an alternative medication available.

Step 2 – Weak opioids
The authors' own experience is that, although theoretically useful, in children the addition of weak opioids to a child who is already on maximum paracetamol and NSAID therapy rarely adds any significant effect. However, in areas where strong opioids are unavailable, it is sensible to try these. Weak opioids have a 'ceiling' or maximum dose.

Step 3 – Strong opioids
Morphine is the strong opioid of choice in children. In many African countries, it is the only available strong opioid. It comes in two formulations:

◆ Immediate release (short acting) form in liquid (cheap)/tablets (expensive)

◆ A sustained release opioid such as MST M/R

Morphine is *very safe*, particularly in children, who tend to be more resilient and have a stronger respiratory drive than in elderly people. It often causes slight sedation for the 1st 24–48 hours. This is partly a drug side effect, but also partly due to the patient finally being able to rest after being kept awake by the pain. Do not fear slight initial sedation – it will pass and is almost part of the therapy. As long as there are no signs of morphine toxicity and it does not last more than 48 hours, you, the child and the family have no need to fear.

Initially, an immediate release morphine preparation should be used. During this period, liquid morphine is administered four hourly (six to eight hourly in infants or renal impairment) with breakthrough doses administered in between as necessary. For breakthrough pain (that occurs before the next regular dose of analgesia) repeat the full previous dose of oral morphine again; and then also give the same dose again at the prescribed time.

In general, one should allow 24 hours before considering a dose increase of oral morphine. Increases should always be based on a percentage of the current dose, e.g. 25% when small improvement is needed, 50% for moderate pain on current dose, 100% increase for pain that is severe.

In some African countries, controlled-release/'long acting' formulations of morphine are available, e.g. a sustained release opioid such as MST, M/R. If available and affordable, the 12-hourly dose is calculated (from the total liquid morphine dose required the previous day, divided by 2) and administered as a controlled release preparation, e.g. MST, M/R tablets or sachets. 'Breakthrough' doses should continue to be calculated as one-sixth of the total 24-hour-oral dose.

If MST is unavailable, or liquid preferred, regular 4-hourly morphine can be continued. *It is important to note that there is no maximum dose for oral morphine, as long as the child is experiencing pain and there are no signs of opioid toxicity.*

Other strong opioids

In some African countries, other strong opioids are available. In practise, there is not a great deal to choose between them in terms of effectiveness, but routes and pharmacology of each vary, and this may give one an advantage over another with any particular child. They include:

Diamorphine: This arguably causes less nausea and hypotension than morphine, but its main advantage is its solubility. This means that smaller volumes can be used (useful in sc infusion) and also that it can be used nasally or buccaly in very small volumes (less than 0.2 ml fluid) as a rapid-acting and painless alternative to injections[42].

Buprenorphine[43]: This has opioid agonist and antagonist properties and may precipitate withdrawal symptoms, including pain, in children dependent on other opioids. However, it has a longer duration of action than morphine (6–8 hours) and can be used sublingually and transdermally. It does not rely on renal excretion and therefore can be used when renal failure is a problem.

Methadone: This is less sedating than morphine and acts for much longer periods. Anecdotally, it seems more effective in neuropathic pain. It may also be useful when morphine causes paradoxical excitation (exacerbation of pain). However, it is quite tricky to convert from morphine (see Chapter 20 – Formulary), and there is a risk of accumulation and overdose if administered more than twice a day long term.

Pethidine: This is fairly widely available across Africa, but it has a short duration of action, is less potent than morphine and is more likely to cause psychiatric side effects.

Tramadol[44]: This is an opioid which also has an effect on serotonergic and adrenergic pathways. It has fewer of the typical opioid side effects (notably, less respiratory depression, less constipation and less addiction potential) but psychiatric reactions have been reported.

Codeine: This is effective for the relief of mild to moderate pain but is too constipating for long-term use. The authors have not found it particularly useful. If paracetamol and NSAIDs do not cover the pain adequately, it has been our experience that it is better to move to a stronger opioid straight away.

Dihydrocodeine: This has an efficacy similar to codeine.

Fentanyl[45]**:** This has been developed in transdermal patches and buccal 'lollipops', which can be very useful in a child with poor oral intake but who is too active for sc infusions to be useful.

Box 5.6 Side effects of opioids

Generally, *opioids are very well tolerated* in children. With the exception of infants, children metabolise opioids faster than adults and are more resistant to respiratory suppression. A few specific issues deserve mention.

- Twitching
- Pin-point pupils
- Confusion/agitation
- Hallucinations
- Initial sedation
- Constipation
- Pruritus.

It is arguable that this should not be classified as an adverse side effect. Imagine how you would feel if you were a child with chronic pain: sleeping poorly, agitated and anxious. A doctor then gives you wonderful pain relief. What are you going to do? Sleep for a couple of days! Is that an adverse or a beneficial effect? If you see sedation in the first 48 hour without the features of morphine toxicity listed above, relax, reassure the family and allow the poor child to catch up on some much needed rest.

- Pruritus: treat with topical treatments (calamine lotion, Eurax®, hydrocortisone creams) or oral antihistamines. Reducing the dose of opioid or changing to an alternative such as fentanyl can also help. It is important to note that pruritus is *not* an allergic reaction and so morphine can and should be continued.

- Urinary retention: can often be treated with carbachol or bethanechol, but catheterization may be required.

- Constipation: consider prescribing mild laxatives if necessary (e.g. stool softeners).

5.8.3 Principles of effective morphine prescribing

- Give immediate release morphine 4 hourly (6 hourly in neonates or in patients with impaired renal function).
- Start at low dose (as per chart below).
- Increase the dose in 30–50% steps (usually after a minimum of two doses) until pain control is achieved.
- If available, convert the immediate release morphine dose to the equivalent 12 hourly sustained release morphine dose by adding the previous days total morphine requirement (regular and breakthrough doses) and dividing by 2.

- Give the last immediate release morphine dose with the first sustained release dose to ensure full analgesic cover.

- Always prescribe immediate release morphine PRN (at a dose equivalent to 4 hourly dose of morphine) to cover breakthrough pain. If breakthrough pain occurs regularly increase the sustained release morphine dose by 30–50%.

- There is no dose limit. The correct dose is the dose that relieves the pain. The authors have experience of children requiring several grams of morphine daily to achieve good pain relief, and without significant side effects.

- If you have facilities, switch to parenteral opioid only when the child is unable to take oral medication.

5.9 Special kinds of pain requiring special treatments

Some pains are not 'typical' and require alternative approaches. Adjuvant analgesics are a group of medications that are analgesic in certain painful conditions but have a primary indication other than pain, e.g. antidepressants, anticonvulsants and corticosteroids. From the section on 'How the Drugs Work' you can see how some adjuvants might work. They can be very helpful for specific pain syndromes.

5.9.1 Neuropathic/nerve pain

Neuropathic (nerve) pain is caused by damage to peripheral nerves/nervous system and does not respond as well to standard medications. It often requires the addition of extra drugs. Examples include peripheral neuropathy due to HIV/ART medications (described as burning pain affecting feet/hand), post-herpetic neuralgia after varicella zoster (shingles) or arm pain due to tumour invasion of brachial plexus nerves. Patients often described it as 'burning', 'shooting', 'pricking', 'cold/numb' or 'electric shocks'.

You should take care in diagnosing neuropathic pain by using the child's pain description alone however. Look for other evidence such as a dermatomal distribution or other neurological symptoms in the affected area. When you examine, look for weakness, numbness, hypersensitivity or allodynia (where a non-painful stimulus such as touch feels like pain). If peripheral neuropathy occurred after the introduction of ARTs, consider changing to a different combination.

It is a common misconception that neuropathic pain does not respond to opioid analgesia. In fact about 70% of the time it does. You should therefore still titrate up the opioid dose as necessary even if you do suspect neuropathic causes. However, sometimes opioid analgesia is not sufficient and the child will require adjuvants such as an anticonvulsant or antidepressant.

In the African setting, the most widely available and effective drug is amitriptyline. Currently evidence of the relative effectiveness of different agents is not strong, but it appears amitriptyline and other tricyclics are more effective and safer than both morphine and drugs such as gabapentin and pregabalin in neuropathic pain[46]. It is given at night in low dosage. Side effects include sedation and dry mouth. Anticonvulsants used for neuropathic pain in children include carbamazepine, phenytoin and gabapentin. Carbamazepine and phenytoin are alternatives. Anticonvulsants require careful titration to an effective dose and regular assessment of side effects.

N.B. For children on antiretroviral medication, both carbamazepine and phenytoin can cause significant drug interactions, by reducing or increasing effect of some ARTs. Valproate is relatively free of significant drug–drug interactions with ARTs.

5.9.2 **Raised intracranial pressure (and tumour compression in other areas)**

Corticosteroids including dexamethasone can help reduce nerve pain due to tumour compression/infiltration, raised intracranial pressure and bone pain, but they are more toxic in children than in adults and should be used with more caution. When steroids are used in acute medical situations (for example in stridor, asthma or lymphocytic interstitial pneumonitis) they are largely safe and well tolerated. When used long term to suppress intracranial pressure, they can be very effective. However, long-term use in this situation can be more problematic. The advantages of using them like this are that they can be rapidly effective at reducing headache, nausea and vomiting, and also in giving a window of relatively symptom-free survival, to allow the child and family time to say their goodbyes and put any affairs in order.

Unfortunately however longer-term use can cause problems including cushingoid side effects, immunosuppression, candidiasis, mood and behaviour problems, weight gain and changes of appearance, reduced mobility, insomnia, dyspepsia and peptic ulceration. Also, if the child's prognosis is likely to be more than a few weeks, then a combination of worsening neurological status with distressing neurological symptoms, such as the loss of sight or hearing, paralysis or cognitive effects and steroid side effects (cushingoid symptoms, psychiatric symptoms, etc.), may adversely affect the balance of benefits and risks of treatment and cause patients to be kept alive for longer, while experiencing worse symptoms (i.e. the inverse of the principles of palliative care).

It is therefore imperative that patients and their families should fully understand the benefits of treating and risks of not treating with steroids. Informed consent must be sought before steroid treatment is started.

The drug of choice is high-dose dexamethasone. If this is unavailable, other steroids such as prednisolone can be used. Use for 4–7 days then reduce slowly until stopped or until symptoms begin to resurface. It is usually possible to stop altogether in 2–3 weeks. In children, some anecdotal evidence suggests that 'pulsing' (i.e. 3 days of treatment followed by 3 days off) may be as beneficial with fewer side effects, but hard evidence for this is lacking.

5.9.3 **Spasticity/increased muscle tone**

HIV encephalopathy occurs in about 20% of children with HIV/AIDS and frequently causes muscle spasms, spasticity and contractures that make positioning and movement very difficult. Physio-therapy where available is helpful and teaching carers useful techniques. Antispasmodics such as baclofen and benzodiazepines may act as muscle relaxants but also have sedative effects. Generally speaking, spasticity in children is difficult to treat pharmacologically and physiotherapeutic approaches are more useful (see Chapter 9 – Neurological symptoms for more details). Physiotherapy can be painful in children with spasticity and some form of pharmacological and non-pharmacological pre-treatment is recommended.

5.9.4 **Bone pain/soft tissue pain**

NSAIDs are often very effective in bone pain. Even in cases where therapeutic radiotherapy is no longer appropriate, pain from bone or soft tissue malignant deposits can be treated with palliative radiotherapy. Bone pain also has a neuropathic component and using adjuvants (e.g. anti-convulsants) may also help.

5.9.5 **Colicky abdominal pain**

Cause must be assessed and treated if possible. Hyoscine butylbromide may be a helpful adjuvant medication for such pain, but can contribute to constipation.

5.9.6 **Anxiety**

Remember many children in pain are also anxious. Anxiety heightens pain perception. This should be addressed with non-pharmacological measures, and if it is not effective then use anxiolytics such as benzodiazepines.

5.9.7 **Procedural pain management**

Health workers often have to perform painful procedures on children in the African setting. These might include suturing of lacerations, fracture setting, lumbar punctures or venesection, bone marrow biopsies and so on. In the authors' experience, procedural pain management in the African setting is almost non-existent.

Yet, as has been made clear, pain suffered by infants has long-lasting effects and should be prevented[47]. As a result of poor pain management, children may feel helpless, anxious, irritable and depressed, and their coping skills may be undermined. Once pain has been undertreated, it becomes harder to treat, even with the same noxious stimulus[48].

5.9.7.1 **The principles of procedural pain management**

It is natural for health workers to dislike performing painful procedures on children and very tempting indeed to rush in and 'get-it-over-with'. Yet, as with most children's palliative care situations, time is the key. Time spent preparing the child and family is so important in preventing trauma for child and family both in the short and longer term. Try and adopt the following approach:

1. Ask yourself: 'Does the child really need this procedure?' If it is a test, ask: 'What am I going to do with the result and is it going to alter anything?' If the answer to either of these questions is no, don't do it.

2. Prepare yourself first: Think through what you are going to have to do, what materials you might need, where you are going to do it, what might go wrong and what you will do if things go wrong. If you do not feel you have the expertise, try and find someone who has. If there is no one available, practise in a mock-up before doing it for real.

3. Get the child and family involved: Find out child's likes and interests. Get him or her to tell you about previous experiences and work out what their fears and expectations are this time. Talk through what is to be done and get their views on the when, where and how. Be thoughtful about when to tell the child: too early and you will leave them hanging on in painful expectation; too late and you will not give them time to prepare and get them into a panic.

4. Encourage the parents to be helpful and supportive: Before you start take them to one side and explain that you don't want them to get cross with the child, unduly restrain them and certainly not shout at or hit them. All of this will only add to the pain and trauma.

5. Carry out the procedure in a child-friendly environment and away from the bed.

6. Use both non-pharmacological and pharmacological interventions to manage pain and anxiety. If it is a first procedure, make even more sure that it is as pain-free as possible: this will reduce anticipatory pain the next time (and make your life easier too).

7. After the event, offer plenty of congratulations on how well they have done and try and instill a sense of achievement.

5.9.7.2 **Specific techniques**

Up to 2 months of age:

◆ Feed or use a pacifier with 15–50% sucrose.

◆ Swaddling and containment of infants.

Older children

◆ Distraction, relaxation or other coping skills in children (see above).

Drugs to use:

◆ Use topical anaesthetic agents if you have them (e.g. EMLA cream).

◆ Use local anaesthetic agents such as subcutaneous lidocaine (but make sure that they are at body temperature and buffer it with sodium bicarbonate to reduce the pain of administration without compromising efficacy)[49,50].

◆ Use nitrous oxide if it is available. But don't use to the point of complete sedation.

◆ If anxiety rather than pain is the major issue: sedate using a benzodiazepine (preferably short acting such as midazolam or lorazepam). Administer long enough in advance that it has time to reach the maximum effect.

◆ If pain is a significant problem: Use opioid analgesia in treatment doses.

5.10 **A practical approach to pain treatment in children**

As mentioned, while it is helpful to know the theory, it is arguably more helpful to know what to do in practise. When confronted with a child in pain, one's memory can become a bit hazy just at the time you need it to be slick and sharp. Half-remembered and unwanted physiological and pathological facts can clutter your mind just at the wrong time. In this situation, 'recipe book medicine' can be just what the doctor ordered!

Table 5.6 A practical approach to managing pain

1	Is the child in pain?	Assess carefully to ensure you are dealing with pain.
2	Is the pain severe?	Before you go any further, *relieve the pain*. Further assessment can wait until the child is comfortable. Give a dose of morphine stat (see doses below).
3	What is the likely cause?	Use the sieve to work out what the cause might be: compression, infiltration, infection, drug side effect, neuropathic, psychological and spiritual. Use the table above to decide which drug might be most effective.
4	Is there a remediable cause?	If there is, remedy it. If the bed is wet, change it. If there is an infection, treat it. If the bone is broken, immobilize it.
5	Is the child properly hydrated, nourished and oxygenated?	Imagine how much worse pain is when you are cold, tired and hungry. Good nutrition, hydration and tissue oxygenation can avoid further stress in a painful situation.
6	Is the child comfortable, comforted and distracted?	Use warmth, swaddling, feeding & reassurance. Handle gently and use supportive positioning to minimize pain from movement. Minimize invasive procedures. Use distraction, relaxation and imagery (see above).

(continued)

Table 5.6 (continued) A practical approach to managing pain

7	Is the pain related to movement?	This suggests musculoskeletal cause. Think of fractures or sprains (immobilize), metastasis (orthopaedic surgery or radiotherapy), soft tissue infection (especially myositis in AIDS) (antibiotics, drainage and immobilization), nerve compression (if neurological features – see below), spasticity (can be very painful, use benzodiazepines).
8	Is the pain due to organ distension?	In organs which cannot easily expand (e.g. brain, liver) think about the use of radiotherapy or steroids (but take care using steroids in children – see below).
9	Are there neuropathic features?	If the pain is shooting/burning, is dermatomal in distribution and is associated with neurological signs, think of using adjuvants, particularly amitriptyline.
10	Is there headache with raised symptoms/signs of raised intracranial pressure?	Consider steroids or radiotherapy, but see the note above regarding steroids.
11	Does the child have a disease/complication that would cause pain in an adult?	If so, try to track down and treat.
12	Is there pain due to muscle spasm?	Use warmth, gentle stretching, splinting and physiotherapy. Try benzodiazepines or baclofen.

But, *remember rule* 4: If in doubt about the cause, treat what you can treat. In this case – give a trial of analgesics and re-assess.

Notes

1 Anand, K.J.S. & The International Evidence-Based Group For Neonatal Pain. (2001). Consensus statement for the prevention and management of pain in the newborn. *Archives of Pediatrics & Adolescent Medicine, 155*, 173–180.

2 Anand, K.J.S. & Hickey, P.R. (1987). Pain and its effects in the human neonate and fetus. *New England Journal of Medicine, 317*, 1321–29.[Medline]

3 Grunau, R.V. & Craig, K.D. (1987). Pain expression in neonates: Facial action and cry. *Pain, 28*, 395–410.

4 Levine, J.D. & Gordon, N.C. (1982). Pain in prelingual children and its evaluation by pain-induced vocalization. *Pain, 14*, 85–93.

5 Williamson, P.S. & Williamson, M.L. (1983). Physiological stress reduction by a local anesthetic during newborn circumcision. *Pediatrics, 71*, 36–40.

6 Anand, K.J.S., Sippell, W.G. & Aynsley-Green, A. (1987). Randomized trial of fentanyl anaesthesia in preterm babies undergoing surgery: Effects on stress response. *Lancet, 1*, 62–6; [Erratum, *Lancet*, 1987; *1*, 234].

7 Marshall, R.E., Stratton, W.C., Moore, J.A. & Boxerman, S.B. (1980). Circumcision: I. Effects upon newborn behavior. *Infant Behaviour Development, 3*, 1–14.

8 Fitzgerald, M. & Anand, K.J.S. (1993). Developmental neuroanatomy and neurophysiology of pain. In N.L. Schechter, C.B. Berde & M. Yaster (Eds.). *Pain in Infants, Children, and Adolescents*. (pp. 11–31) Williams & Wilkins, Baltimore.

9 Schechter, N.L. & Allen, D. (1986). Physicians attitudes toward pain in children. *Journal of Developmental and Behavioral Pediatrics, 7*, 350–54.

10 Morrison, R.A. (1991). Update on sickle cell disease: Incidence of addiction and choice of opioid in pain management. *Pediatrics Nursing, 17*, 503.

11 Pegelow, C.H. (1992). Survey of pain management therapy provided for children with sickle cell disease. *Clinic Pediatrics, 31*, 211–4.

12 Berde, C.B., Lehn, B.M., Yee, J.D., Sethna, N.F. & Russo, D. (1991). Patient-controlled analgesia in children and adolescents: A randomized, prospective comparison with intramuscular administration of morphine for postoperative analgesia. *Journal of Pediatrics, 118*, 460–6.

13 Mechanic, D. (1980). The experience and reporting of common physical complaints. *Journal of Health Social Behaviour, 21*, 146–55.

14 Larochette, A., Chambers, C. & Craig, K. (2006). Genuine, suppressed and faked facial expressions of pain in children. *Pain, 126*(Issue 1–3), 64–71A.

15 BMJ Publishing group. (1995). Managing Acute Pain in Children. *Drug and Therapeutics Bulletin, 33*, 41–4. doi:10.1136/dtb.1995.33641.

16 Nolan, K. (1993). Ethical issues in pediatric pain management. In N.L. Schechter, C.B. Berde & M. Yaster (Eds.) *Pain in Infants, Children, and Adolescents.* (pp. 11–31). Williams & Wilkins, Baltimore.

17 Schechter, N.L., Allen, D.A. & Hanson, K. (1986). Status of pediatric pain control: A comparison of hospital analgesic usage in children and adults. *Pediatrics, 77*, 11–5.

18 Hammond D. (1979). Unnecessary suffering: Pain and the doctor–patient relationship. *Perspective in Biology and Medicine, 23*, 152–60.

19 Mcgrath, P.J. & Craig, K.D. (1989). Developmental and psychological factors in children's pain. *Pediatric Clinics in North America, 36*, 823–36.

20 Gharaibeh, M. & Abu-Saad, H. (2002).Cultural validation of pediatric pain assessment tools: Jordanian perspective. *Journal of Transcultural Nursing, 13*(1), 12–8.

21 Newman, C. J., Lolekha, R., Limkittikul, K., et al. (2005). A comparison of pain scales in Thai children. *Archive of Disease in Children, 90*, 269–70.

22 Robin, I., Luffy, M.S.N., R.N, C.P.N.P. (Jan 2003). Examining the validity, reliability, and preference of three pediatric pain assessment tools in African-American children. *Paediatric Nursing.*

23 'Play Therapy Boosts HIV Children' In *Staff at Groote Schuur Hospital in Cape Town are Using Play Therapy to Help Mothers and Their Children to Cope with HIV.* Available online at BBC Website http://www.bbc.co.uk/News.

24 Mmola, Z.F. (2002). Play therapy to reduce the psychosocial impact of AIDS on children. International Conference on AIDS (July 7–12). 14, Abstract No. Wepef6592

25 The Association for Children's Palliative Care (ACT) Charter. (1997). ACT, London Available online at http:// www.act.org.

26 Eland, J.M. (1985). Pediatrics. In *Pain.* Springhouse Corporation, Springhouse, PA.

27 Hockenberry, M.J., Wilson, D. & Winkelstein, M.L. (2005).*Wong's Essentials of Pediatric Nursing* (7th Edition). (p. 1259). Mosby, St. Louis. (Used with permission. Copyright).

28 Merkel, S. & Others. The FLACC: A behavioral scale for scoring postoperative pain in young children. *Pediatric Nurse, 23*(3), 293–7. (Copyright 2002 By Jannetti Co. University of Michigan Medical Center).

29 Watson, M.S., Lucas, C., Hoy, A. et al. (Eds.) (2005). Management of pain. In *Oxford Handbook of Palliative Care.* Oxford University Press, Oxford.

30 Breitbart, W. (1998). Pain in AIDS: An overview. *Pain Reviews, 5*(4), 247–72.

31 Katabrira, Elly et al. (2000). *HIV Infection Diagnosis and Treatment Strategies for Health Care Workers* (2nd Edition). Makarere University Printery, Kampala, Uganda.

32 O'Neill, J. et al. (2003). *A Clinical Guide for Supportive and Palliative Care for HIV/AIDS.* US Health Resources and Services (HRSA) Administration Information Centre. Available online at http://hab.hrsa.gov/tools/palliative.

33 Strafford, M., Cahill, C., Schwartz, T. et al. (1991). Recognition and treatment of pain in pediatric patients with AIDS (Abstract). *Journal of Pain and Symptom Management, 6*, 146.

34 Hewitt, D., Mcdonald, M., Portenoy, R., et al. (1997). Pain syndromes and etiologies in ambulatory AIDS patients. *Pain, 70,* 117–23.

35 Cherny, N.I., Coyle, N. & Foley, K.M. (1994). Suffering in the advanced cancer patient: A definition and taxonomy. *Journal of Palliative Care, 10,* 57–70.

36 Foley, K.M. (1996). Pain syndromes in patients with cancer. In R. Portenoy & R.M. Kranner (Eds.) *Pain Management: Theory and Practice.* (p. 191). FA Davis, Philadelphia.

37 Texas Children's Cancer Centre, Texas Children's Hospital, Houston, Texas. Available online at http://www.childcancerpain.org.

38 Uman, L.S., Chambers, C.T. Mcgrath, P.J. & Kisely. (2006). *Psychological Interventions for Needle-Related Procedural Pain and Distress in Children and Adolescents,* Cochrane Review. Available online at http://www.cochrane.org/Reviews/En/Ab005179.html.

39 French, G., Painter, E. & Coury, D. (1994). Blowing away shot pain: A technique for pain management during immunization. *Pediatrics.*

40 Spiegel, D. (2003). Self-regulation skills training for adults including relaxation. In H. Breivik, W. Campbell & C. Eccleston (Eds.) *Clinical Pain Management: Practical Applications and Procedures.* (pp. 113–20). Arnold, London.

41 Von Baeyer, C.L., Marche, T.A., Rocha, E.M. & Salmon, K. (2004). Children's memory for pain: Overview and implications for practice. *The Journal of Pain, 5*(5), 241–9.

42 Wilson, J.A. & Kendall, J.M. (1997). P Cornelius intranasal diamorphine for paediatric analgesia: Assessment of safety and efficacy. *Journal of Accident and Emergency Medicine, 14,* 70–2. doi:10.1136/emj.14.2.70, BMJ Publishing.

43 Khan, F.A., Memon, G.A. & Kamal, R.S. (2002). Effect of route of buprenorphine on recovery and postoperative analgesic requirement in paediatric patients. *Paediatric Anaesthesia, 12*(9), 786–90.

44 Ozalevli, M., Unlugenc, H., Tuncer, U. et al. (2005). Comparison of morphine and tramadol by patient-controlled analgesia for postoperative analgesia after tonsillectomy in children. *Paediatric Anaesthesia, 15*(11), 979–84. [Abstract]

45 Finkel, J.C., Finley, A., Greco, C. et al. (2005). Transdermal fentanyl in the management of children with chronic severe pain: Results from an international study. *Cancer, 104*(12), 2847–57.

46 Finnerup, N., Otto, M. , Mcquay, M., Jensen,T. & Sindrup, S. (2007). Algorithm for neuropathic pain treatment: An evidence based proposal. *Pain, 118*(Issue 3), 289– 305.

47 Taddio, A. (1999). Effects of early pain experience: The human literature. Chronic and recurrent pain in children and adolescents. In P.J. Mcgrath & G.A. Finley (Eds.) *Progress in Pain Research and Management.* (pp. 57–74). IASP Press, Seattle.

48 Weisman, S.J., Bernstein, B. & Schechter, N.L. (1998). Consequences of inadequate analgesia during painful procedures in children. *Archives of Pediatrics and Adolescent Medicine, 152*(2), 147–9.

49 Fatovich, D.M. & Jacobs, I.G. (1999). A randomized controlled trial of buffered lidocaine for local anesthetic infiltration in children and adults with simple lacerations. *Journal of Emergency Medicine, 17*(2), 223–8.

50 Davies, R.J. (2003). Buffering the pain of local anaesthetics: A systematic review. *Emergency Medicine, 15*(1), 81–8.

Chapter 6

Respiratory symptoms

Justin Amery and Michelle Meiring

Key points

- *Don't panic*: Breathing symptoms are frightening for everyone, including you. Mostly you have more time than you think, and symptoms tend to respond well to treatment.

- *Hope for the best, prepare for the worst*: There are two life-threatening situations in this area: acute airway obstruction and massive haemoptysis. Both need forward planning to ensure that, if they happen, you and your team can be calm, efficient and effective. Make sure you have rapid access to drugs to enable rapid and complete sedation. Don't duck it, *do it now*.

- Non-pharmacological methods are very effective.

- Most distressing respiratory symptoms will respond to low dose opioids and/or benzodiazepines.

6.1 Assessment of the respiratory system in children's palliative care

Full respiratory system assessment is beyond the scope of this book, but the following tips might be helpful.

In all children:

- Is the child blue?
  - With HIV/AIDS: Think lower respiratory tract infections and LIP.
  - If not, think of obstruction (e.g. inhaled material, upper airway obstruction, bronchospasm) or hypoventilation (e.g. debility, weakness).
- Fever?
  - Think of infection.
- Stridor or a rasping sound from the upper airway?
  - Think of inhaled foreign body or acute upper airway obstruction from disease.
- Facial oedema or neck vein distension?
  - Think of superior vena cava (SVC) obstruction.
- Orthopnoea (breathlessness on lying flat) and basal lung crackles?
  - Think of left ventricular failure.

- ◆ Hyper-resonance and reduced air entry in the upper zones?
  - Think of pneumothorax.
- ◆ Dullness and reduced air entry in the base?
  - Think of a pleural effusion.
- ◆ Audible expiratory wheezing?
  - Think of bronchospasm/asthma.

In children with known or suspected HIV/AIDS[1]

- ◆ Chronic cough, loss of appetite, loss of weight, history of TB contact, constitutional symptoms
  - Think TB.
- ◆ Marked cyanosis, respiratory distress and a clear sounding chest?
  - Think PCP.
- ◆ Clubbing and recurrent fevers?
  - Think of bronchiectasis.
- ◆ Clubbing and no or low fever, lymphadenopathy or parotid enlargement?
  - Think of lymphoid interstitial pneumonitis.

6.2 Breathlessness

6.2.1 Background

Breathlessness is common, frightening and not always easy to treat. It occurs in 70% of patients with cancer in the West[2]. In AIDS the incidence of breathlessness is between 11% and 48%[3]. Simple measures are very helpful but often overlooked.

6.2.2 Causes

The causes of breathlessness are not entirely clear, but it is known that the brain stem regulates the frequency of breathing, and this is stimulated by chemoreceptors (which pick up changes in oxygen and carbon dioxide levels in the blood) and stretch-receptors in the lung. It follows that

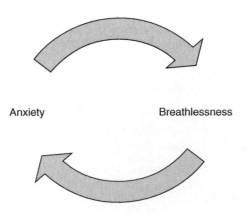

Anxiety   Breathlessness

Fig. 6.1 Dyspnoea and anxiety.

problems which cause reduction in blood levels of oxygen, increases in carbon dioxide or that stretch the receptors in the lung (e.g. by fluid, tumour or infection) will generate a sensation of breathlessness. However, there is also a strong cerebral component to breathlessness, which can be exacerbated significantly by anxiety. A vicious circle of breathlessness leading to anxiety which in turn exacerbates breathlessness is established and this needs to be broken. For this reason, simple, non-pharmacological approaches to reduce anxiety are very important in the management of breathlessness.

In the sub-Saharan African setting, breathlessness in children's palliative care is most likely to be:

- Related to cancer or AIDS
  - Leading to effusion, consolidation, ascites, lung destruction cancer (e.g. Kaposi's sarcoma), lymphangitis, chronic interstitial pneumonitis.
- Related to treatment
  - Post-radiation fibrosis, post-pneumonectomy (uncommon).
- Related to debility
  - Caused by anaemia, pneumonia, CMV, encephalopathy.
- Unrelated to cancer or treatment
  - e.g. asthma, cardiac failure.

6.2.3 Management

Table 6.1 Practical management of breathlessness

Condition	Management
All patients: non-pharmacological management	◆ Sit the child up if possible ◆ Ensure some air flow across the child's face (using an open window, or fan) ◆ Reassure the child as much as possible ◆ Try and help the child relax using the techniques described in the chapter on pain ◆ Try and use the distraction techniques described in the chapter on pain
All patients: pharmacological management	◆ Give morphine and/or benzodiazepine if the breathlessness is severe. (Oral/rectal diazepam works as fast as parenteral – you can use injectable diazepam rectally.) ◆ If already on morphine, increase dose by $1/3$ rd
Acute stridor or upper airway obstruction	◆ *Don't panic*: Try and keep calm ◆ *Treat what you can treat*: Try and clear airway but be careful of pushing foreign bodies in deeper ◆ Heimlich manoeuvre for foreign bodies in older children, back blows and chest thumps for children less than 2 years ◆ Administer oxygen ◆ Consider nebulization with adrenaline which will address many inflammatory causes of acute stridor ◆ Consider tracheostomy (hospital setting) if overall prognosis allows ◆ Consider dexamethasone high dose IV over 2 minutes

(continued)

Table 6.1 (continued) Practical management of breathlessness

Condition	Management
	♦ Give parenteral morphine and/or benzodiazepine if the breathlessness is severe. (Oral/rectal diazepam works as fast as parenteral – you can use injectable diazepam rectally.) ♦ Consider referral for surgery or radiotherapy or chemotherapy if available
Pneumothorax	♦ Symptomatic or if >30% consider chest drain
Acute heart failure	♦ Oxygen ♦ Loop diuretic (e.g. furosemide) ♦ Start or increase morphine
Chronic heart failure and Cor Pulmonale	♦ Low-dose oxygen ♦ Diuretics ♦ ACE inhibitors ♦ ART reduces episodes of intercurrent lower respiratory tract infections. ♦ Consider digoxin
Bronchospasm (e.g. asthma)	♦ Oxygen high dose ♦ Bronchodilator nebulized or at least 10 puffs of metered-dose inhaler through a spacer device (1 liter plastic bottles with hole cut for inhaler will work) ♦ Parenteral or oral steroids
Pleural effusion	♦ Pleural drainage is effective in the short term, but fluid recollects unless pleurodesis is carried out. Therefore, you need to consider benefit verses burden, especially with malignant effusions.
HIV pneumonia	♦ Unknown organism: chloramphenicol; or ampicillin, flucloxacillin and gentamicin; or cefalosporins ♦ PCP: high-dose co-trimoxazole (Septrin®), oxygen, steroids
Lymphoid interstitial pneumonitis	♦ Physiotherapy, pulsed steroids, bronchodilators, oxygen and ARTs

6.3 **Cough**

Cough is a common symptom in AIDS, reported by 19–34% of patients in surveys of symptom prevalence in HIV disease[4,5].

6.3.1 **Causes**

♦ Infection: Secondary bronchial infection, tuberculosis, pneumonia or an abscess in a necrotic tumour

♦ Lymphoid interstitial pneumonitis

♦ Tuberculosis

♦ Bronchospasm

♦ Post-nasal drip

♦ Unrecognized oesophageal reflux with aspiration

♦ Drugs and inhaled irritants: e.g. cigarette smoke or indoor air pollution at home

♦ Airway tumours: From a primary tumour or mediastinal mass, most commonly enlarged mediastinal glands.

6.3.2 Management

Table 6.2 Practical management of cough

Condition	Management
All children	♦ Explanation ♦ Sit up ♦ Manage breathlessness if present ♦ Humidify air as much as possible ♦ Stop smoking in the room and also reduce the use of stoves, kerosene lamps, etc. in the house
Infections	♦ See above
Bronchospasm	♦ See above
Lymphoid interstitial pneumonitis	♦ See above
Recurrent aspiration and/or reflux	♦ See management of dysphagia and reflux in Chapter 8 – Gastrointestinal symptoms
Post-nasal drip	♦ Position child upright ♦ Consider antihistamines ♦ Consider nasal steroid drops or spray
If no better after above	♦ Consider cough suppressants such as low-dose morphine or codeine ♦ Consider nebulized local anaesthetics (e.g. lidocaine) if airway tumours (can inhibit gag reflex so do not feed for 1 hour before and after to reduce risk of aspiration)

Table 6.3 Use of cough suppressants and the cough ladder

Indications for cough suppressants	The cough ladder
♦ Severe cough paroxysms ♦ Cough interfering with feeding ♦ Cough interfering with sleep ♦ Cough leading to exhaustion	1. Simple linctus 2. Codeine linctus 3. Morphine or diamorphine Linctus 4. Codeine phosphate 5. Morphine sulphate

6.4 Haemoptysis

6.4.1 Background

This is a very frightening event for the patient, the family and the professional. The *don't panic* rule applies very strongly here. It is actually quite unusual for someone to bleed to death through the lungs. For a start, most causes of apparent haemoptysis are due to non-serious bleeding from the nose, pharynx or upper oesophagus. Also, even true haemoptysis is not usually life-threatening and will often settle once the cause of the bleeding is managed and the cough is suppressed (coughing generates tearing forces in the airways).

That said, catastrophic haemoptysis does happen rarely. About 3% of adult lung cancer patients suffer with this, and some of these occur without warning[6]. Therefore, in order to minimize upset and trauma, it is also important to *hope for the best, plan for the worst*, where haemoptysis is a possibility.

6.4.2 **Causes**

- Infections, such as bronchitis or tuberculosis
- Tumours invading blood vessels
- Pulmonary embolism
- Clotting disorders.

6.4.3 **Management**

Table 6.4 Practical management of haemoptysis

Condition	Management
In all patients	• *Don't panic*: Take a deep breath and try to stay calm • *Hope for the best*: Explain what is happening and that the bleeding is unlikely to be life-threatening • *Prepare for the worst*: Arrange for the family to have dark towels and rapid sedation to hand • Ensure that all team members know what to do in the event of catastrophic bleed • *Treat what you can treat*: Try to suppress coughing using morphine
Upper airway or upper GI bleeding	• Manage cause
Infections	• Treat infection and use cough suppressant (see above)
Clotting disorders	• Treat haematological abnormalities if possible
Mild/moderate bleeding	• May need to hospitalize for transfusion (if available and appropriate) • If available, tranexamic acid can be helpful • Refer for radiotherapy if appropriate and available
Catastrophic haemoptysis	• Aim for rapid and complete sedation with benzodiazepines and/or opioids • If available, use parenteral routes. If not, and if the child is still able to swallow, give double usual dose of morphine +/− diazepam • If child is not able to swallow, give large (rapidly sedative) doses of morphine and diazepam rectally, or lorazepam or midazolam buccally (if available) • Try to keep patient clean by using receptacles and changing materials soiled with blood

Box 6.1 Case scenario – Beatrice

Beatrice is a 7-year-old girl with advanced and incurable leukaemia. She has known hilar lymphadenopathy. She is staying at home with her mother Gloria and older sisters (Sarah aged 10 and Josephine aged 12). During your visit she starts coughing up large volumes of bright red blood and starts to become weak and faint.

- What might be the causes of the haemoptysis?
- How will you manage this situation?

6.5 **Hiccup**

Hiccup is quite common and is often overlooked as a cause of distress. It can cause considerable interruption to normal activity and may cause low mood, sleep and feeding disturbances[7].

6.5.1 **Causes**

- ◆ Phrenic nerve or diaphragmatic irritation by tumour, chest infection
- ◆ Vagus nerve irritation: e.g. gastro-oesophageal reflux, oesophagitis, hiatus hernia, acsites, hepatic tumour
- ◆ Metabolic disturbances: uraemia, hyponatremia
- ◆ CNS tumours (especially brainstem)
- ◆ Drugs: benzodiazepines, corticosteroids and barbiturates.

6.5.2 **Management**

Table 6.5 Practical management of hiccup

Condition	Management

All patients	◆ Stimulate the pharynx (e.g. swallowing dry bread)
	◆ Stimulate the vagus
	  • Try re-breathing through paper bag
	  • Drink cold drinks
	◆ Give small frequent meals to reduce gastric distension

Metabolic disturbances	◆ Correct if possible
Oesophagitis and reflux	◆ See Chapter 8 – Gastrointestinal symptoms
Reduce vagus nerve irritation by reducing gastric distention	◆ Prokinetics such as domperidone or metoclopramide ◆ Antacids and antiflatulents
Relaxing smooth muscle	◆ Nifedipine ◆ Baclofen
Central suppression	◆ Chlorpromazine or promazine or haloperidol

6.6 **Noisy secretions ('death rattle')**

6.6.1 **Background**

Noisy secretions are caused because the child is no longer able to cough or swallow secretions in the large airways, usually because the child's conscious level is dropping prior to death. It can be very distressing to the family, who can think that their child is choking or drowning in his/her own secretions[8]. In fact, it is unlikely to be a cause of distress for the child, and this needs to be explained.

6.6.2 **Management**

Table 6.6 Practical managements of noisy secretions

Condition	Management
All patients	◆ Position the child with his or her head low, so that secretions can drain from the mouth ◆ Ensure that pulmonary oedema is excluded or treated with furosemide ◆ If you suspect that the child is distressed or breathless, treat with opioids and/or benzodiazepines as per the instructions in the section on breathlessness
Where secretions remain a problem	◆ Consider using hyoscine butylbromide (Buscopan®) subcutaneously to reduce the production of secretions ◆ Review after 30 minutes and repeat ◆ You can repeat the doses every 4 hours ◆ Only use suction in unconscious children and only very gently

6.7 **Question for you**

◆ Have you ever had to manage a child with frightening breathing difficulties? If so reflect back. How did you cope? What went well and what did not go so well? Having read this chapter, what would you do differently if it happened again?

Notes

1 Gwyther, L., Merriman, A., Mpanga Sebuyira L. & Schietinger H. (Eds) (2006). *A Clinical Guide to Supportive and Palliative Care for HIV/AIDS in Sub-Saharan Africa.* Foundation for Hospices in Sub-Saharan Africa. Available online at http:// www.fhssa.org

2 Reuben, D.B., Mor, V. & Hiris, J. (1988). Clinical symptoms and length of survival in patients with terminal cancer. *Archives of Internal Medicine, 148*(7), 1586.

3 Alexander, C.S. (2001). Palliative and end of life care. In J.R. Anderson (Ed.) *A Guide to the Clinical Care of Women with HIV.* (pp. 349–82). US Department of Health and Human Services Health Resources and Services Administration, Rockville, MD.

4 Alexander, C.S. (2001). Palliative and end of life care. In J.R. Anderson (Ed.) *A Guide to the Clinical Care of Women with HIV.* (pp. 349–82). US Department of Health and Human Services Health Resources and Services Administration, Rockville, MD; Pulmonary Symptoms.

5 Gwyther, L., Adams, V., Wilson, D. & Mandwa, D. (2006). Pulmonary Symptoms. In Gwyther, L., Merriman, A., Mpanga Sebuyira L. & Schietinger H. (Eds) *A Clinical Guide to Supportive and Palliative Care for HIV/AIDS in Sub-Saharan Africa.* Foundation for Hospices in Sub-Saharan Africa. Available online at www.fhssa.org.

6 Watson, M., Lucas, C., Hoy, A. & Back, I. (Eds). (2005). *Oxford Handbook of Palliative Care.* (pp. 404). Oxford University Press, OUP.

7 Walker, P., Watanabe, S., Brurera, E. & Baclofen. (1998). A treatment for chronic hiccup. *Journal of Pain and Symptom Management, 16*, 125–32.

8 Wee, Bee, L., Coleman, P.G., Hillier, R. & Holgate, S.H. (2006). The sound of death rattleII: How do relatives interpret the sound? *Palliative Medicine, 20*(3), 177–81.

Chapter 7

Feeding and hydration problems

Justin Amery

Key points

+ Imagine how rotten you feel if you are hungry or thirsty.

+ Eating and drinking are very powerful statements to ourselves and to others that we are alive and well.

+ Feeding one's child is also a very powerful maternal (and paternal) drive.

+ Malnutrition is common but poorly managed in children with AIDS and/or cancer in Africa: perhaps familiarity breeds contempt.

+ Malnutrition is a social problem with medical consequences: to treat it only using medical approaches is to miss the point. We need to address the social issues that caused it, or it will simply return.

+ Management of terminal loss of appetite and thirst is guided largely by what the child wants: if he/she is thirsty or hungry, then drink and food should be given. If not, the situation is less clear.

It may seem obvious, but eating and drinking, along with breathing, are very powerful statements to ourselves and to others that we are alive and well. Food and drink are basic survival needs, but they are also used for pleasure, socializing, habit, comfort or even boredom. Feeding one's child is also a very powerful maternal (and paternal) drive. For all these reasons, problems with childhood nutrition and hydration are often found to be such distressing problems in children's palliative care, particularly for parents.

This seems to be an area that tends to be overlooked in the African children's palliative care setting, perhaps because malnutrition is so common in children with AIDS and/or cancer in Africa. Perhaps familiarity breeds contempt.

However, by focusing only on 'illnesses' and 'treatments', we risk missing very distressing and often easily manageable problems, such as being unable to eat or drink properly. But stop for a second. Imagine how rotten you feel if you are hungry or thirsty. A child's quality of life can be improved a great deal by simply being cuddled, kept warm, well fed and well hydrated.

7.1 Causes of feeding problems

In African children's palliative care many children are hungry simply because they do not have enough to eat. In a Hospice Africa Uganda study, over two-thirds of children in the study received basic needs support and 68% mentioned food as one of the best things about the service (third only after medication and play services)[1].

Apart from poverty, there can be a number of reasons why children don't eat, including

- Under-provision for other reasons (neglect, ignorance, etc.)
- Anorexia
- Sore mouth
- Dysphagia
- Nausea and vomiting
- Squashed stomach syndrome.

We will deal with these in the following sections.

7.2 Assessment of children who are not eating

Table 7.1 Assessment of children who are not eating

Cause	Management
1. Is the child hungry?	• This is a crucial question: a child with cachexia will rarely be hungry, whereas a child with mild or moderate malnutrition will be. Take care though. Most children with severe malnutrition have lost their appetite. • Use the WHO criteria of weight for height and height for age to determine degree of malnutrition. • If the child is hungry, help him or her feed and drink. See the section below for management of children with malnutrition.

2. If the prognosis is short	• Give food or drink for pleasure, but not if the child resists.
	• Remember families may often be reluctant to withdraw feeding even well after they have agreed to withdraw all other interventions and treatments.
	• You might (or probably will) feel under pressure from the parents or family to continue feeding[2].
	• Use compassion, skill and patience to help the family understand that
	  • feeding is pointless (it won't prolong life);
	  • the child is not feeling hungry (so there is no question of the child suffering);
	  • forced feeding will cause suffering.

3. Manage treatable causes	• Manage sore mouth, swallowing problems, nausea, squashed stomach and breathlessness (see relevant sections for treatment), pain, renal or liver failure, chronic infection, etc. • Think about disability (a child may need help with feeding and positioning to eat properly).
4. Are you dealing with drug side effects?	• Think of opioids, metronidazole, co-trimoxazole, NSAIDs, chemotherapy, some antibiotics. • Change drugs if possible.
5. Are there problems with the food?	• Check that food being offered is known and liked by the child and is culturally acceptable. • Try using low bulk and high energy/high protein foods (if available). • Ensure that the child can sit up and has company around the bed. • Avoid strong odours that may cause nausea. Also avoid overly spicy or fatty foods.

Table 7.1 (Continued) Assessment of children who are not eating

Cause	Management
	◆ Do not pressurize the child but tempt him or her with small helpings of favourite foods on the smallest plate available. ◆ Be ready to permit and encourage any bizarre fancy the patient may have[3].
6. Is appetite stimulation available or appropriate?	◆ You can try low-dose dexamethasone (but caution in children).
7. If still no better, treat symptomatically	◆ For feeding (or as an alternative to non-oral hydration) consider tube feeding (either nasogastric or gastrostomy if available).

7.3 **Cachexia**

Health workers frequently confuse malnutrition with cachexia in children's palliative care. It is important to tell the difference as the treatment approaches are significantly different.

> Cachexia is not associated with hunger or thirst, nor will it improve by forced feeding or hydration.

7.3.1 **Assessment**

Cachexia is a syndrome of weight loss (fat and skeletal muscle), anorexia, anaemia, fatigue and oedema which results from inflammatory mediators (cytokines) being released either by or in response to the underlying pathological condition. It is particularly seen in cancer, AIDS, heart failure, rheumatoid arthritis, chronic respiratory disease and liver cirrhosis[4–8].

7.3.2 **Management**

Although there is some evidence that cachexia can be modified by large doses of the fatty acid eicosapentaenoic acid (EPA)[9] (found in omega-3 fish oils), in practise this is not a realistic alternative in the African children's palliative care setting. It can therefore only be treated by treatment of the underlying condition. HIV-related cachexia usually improves with ART, but of course, in advanced cancers, successful treatment of the underlying condition is rarely possible. The body changes associated with cachexia can be distressing to both the child and family, but it is important to note that cachexia is not associated with hunger or thirst, nor will it improve by forced feeding or hydration. Over-feeding itself may have adverse consequences: abdominal distension, re-feeding diarrhoea and malabsorption.

Table 7.2 Case study – Naledi

Naledi is a 6-year-old girl who lives with her aunty in rural Zimbabwe. The aunty looks after other children, all of whom are healthy and well-noursihed, and it seems that Naledi was healthy until only a few months ago. She now looks very wasted and, when you assess her, you find her to be underweight for her height (2 SD) and also short for her age (2 SD). You also find a large abdominal mass arising from the right upper quadrant of the abdomen which later turns out to be an inoperable renal tumour. She has however no other signs of infection, her blood film is clear, her HIV status is negative, her urine and faecal cultures are negative and her blood is normal except for a slightly low haemoglobin level.

(continued)

Table 7.2 (continued) Case study – Naledi

She has no appetite and will hardly touch food even when offered her favourite foods. You treat all of the conditions you can treat and make sure not to give her drugs that will interfere with her appetite. However, her weight continues to fall as her tumour continues to enlarge. She does not seem distressed by her lack of food intake, although her aunt gets increasingly upset, as do some of your nursing colleagues. One of them asks if you should start nasogastric feeding.

- What do you think is going on here?
- What are the options open to you?
- How will you manage this situation?

7.4 **Malnutrition**

7.4.1 **Causes**

Childhood malnutrition is very prevalent in children's palliative care in Africa, particularly in children with cancers and HIV[10]. The reasons for this are as follows :

- poverty
- anorexia associated with illness, mouth ulcers, oral thrush
- nutrient loss from malabsorption, diarrhoea or HIV enteropathy
- increased metabolic rate because of cancer and opportunistic infections
- in cancer and AIDS, the release of cytokines (TNF alpha, cachetin) results in anorexia, which worsens underlying malnutrition
- HIV-positive mothers have higher rates of low-birth-weight babies and premature birth.

Malnutrition can be either micronutrient malnutrition[i], which can reduce immunity further and predispose children to worsening infections; or macronutrient malnutrition. Marasmus is more common than kwashiorkor among HIV-infected children.

The rest of this section is adapted from the WHO Manual for Physicians and Other Health Workers[11].

7.4.2 **Overview**

Malnutrition is effectively a social not a medical disorder, although of course it causes medical problems. It is a result of chronic nutritional deprivation due to:

- poverty
- poor understanding of child feeding
- family problems
- abuse, deprivation and neglect.

Unless such underlying social problems are addressed, medical treatment will be pointless: the child will simply become malnourished again once he or she returns home.

The stages of medical treatment for malnutrition include

- Stage 1 – Initial treatment: life-threatening problems are identified and treated (ideally in a hospital or a residential care facility, specific deficiencies are corrected, metabolic abnormalities are reversed and feeding is begun).
- Stage 2 – Rehabilitation: intensive feeding is given to recover most of the lost weight, emotional and physical stimulation are increased, the mother or carer is trained to continue care at home, and preparations are made for discharge of the child.

---

[i] Particularly zinc, selenium, vitamins, A, E, B6, B12 and C

◆ Stage 3 – Follow-up: after discharge, the child and the child's family are followed to prevent relapse and assure the continued physical, mental and emotional development of the child. A typical time frame for the management of a child with severe malnutrition* is shown in Table 7.7.

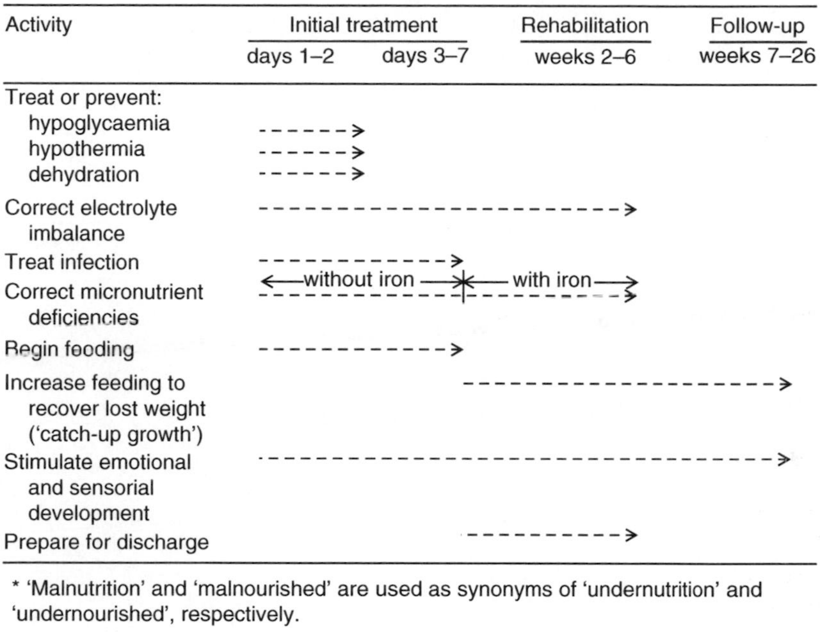

Activity	Initial treatment		Rehabilitation	Follow-up
	days 1–2	days 3–7	weeks 2–6	weeks 7–26
Treat or prevent:				
hypoglycaemia	- - - - - ->			
hypothermia	- - - - - ->			
dehydration	- - - - - ->			
Correct electrolyte imbalance	- ->			
Treat infection	- - - - - - - - - - - ->			
Correct micronutrient deficiencies	<—without iron —>*<— with iron—> ->			
Begin feeding	- - - - - - - - - - - ->			
Increase feeding to recover lost weight ('catch-up growth')			- ->	
Stimulate emotional and sensorial development	- ->			
Prepare for discharge			- - - - - - - - - ->	

* 'Malnutrition' and 'malnourished' are used as synonyms of 'undernutrition' and 'undernourished', respectively.

Fig. 7.1 Timeframe for managing severe malnutrition.

7.4.3 Assessment of the degree of malnutrition

Up until recently, the Wellcome classification of malnutrition has been the most widely used system, but this has now been adapted and replaced by the WHO system (see table below).

Table 7.3 WHO classification of malnutrition[12,]*

Evidence of malnutrition	Moderate	Severe (type)
Symmetric oedema	No	Yes (oedema PEM)*
Weight for height[†]	SD[‡] score between −2 and −3(70–90%)[§]	SD score <−3 (i.e. severe wasting[ǁ]) (<70%)
Height for age	SD score between −2 and −3(85–89%)	SD score <−3 (i.e. severe stunting) (<85%)

*Includes KW and KW marasmus (presence of oedema always indicates serious PEM)

[†] Standing height should be measured in children taller than 85 cm, and supine length should be measured in children shorter than 85 cm or in children who are too sick to stand. Generally, the supine length is considered to be 0.5 cm longer than the standing height; therefore, 0.5 cm should be deducted from the supine length measured in children taller than 85 cm who are too sick to stand.

[‡] Below the median National Center for Health Statistics (NCHS)/WHO reference: The standard deviation (SD) score is defined as the deviation of the value for an individual from the median value of the reference population divided by the standard deviation of the reference population, ie, SD score = (observed value − median reference value) ÷ standard deviation of reference population.

[§] Percentage of the median NCHS/WHO reference

[ǁ] This corresponds to marasmus (without oedema) in the Wellcome clinical classification and to grade III malnutrition in the Gomez system. However, to avoid confusion, the term severe wasting is preferred.

Table 7.4 Assessment of a malnourished child

Medical history	
Usual diet before current episode of illness	Look for clues as to type and extent of malnutrition
Breastfeeding history	If not, what else is being fed?
Food and fluids taken in past few days	Try to assess recent intake
Thirst	Drinking eagerly suggests dehydration, but in infants this may be expressed as restlessness. Thirst is *not* a symptom of septic shock
Urine flow	Diminishes as dehydration or septic shock worsens. In severe dehydration or fully developed septic shock, no urine is formed
Recent sinking of eyes	Suggesting dehydration but only when the mother says the sunken appearance is recent
Duration and frequency of vomiting or diarrhoea, appearance of vomit or diarrhoeal stools	A child with dehydration should have a history of watery diarrhoea. Small mucoid stools are commonly seen in severe malnutrition, but do not cause dehydration. A child with signs of dehydration, but without watery diarrhoea, should be treated as having septic shock
Time when urine was last passed	Suggesting dehydration
Contact with people with measles or tuberculosis	Think of suprainfection
Any deaths of siblings	Due to malnutrition or communicable disease
Birth weight	To assist charting and progress assessment
Milestones reached (sitting up, standing, etc.)	To assist in developmental assessment
Immunizations	
Physical examination	
Weight and length or height	Chart against normal ranges
Oedema	Suggesting protein deficiency, cardiac failure, etc.
Enlargement or tenderness of liver, jaundice	Think of hepatitis, haemolytic disease (e.g. malaria, etc.)
Abdominal distension, bowel sounds	Look for 'abdominal splash' (a splashing sound in the abdomen) suggesting bowel stasis
Weak or absent radial pulse	*Suggesting* shock, from either severe dehydration or sepsis. As hypovolaemia develops, the pulse rate increases and the pulse becomes weaker. If the pulse in the carotid, femoral or brachial artery is weak, the child is at risk of dying and must be treated urgently
Severe pallor	Suggesting anaemia
Cold hands and feet, weak radial pulse, diminished consciousness	Signs of circulatory collapse
Temperature	Look for hypothermia or fever. Hypothermia is a sign of serious infection, including septic shock. It is not a sign of dehydration.

Table 7.4 (continued) Assessment of a malnourished child

Physical examination	
Thirst	Urine flow diminishes as dehydration or septic shock worsens. In severe dehydration or fully developed septic shock, no urine is formed
Eyes	Corneal lesions indicative of vitamin A deficiency
Ears, mouth, throat	Evidence of infection
Skin	Evidence of infection or purpura (suggesting clotting/platelet disorders)
Respiratory rate and type of respiration	Chronic malaria, other signs of pneumonia or heart failure
Appearance of faeces	Any blood, pus, mucus suggesting GI infection or inflammation

7.4.4 Clinical assessment of the malnourished child

Table 7.5 Comparison of clinical signs of dehydration and septic shock in the malnourished child

Clinical sign	Some dehydration	Severe dehydration	Incipient septic shock	Developed septic shock
Watery diarrhoea	Yes	Yes	Yes or no[a]	Yes or no[a]
Thirst	Drinks eagerly[b]	Drinks poorly	No[a]	No[a]
Hypothermia	No	No	Yes[a] or no	Yes[a] or no
Sunken eyes	Yes[b, c]	Yes[b, c]	No	No[a]
Weak or absent radial pulse	No[b]	Yes	Yes	Yes
Cold hands and feet	No[b]	Yes	Yes	Yes
Urine flow	Yes	No	Yes	No
Mental state	Restless irritable[b]	Lethargic comatose	Apathetic[a]	Lethargic
Hypoglycaemia	Sometimes	Sometimes	Sometimes	Sometimes

[a] Signs that may be useful in diagnosing septic shock.

[b] Signs that may be useful in diagnosing dehydration

[c] If confirmed as recent by the mother.

7.4.5 Investigation of the malnourished child

Table 7.6 Investigation of the malnourished child

Investigation	Interpretation
Blood glucose	Glucose concentration 54 mg/dl (3 mmol/l) is indicative of hypoglycaemia
Examination of blood smear	Malaria parasites
Haemoglobin or packed-cell	Haemoglobin <40 g/l or packed-cell volume <12% is volume indicative of very severe anaemia
Examination and culture of urine	Presence of bacteria on microscopy (or >10 leukocytes specimen per high-power field) is indicative of infection
Examination of faeces by microscopy	Blood (suggests dysentery), Giardia cysts or trophozoites

(continued)

Table 7.6 (continued) Investigation of the malnourished child

Investigation	Interpretation
Chest X-ray	Shadowing suggesting infection (but remember pneumonia causes less shadowing of the lungs in malnourished children than in well-nourished children) vascular engorgement (heart failure), bone (rickets or fractures of the ribs)
Skin test for tuberculosis	Often negative in children with tuberculosis or those previously vaccinated with BCG vaccine

7.4.6 Initial treatment of the malnourished child

This usually lasts from the first treatment until the child's condition is stable and his or her appetite has returned (usually after 2–7 days). If longer than 10 days, the child is failing to respond and additional measures are required.

Table 7.7 Initial management of the malnourished child

Aim	Notes
Treat or prevent hypoglycaemia	Conscious/rousable?
	◆ 50 ml of 10% glucose or sucrose, or give F-75 diet, by mouth.
	◆ Stay with the child until he or she is fully alert.
	Losing consciousness, cannot be aroused or has convulsions?
	◆ 5 ml/kg of body weight of sterile 10% glucose intravenously (IV), followed by 50 ml of 10% glucose or sucrose by nasogastric (NG) tube.
	◆ If IV glucose cannot be given immediately, give the NG dose first.
	◆ When the child regains consciousness, immediately begin giving F-75 diet or glucose in water (60 g/l).
	◆ Continue frequent oral or NG feeding with F-75 diet to prevent a recurrence.
	All malnourished children with suspected hypoglycaemia should also be treated with broad-spectrum antimicrobials for serious systemic infection.
Treat or prevent hypothermia	◆ Use 'kangaroo technique' by placing the child on the mother's bare chest or abdomen (skin-to-skin) and covering both of them.
	◆ If not possible, clothe the child well (including the head), cover with a warmed blanket and place an incandescent lamp over, but not touching, the child's body. Fluorescent lamps are of no use and hotwater bottles are dangerous.
	◆ Monitor rectal temperature every 30 minutes during rewarming (might rapidly become hyperthermic). Underarm temperature is not a reliable guide.
Treat or prevent dehydration and restore electrolyte balance	Use ReSoMal (see below): Severely malnourished children are deficient in potassium and have abnormally high levels of sodium; the oral rehydration salts (ORS) solution should contain less sodium and more potassium than the standard.
	How much and how fast?
	Give ReSoMal at 70 to 100 ml/kg over 12 hours. Start with 5 ml/kg every 30 minutes (orally or NG) for 2 hours, and then 5–10 ml/kg per hour. The exact amount to give should be determined by how much the child will drink, the amount of ongoing losses in the stool, and whether the child is vomiting and has any signs of overhydration, especially signs of heart failure. ReSoMal should be stopped if respiratory and pulse rates increase, the jugular veins become engorged or there is increasing oedema (e.g. puffy eyelids). Rehydration is completed when the child is no longer thirsty, urine is passed and any other signs of dehydration have disappeared.

Table 7.7 (continued) Initial management of the malnourished child

Aim	Notes
	Intravenous rehydration
	Only if the child has circulatory collapse due to severe dehydration or septic shock. Use one of the following solutions (in order of preference):
	◆ Half-strength Darrow's solution with 5% glucose (dextrose)
	◆ Compound sodium lactate (Ringer's lactate) solution with 5% glucose
	◆ 0.45% sodium chloride (half-normal saline) with 5% glucose
	Give 15 ml/kg IV over 1 hour and monitor the child carefully for signs of overhydration. While the IV drip is being set up, also insert an NG tube and give ReSoMal through the tube (10 ml/kg per hour).
	Reassess the child after 1 hour. If the child is severely dehydrated, there should be an improvement with IV treatment and his or her respiratory and pulse rates should fall.
	In this case, repeat the IV treatment (15 mg/kg over 1 hour) and then switch to ReSoMal orally or by NG tube (10 ml/kg per hour) for up to 10 hours.
	If the child fails to improve after the first IV treatment and his or her radial pulse is still absent, then assume that the child has septic shock and treat accordingly.
	Feeding during rehydration
	Breastfeeding should not be interrupted during rehydration. Begin to give the F-75 diet as soon as possible, orally or by NG tube, usually within 2–3 hours after starting rehydration (see Section 7.4.5). If the child is alert and drinking, give the F-75 diet immediately, even before rehydration is completed. Usually the diet and ReSoMal are given in alternate hours. If the child vomits, give the diet by NG tube.
Treat incipient or developed septic shock, if present	Every child with septic shock should *immediately* be given broad-spectrum antibiotics and kept warm to prevent or treat hypothermia. The child should not be handled, washed or bathed any more than is essential for treatment. Iron supplements should *not* be given.
	Treatment of **septic shock**
	◆ Feed promptly to prevent hypoglycaemia by NG tube.
	◆ Begin IV rehydration immediately (15 ml/kg per hour).
	◆ Observe the child carefully (every 5–10 minutes) for signs of overhydration and congestive heart failure.
	◆ As soon as the radial pulse becomes strong and the child regains consciousness, continue rehydration orally or by NG tube.
	◆ If signs of congestive heart failure develop or the child does not improve after 1 hour of IV therapy, give a blood transfusion (10 ml/kg slowly over at least 3 hours). If blood is not available, give plasma.
	◆ If there are signs of liver failure (e.g. purpura, jaundice, enlarged tender liver), give a single dose of 1 mg of Vitamin K1 intramuscularly.
	◆ During the blood transfusion, nothing else should be given, so as to minimize the risk of congestive heart failure.
	◆ If signs of congestive heart failure continue give a diuretic and slow the rate of transfusion.
	Steroids, adrenaline or nikethamide are of no value and should *never* be used.
	After the transfusion, begin to give F-75 diet by NG tube (see section 4.5). If the child develops increasing abdominal distension or vomits repeatedly, give the diet more slowly.
	If vomiting continues, stop feeding the child and return to IV hydration at a rate of 2–4 ml/kg per hour. Also give 2 ml of 50% magnesium sulfate solution intramuscularly (IM).

(continued)

Table 7.7 (continued) Initial management of the malnourished child

Aim	Notes
Start to feed the child	Severely malnourished children usually have infections, electrolyte imbalance, impaired liver and intestinal function, and so are unable to tolerate usual intakes of protein, fat and sodium. Early feeding is therefore with high carbohydrate and low protein/fat/sodium.
	Two formula diets, F-75 and F-100, are commonly used:
	◆ F-75 (75 kcal /315 kJ/100 ml): for initial phase
	◆ F-100 (100 kcal/420 kJ/100 ml): for rehabilitation (i.e. after appetite has returned)
	These formulas can easily be prepared from the basic ingredients: dried skimmed milk, sugar, cereal flour, oil, mineral mix and vitamin mix. They are also commercially available as powder formulations that are mixed with water.
	The mineral mix supplies potassium, magnesium and other essential minerals (see Table 8); it *must* be added to the diet. The potassium deficit, present in all malnourished children, adversely affects cardiac function and gastric emptying. Magnesium is essential for potassium to enter cells and be retained. The mineral mix does not contain iron as this is withheld during the initial phase.
Feeding on admission	To avoid overloading the intestine, liver and kidneys, it is essential that food be given frequently and in small amounts. Children who are unwilling to eat should be fed by NG tube (do *not* use IV feeding). Children who can eat should be given the diet every 2, 3 or 4 hours, day and night. If vomiting occurs, both the amount given at each feed and the interval between feeds should be reduced.
	The F-75 diet should be given to all children during the initial phase of treatment. The child should be given at least 80 kcal/kg or 336 kJ/kg, but no more than 100 kcal/kg or 420 kJ/kg per day. If less than 80 kcal or 336 kJ/kg per day are given, the tissues will continue to be broken down and the child will deteriorate. If more than 100 kcal or 420 kJ/kg per day are given, the child may develop a serious metabolic imbalance.
	Table 9 shows the amount of diet needed at each feed to achieve an intake of 100 kcalh or 420 kJ/kg per day. For example, if a child weighing 7.0 kg is given the F-75 diet every 2 hours, each feed should be 75 ml. During the initial phase of treatment, maintain the volume of F-75 feed at 130 ml/kg per day, but gradually decrease the frequency of feeding and increase the volume of each feed until you are giving the child feeds 4 hourly (6 feeds per day). Nearly all malnourished children have poor appetites when first admitted to hospital. Patience and coaxing are needed to encourage the child to complete each feed. The child should be fed from a cup and spoon; feeding bottles should *never* be used, even for very young infants, as they are an important source of infection. Children who are very weak may be fed using a dropper or a syringe. While being fed, the child should always be held securely in a sitting position on the attendant's or mother's lap. Children should never be left alone in bed to feed themselves.
Nasogastric feeding	Despite coaxing and patience, many children will not take sufficient diet by mouth during the first few days of treatment. Common reasons include a very poor appetite, weakness and painful stomatitis. Such children should be fed using a NG tube. However, NG feeding should end as soon as possible. At each feed, the child should first be offered the diet orally. After the child has taken as much as he or she wants, the remainder should be given by NG tube. The NG tube should be removed when the child is taking three-quarters of the day's diet orally, or takes two consecutive feeds fully by mouth. If over the next 24 hours the child fails to take 80 kcal or 336 kJ/kg, the tube should be reinserted. If the child develops abdominal distension during NG feeding, give 2 ml of a 50% solution of magnesium sulfate IM. The NG tube should always be aspirated before fluids are administered. It should also be properly fixed so that it cannot move to the lungs during feeding. NG feeding should be done by experienced staff.

Table 7.7 (continued) Initial management of the malnourished child

Aim	Notes
Feeding after the appetite improves	If the child's appetite improves, treatment has been successful. The initial phase of treatment ends when the child becomes hungry. This indicates that infections are coming under control, the liver is able to metabolize the diet and other metabolic abnormalities are improving. The child is now ready to begin the rehabilitation phase. This usually occurs after 2–7 days. Some children with complications may take longer, whereas others are hungry from the start and can be transferred quickly to F-100. Nevertheless, the transition should be gradual to avoid the risk of heart failure which can occur if children suddenly consume large amounts of feed. Replace the F-75 diet with an equal amount of F-100 for 2 days before increasing the volume offered at each feed. It is important to note that it is the child's appetite and general condition that determine the phase of treatment and *not* the length of time since admission.
Anti-microbial treatment	**All children should receive anti-microbial treatment**
	If the child is well with no apparent signs of infection and no complications, give co-trimoxazole orally twice daily for 5 days.
	If the child has complications (septic shock, hypoglycaemia, hypothermia, skin infections, respiratory or urinary tract infections, or who appear lethargic or sickly), give ampicillin plus gentamicin IM or IV 2 days, followed by amoxicillin orally plus gentamicin IM or IV once daily for 7 days.
	If the child fails to improve within 48 hours: *Add* chloramphenicol every 8 hours (or every 6 hours if meningitis is suspected) for 5 days.
	Disease-specific therapy should be given if indicated (e.g. dysentery, candidiasis, malaria or intestinal helminthiasis)
Severe anaemia	If the haemoglobin concentration is less than 40 g/l or the packed-cell volume is less than 12%, the child has very severe anaemia, which can cause heart failure. Children with very severe anaemia need a blood transfusion. Give 10 ml of packed red cells or whole blood per kg of body weight *slowly* over 3 hours. Where testing for HIV and viral hepatitis B is not possible, transfusion should only be given when the haemoglobin concentration falls below 30 g/l (or packed-cell volume below 10%), or when there are signs of life-threatening heart failure. Do *not* give iron during the initial phase of treatment, as it can have toxic effects and may reduce resistance to infection.
Congestive heart failure	Usually a complication of overhydration (IV infusion or standard ORS solution), severe anaemia, blood/plasma transfusion or high sodium diet.
	Early signs: Fast breathing (50 breaths per minute from age 2 months to 12 months; 40 breaths per minute aged 12 months up to 5 years).
	Later signs: Respiratory distress, rapid pulse, jugular engorgement, cold hands and feet, peripheral cyanosis.
	Differential diagnosis: Respiratory infection and septic shock (usually within 48 hours of admission).
	Management: Stop *all* oral intake and IV fluids until heart failure is improved, even if this takes 24–48 hours. Give a diuretic IV (e.g. furosemide 1 mg/kg)
Treatment of clinical vitamin A deficiency	Severely malnourished children are at high risk of developing blindness due to vitamin A deficiency. A large dose of vitamin A should be given routinely to all malnourished children on day 1, as follows:
	◆ Infants <6 months of age: 50 000 IU orally
	◆ Infants 6–12 months of age: 100 000 IU orally
	◆ Children >12 months of age: 200 000 IU orally
	If there are any clinical signs of vitamin A deficiency (e.g. night blindness, conjunctival xerosis with Bitot's spots, corneal xerosis/ulceration or keratomalacia), the doses above should be repeated on day 2 and again on day 14. IM treatment should be given unless it cannot be tolerated.

(continued)

Table 7.7 (continued) Initial management of the malnourished child

Aim	Notes
	If there is ocular inflammation or ulceration, corneal perforation is possible. Take great care when handling the eyes and protect the eyes with pads soaked in 0.9% sodium chloride. Also give tetracycline eye drops (1%) and atropine eye drops (0.1%) four times daily until symptoms resolve
Other vitamin deficiencies	All malnourished children should receive 5 mg of folic acid orally on day 1 and then 1 mg orally per day thereafter. Many malnourished children are also deficient in riboflavin, ascorbic acid, pyridoxine, thiamine and the fat-soluble vitamins D, E and K. All diets should be fortified with these vitamins by adding the vitamin mix.

Table 7.8 Composition of ReSoMal

Component	Concentration (mmol/l)
Glucose	125
Sodium	45
Potassium	40
Chloride	70
Citrate	7
Magnesium	3
Zinc	0.3
Copper	0.045
Osmolarity	300

Permission 5: Reproduced with permission from BNF for Children © BNF

Table 7.9 Preparation of F-75 and F-100 diets

Ingredient	Amount	
	F-75[1-3]	F-100[4,5]
Dried skimmed milk	25 g	80 g
Sugar	70 g	50 g
Cereal flour	35 g	—
Vegetable oil	27 g	60 g
Mineral mix[6]	20 ml	20 ml
Vitamin mix[7]	140 mg	140 ml
Water to make	1000 ml	1000 ml

Permission 6: Reproduced with permission from BNF for Children © BNF

[1] To prepare the F-75 diet, add dried skimmed milk, sugar, cereal flour and oil to warm water and mix. Boil for 5–7 minutes. Allow to cool, then add the mineral mix and vitamin mix again. Make up the volume to 1000 ml with water.

[2] A compatible formula can be made from 35 g of whole dried milk, 70 g of sugar, 35 g of cereal flour, 17 g of oil, 20 ml of mineral mix, 140 mg of vitamin mix and water to make 1000 ml. Alternatively, use 500 ml of fresh cows' milk, 70 g of sugar, 35 g of cereal flour, 17 g of oil, 20 ml of mineral mix, 140 mg of vitamin mix and water to make 1000 ml.

[3] Isotonic versions of F-75 (230 mOsmol/l), which contain maltodextrin instead of cereal flour and some of the sugar and include all the necessary micronutrients, are available commercially.

[4] If normal flour is not available or there are no cooking facilities, a comparable formula can be made from 25 g of dried skimmed milk, 100 g of sugar, 27 g of oil, 20 ml of mineral mix, 140 mg of vitamin mix and water to make 1000 ml. However, this formula has a high osmolarity (415 mOsmol/l) and may not be well tolerated by all children, especially those with diarrhoea.

[5] To prepare the F-100 diet, add the dried skimmed milk, sugar and oil to some warm boiled water and mix. Add the mineral mix and vitamin mix and mix again. Make up the volume to 1000 ml with water.

[6] A comparable formula can be made from 110 g of whole dried milk, 50 g of sugar, 50 g of oil, 20 ml of mineral mix, 140 mg of vitamin mix and water to make 1000 ml. Alternatively, use 350 ml of fresh cow's milk, 75 g of sugar, 20 g of oil, 20 ml of mineral mix, 140 mg of vitamin mix and water to make 1000 ml.

[7] See Appendix 4. If only small amounts of food are being prepared, it will not be feasible to prepare the vitamin mix because of the small amounts involved. In this case, give a proprietary multivitamin supplement. Alternatively, a combined mineral and vitamin mix for malnourished children is available commercially and can be used in the above drink.

Table 7.10 Composition of F-75 and F-100 diets

Constituent	Amount per 100 ml	
	F-75	F-100
Energy	75 kcal (315 kJ)	100 kcal (420 kJ)
Protein	0.9 g	2.9 g
Lactose	1.3 g	4.2 g
Potassium	3.6 mmol	5.9 mmol
Sodium	0.6 mmol	1.9 mmol
Magnesium	0.43 mmol	0.73 mmol
Zinc	2.0 mg	2.3 mg
Copper	0.25 mg	0.25 mg
Percentage of energy from:		
protein	5%	12%
fat	32%	53%
Osmolarity	333 mOsmol/1	419 mOsmol/1

Table 7.11 The amount of diet to give at each feed to achieve a daily intake of 100 kcal/kg

Weight of child (kg)	Volume of F-75 per feed (ml)*		
	Every 2 hours (12 feeds)	Every 3 hours (8 feeds)	Every 4 hours (6 feeds)
2.0	20	30	45
2.2	25	35	50
2.4	25	40	55
2.6	30	45	55
2.8	30	45	60
3.0	35	50	65
3.2	35	55	70
3.4	35	55	75
3.6	40	60	80
3.8	40	60	85
4.0	45	65	90
4.2	45	70	90
4.4	50	70	95
4.6	50	75	100
4.8	55	80	105
5.0	55	80	110
5.2	55	85	115
5.4	60	90	120
5.6	60	90	125
5.8	65	95	130
6.0	65	100	130

(continued)

Table 7.11 (continued) The amount of diet to give at each feed to achieve a daily intake of 100 kcal/kg

Weight of child (kg)	Volume of F-75 per feed (ml)*		
	Every 2 hours (12 feeds)	Every 3 hours (9 feeds)	Every 4 hours (6 feeds)
6.2	70	100	135
6.4	70	105	140
6.6	75	110	145
6.8	75	110	150
7.0	75	115	155
7.2	80	120	160
7.4	80	120	160
7.6	85	125	165
7.8	85	130	170
8.0	90	130	175
8.2	90	135	180
8.4	90	140	185
8.6	95	140	190
8.8	95	145	195
9.0	100	145	200
9.2	100	150	200
9.4	105	155	205
9.6	105	155	210
9.8	110	160	215
10.0	110	160	220

* Rounded to the nearest 5 ml

7.4.7 Rehabilitation

7.4.7.1 Criteria for transfer to a rehabilitation phase

The child can move into the rehabilitation phase when

- Eating well
- Mental state has improved: smiles, responds to stimuli, interested in surroundings
- Sits, crawls, stands or walks (depending on age)
- Normal temperature (36.5–37.5°C)
- No vomiting or diarrhoea
- No oedema
- Gaining weight: >5 g/kg of body weight per day for 3 successive days.

7.4.7.2 **Nutritional rehabilitation**

The most important determinant of the rate of recovery is the amount of energy consumed. During rehabilitation most children take between 150 and 220 kcalth/kg (630–920 kJ/kg) per day. If intake is below 130 kcalth or 540 kJ/kg per day, the child is failing to respond. At the start of the rehabilitation phase, the child is still deficient in protein and various micronutrients, including potassium, magnesium, iron and zinc. These must also be given in increased amounts. Infants under 24 months can be fed exclusively on liquid or semi-liquid formulas. It is usually appropriate to introduce solid foods for older children.

7.4.7.3 **Feeding children under 24 months**

You should spend sufficient time to enable the child to finish each feed and be gently and actively encouraging

- F-100 diet should be given every 4 hours, night and day.
- Increase the amount of diet given at each feed by 10 ml until the child refuses to finish the feed.
- When a feed is not finished, the same amount should be offered at the next feed.
- If that feed is finished, the amount offered for the following feed should be increased by 10 ml.
- Continue this process until some food is left after most feeds.
- Record amounts of each feed offered and taken on the feeding.
- F-100 should be continued until the child achieves −1 SD (90%) of the median NCHS/WHO reference values for weight-for-height, at which stage discharge can be planned.

7.4.7.4 **Feeding children over 24 months**

- Feed every 4 hours (six feeds per 24 hours).
- This can be reduced to five feeds when they are growing well and no longer at risk of hypothermia or hypoglycaemia.
- You can use the same diet and regimen as for children under 24 months.
- It is appropriate to introduce solid food for older children but you need to fortify local foods with energy (to at least 1 kcal or 4.2 kJ/g) minerals and vitamins by using oil, dried skimmed milk mineral and vitamin mixes.
- F-100 should be given between feeds of the mixed diet. For example, if the mixed diet is given three times daily, F-100 should also be given three times daily, making six feeds a day.
- Water intake is not usually a problem in children over 2 years because they can ask for it when they are thirsty.

7.4.7.5 **Folic acid and iron**

Iron (3 mg/kg per day in two divided doses, up to a maximum of 200 mg daily, for 3 months) must be given during the rehabilitation phase. Iron should only be given orally, never by injection. For folic acid see Formulary, Chapter 20, p. 391.

7.4.7.6 **Assessing progress**

The child should be weighed daily and the weight plotted on a graph, marking the point that is equivalent to −1 SD (90%) of the median NCHS/WHO reference values for weight-for-height on the graph (this is the target weight for discharge). Usual weight gain is about 10–15 g/kg per day and most children are ready for discharge after 2–4 weeks. A child who does not gain *at least* 5 g/kg per day for 3 consecutive days is failing to respond to treatment.

7.4.7.7 Play and stimulation

Severely malnourished children have delayed mental and behavioural development which requires emotional and physical stimulation through play programmes that start during rehabilitation. Care must be taken to avoid sensory deprivation and the mother (or carer) must be with her child to feed, hold, comfort and play as much as possible. The environment should be bright, warm and stimulating with toys and play facilities available. Painful procedures should be carried out using the distraction techniques described in Chapter 5 – Pain.

7.4.7.8 Teaching parents how to prevent malnutrition from recurring

The parents have much to learn; teaching them should not be left until a few days before the child is discharged. Helping, teaching, counselling and befriending the mother are an essential part of the long-term treatment of the child. The mother (or carer) should spend as much time as possible at the nutrition rehabilitation centre with her child. This may be facilitated by providing the mother with money for transportation and meals. The mother, in turn, should help prepare her child's food, and feed and look after her child. A rotation of mothers may also be organized to help with general activities on the ward, including play, cooking, feeding, bathing and changing the children, under supervision. This will enable each mother to learn how to care for her child at home; she will also feel that she is contributing to the work of the centre. Teaching of mothers should include regular sessions at which important parenting skills are demonstrated and practised.

Ensure that the parents or carers understand

- the causes of malnutrition and how to prevent its recurrence
- how to stimulate the child's mental and emotional development
- how to treat, or obtain treatment for, diarrhoea and other infections
- the importance of regular (every 6 months) treatment for intestinal parasites
- the play activities that are appropriate for her child.

If possible, the child's home should be visited by a social worker or nurse before discharge to ensure that adequate home care can be provided. If the child is abandoned or conditions at the child's home are unsuitable, often because of death or absence of a carer, a foster home should be sought.

7.4.8 Discharge

7.4.8.1 Criteria for discharge

A child may be considered to have recovered and be ready for discharge when the child's weight-for-height has reached −1 SD (90%) of the median NCHS/WHO reference values. After reaching −1 SD of the median NCHS/WHO reference values, the child should be fed at least three times daily at home. Adjustment to this change in frequency of feeding should take place under supervision before discharge.

Before discharge, the mother (or carer) must practise preparing the recommended foods and feeding them to the child. It is essential that the mother demonstrates that she is able and willing to do these tasks, and that she understands the importance of continued correct feeding for her child.

Appropriate mixed diets are the same as those normally recommended for a healthy child. They should provide at least 110 kcal or 460 kJ/kg per day and also sufficient vitamins and minerals to support continued growth.

Breast-feeding should be continued; animal milk is also an important source of energy and protein.

Solid foods should include a well-cooked staple cereal, to which vegetable oil should be added (5–10 ml for each 100 g serving) to enrich its energy content. The cereal should be soft and mashed; for infants use a thick pap.

A variety of well-cooked vegetables, including orange and dark-green leafy ones, should be given.

If possible, include fruit, meat, eggs or fish. The mother should be encouraged to give the child extra food between meals.

7.4.8.2 Immunization

Before discharge, the child should be immunized in accordance with national guidelines. The mother should be informed of where and when to bring the child for any required booster doses.

7.4.8.3 Planning follow-up

Before discharge, make an appointment to see the child 1 week after discharge. Follow up visits should preferably take place at a special clinic for malnourished children, not at a general paediatric clinic. If possible, arrange for a health worker or field nurse trained to provide practical advice on health and nutrition to visit the family at home. Also arrange for a social worker to visit the family, in order to find a way of solving the family's social and economic problems.

Table 7.12 Criteria for discharge home

	Criteria
Child	Weight-for-height has reached −1 SD (90%) of NCHS/WHO median reference values
	Eating an adequate amount of a nutritious diet that the mother can prepare at home
	Gaining weight at a normal or increased rate
	All vitamin and mineral deficiencies have been treated
	All infections and other conditions have been or are being treated, including anaemia, diarrhoea, intestinal parasitic infections, malaria, tuberculosis and otitis media.
	Full immunization programme started
Mother or carer	Able and willing to look after the child
	Knows how to prepare appropriate foods and to feed the child
	Knows how to make appropriate toys and to play with the child
	Knows how to give home treatment for diarrhoea, fever and acute respiratory infections, and how to recognize the signs that mean she must seek medical assistance
Health worker	Able to ensure follow-up of the child and support for the mother

7.5 **Dehydration**

As children head towards death, it is common for their desire to eat and drink to decline. As a result, dehydration towards the end of life is commonplace.

The evidence regarding the incidence, effects and management of dehydration in the palliative care situation is sparse and often contradictory and therefore often unhelpful (for an excellent and fuller discussion, please read Dunphy et al.[13] or Burge et al.[14]). Therefore, the decision about whether to use articificial hydration when a patient is not complaining of thirst is a tricky one.

Dehydration in normal (i.e. non-palliative) situations can be a distressing condition[15], associated with thirst, dry mouth, irritability, cramps, headaches, vomiting, nausea, changes in electrolyte balance and ultimately confusion, convulsions and death. It is therefore natural to assume that it should be treated, right up until the moment of death. However, in the terminal phases, dehydration may have benefits too[16], such as reduction in urine output which will lessen incontinence, a decrease in gastrointestinal and pulmonary secretions which can lessen vomiting, coughing and pulmonary congestion and a reduction in the oedematous reaction surrounding tumours resulting in reduced pain.

Fainsinger[17] advocated artificially rehydrating dying patients because he claimed that dehydration can cause confusion and irritability; renal failure from dehydration might cause accumulation of opioid metabolites (with resulting adverse effects); dehydration exacerbates constipation and may increase the risk of pressure sores. However, other studies have not supported all of these claims. McCann[18]et al. (1994) showed that hunger, thirst and dry mouth can be well managed simply with sips of water or mouth care; and opiod side effects can be minimized simply by titrating down the dose if renal failure develops.

There is more evidence for the association of dehydration with terminal restlessness/delirium. Fainsinger also found that the need for sedation in terminal delirium declined if artificial hydration was used. Bruera[19] suggested that relatively low volumes of hydration each day may assist to prevent development of agitated delirium. On the other hand, terminal agitation/delirium can be managed with drugs which are less intrusive than IV lines.

There are also important social and psychological factors at play. The taking of fluids may be seen as a 'symbol of life'[20]. On the other hand, the equipment and monitoring processes associated with artificial hydration can impose a barrier between the patient and his/her family. Food and drink carry a strong social, cultural and religious significance, which is increased when someone is ill[21] but in some (particularly Western) cultures, the quality of life is often seen as the overarching goal[22].

Legally speaking, most countries classify artificial hydration as a medical treatment rather than a fundamental human right, and so, by the principle of double effect (see Chapter 17 – Ethics and Law) a clinician is usually in their rights to withhold or withdraw artificial hydration if it is felt to be ethically justifiable to do so. However, as discussed in the chapter on ethics, it is a very foolish clinician who stands by ethical principles alone against the wishes of a child and family. If such a situation arises, we would always advise individual clinicians to seek advice from their own legal representatives or their organisation's (or government's) legal advisers'.

Ultimately, given that the evidence is unconvincing in either direction, the decision as to whether to use artificial hydration must be one that is openly discussed with the child, family and all relevant stakeholders. Most importantly, the choice should always focus on the needs of the particular child at the particular time, taking physical, psychological and social aspects into account. In other words, it may be ethically acceptable to make different decisions in different children with similar clinical problems. Ultimately, you must assess carefully, balance the benefits and the burdens, make sure that the child and family understand them all and respect their autonomy by allowing them to choose.

Box 7.1 Case study – Adebayo

Adebayo is a 3-year-old boy, looked after by a 13-year-old sister. There are also three other siblings. The parents have died and the family live in very poor shanty accommodation on the edge of town. None of them is in regular schooling and they make their living by begging. Adebayo is very wasted, more than 3 SD below WHO weight for height and height for age tables. He is lethargic, not interested in feeding and looks very pale. His core temperature is 36.1°C. The other siblings also look very thin, but none as bad as Adebayo. His sister says he has been getting progressively worse for the last 2–3 weeks. You examine him and find a slightly enlarged liver and spleen, and a rattly, wheezy chest. His investigations reveal malaria parasites on his blood film, haemoglobin of 40 g/l and a non-specifically hazy chest X-ray.

- What do you think might be going on here?
- What treatments would you start as a matter of urgency?

After putting up an IV infusion you start antibiotics as per WHO guidelines and also transfuse him. He begins to perk up and starts to tolerate F75 feeds orally. Your volunteer support worker proves an excellent friend to him and gently coaxes and encourages his feeding until he begins to start taking some feeds himself. Within 3–4 days he is up and about and managing F100 diet with multiviatmins and minerals. Within two weeks you feel he is able to go home.

- What might happen if you discharge him now?
- What can you do to ensure you don't have to readmit him again in a few weeks or months from now?

7.5.1 Assessment of dehydration

Remember a neonate is 80% water, whereas a 1-year-old is 60% water. The younger the child, the more vulnerable they are to water loss. It is also important to note that oral rehydration therapy will be successful in most cases.

A systematic review has suggested that capillary refill time, abnormal skin turgor and abnormal respiratory pattern are the most useful signs for detecting dehydration. The study authors concluded that initial assessment of dehydration in young children should focus on estimating capillary refill time, skin turgor and respiratory pattern and using combinations of other signs[23].

Signs of 5% dehydration:

- loss of body weight of 5%
- decreased skin turgor
- dry mucous membranes
- fontanelle – may be slightly depressed
- eyes – slightly sunken
- pulses – normal
- respiratory pattern – may be abnormal
- mental state – may be normal.

Signs of 10% dehydration:

- loss of 10% of body weight
- decreased turgor with poor capillary return
- increased capillary filling time

- dry mucous membranes
- fontanelle – depressed
- eyes – sunken
- pulses – poor volume
- respiratory pattern – abnormal
- mental state – lethargic
- oliguria may be noted

Signs of >10% dehydration

- acidotic breathing
- shock – falling blood pressure with tachycardia
- coma
- anuria
- (also all the above signs as well).

7.5.2 Management of children who are not drinking

Table 7.13 Practical management of children who are not drinking

Cause	Management
1. Is the child thirsty?	• If so, give fluids either orally if possible, or by SC, IV or by tube.
2. Is the prognosis short and the child either comfortable or unconscious without agitation?	• It is unlikely that a comfortable or unconscious child is suffering as a result of not drinking, so there is no ethical reason to give fluids. • The family may well feel uncomfortable about not giving fluids and will need compassionate and patient explanation and support[24]. • Treat with good mouthcare (see above).
3. Is the child is uncomfortable, agitated or confused?	• Consider the ethics of non-oral routes: artificial hydration may reduce terminal agitation, but not always. • Check the laws of your own country to discover whether artificial hydration and feeding are viewed as medical treatments or basic human rights. • If the law is unclear or designates artificial hydration as an artificial treatment, decide with the child, family and colleagues whether the benefits outweigh the burdens or vice versa (see the chapter on Ethics for more details). • A pragmatic approach, if the family insists that feeding and/or hydration should continue, is to artificially hydrate (as refusal may reasonably be argued to risk complicating their bereavement, while SC or tube rehydration is unlikely to cause significant discomfort to the child).

7.5.3 Practical aspects

There are a number of options for fluid administration[25] in the terminal phase of a child's life.

- Intravenous infusions are often not appropriate for terminally ill patients due to potential complications.

◆ Hypodermoclysis/infusion of fluids into the subcutaneous space/easier to manage in the home setting.

◆ Nasogastric tube can be useful in short term but can also be distressing.

◆ Proctoclysis (rectal administration) can also be useful.

7.5.3.1 Hypodermoclysis

Trying to get IV lines into small children is difficult and distressing (for the child, family and also for you!). IV lines often last only 2–3 days. In the West, health workers are gradually realizing the benefits of subcutaneous hydration (hypodermoclysis)[26]. Care must be taken if the child is very wasted and the skin friable; but (with care) even these cases can benefit. The suprascapular area is safe, convenient and up to 100 ml/hour can be infused without hyaluronidase[27–29]. Unlike the intravenous route, subcutaneous cannulae can be left in place for 7–10 days without problems.

7.6 Questions for you

1. How can you tell the difference between cachexia, malnutrition and combined cachexia and malnutrition?

2. Apart from simple lack of access to food, what are the main reasons children end up malnourished? How will this knowledge affect how you manage malnourished children?

3. Do you feel artificial feeding and hydration are a human right or a medical treatment that can be withheld in certain situations? Try arguing both sides. How will this effect your management of children in the future?

Notes

1 Amery, J.M. & Rose, C.J. (2008). Quantitative evaluation of children's palliative care service in Uganda. *4th International Cardiff Conference on Paediatric Palliative Care,* http://www.cardiff.ac.uk/medic/aboutus/departments/childhealth/oursearch/paediatricpalliativecare/conferences/index.html

2 Parkash, R. & Burge, F. (1997). The family's perspective on issues of hydration in terminal care. *Journal of Palliative Care, 13*(4), 23–7.

3 Merriman, A. (2006). *Pain and Symptom Control in the Cancer and/or Aids Patient in Uganda and Other African Countries.* (4th Edition). Hospice Africa Uganda. ISBN 9970-830-01-0.

4 Anker, S. & Sharma, R. (2002). The syndrome of cardiac cachexia. *International Journal of Cardiology, 85*(1), 51.

5 Berry, C. & Clark, A.L. (2000). Catabolism in chronic heart failure. *European Heart Journal, 21*(7), 521–32.

6 Walsmith, J. & Roubenoff, R. (2002). Cachexia in rheumatoid arthritis. *International Journal of Cardiology, 85*(1), 89.

7 Plauth, M. & Schütz, E. (2002). Cachexia in liver cirrhosis. *International Journal of Cardiology, 85*(1), 83.

8 Schols, A. (2002). Pulmonary Cachexia. *International Journal of Cardiology, 85*(1), 101.

9 Barber, M.D., Fearon, K.C., Tisdale, M.J., Mcmillan, D.C. & Ross, J.A. (2001). Effect of a fish oil-enriched nutritional supplement on metabolic mediators in patients with pancreatic cancer cachexia. *Nutrition and Cancer, 40*(2), 118–24.

10 Tindyebwa, D., Kayita, J., Musoke, P., et al. (Eds.). *African Network for Care of Children Affected by HIV/AIDS (ANECCA) Handbook on Paediatric AIDS in Africa.* (Revised Edition 2006). Available online at www.Anecca.Org.

11 World Health Organization. (1999). Management of Severe Malnutrition: A manual for physicians and other senior health workers. WHO, Geneva. ISBN 92-4-154511-9. Available online at www.who.int/nutrition/publications/malnutrition/en/index.html.

12 World Health Organization. (1996). *WHO Global Database on Child Growth and Malnutrition*. WHO, Geneva.

13 Dunphy, K., Finlay, I., Rathbone, G., Gilbert, J. & Hicks, F. (1995). Rehydration in palliative and terminal care: If not – why not? *Palliative Medicine, 9*(3), 221–8.

14 Burge, F.I. (1996). Dehydration and provision of fluids in palliative care. What Is The Evidence? *Canadian Family Physician, 42*, 2383–8.

15 Bruera, E., Belzile, M., Watanabe, S. & Fainsinger, R.L. (1996). Volume of hydration in terminal cancer patients. *Supportive Care in Cancer, 4*(2), 147–50.

16 Burge, F.I. (1993). Dehydration symptoms of palliative care. *Journal of Pain and Symptom Management, 8*(7), 454–64.

17 Fainsinger, R.L. & Bruera, E. (1994). The management of dehydration in terminally ill patients. *Journal of Palliative Care, 10*, 55–9.

18 McCann, R.M., Hall, W.J. & Groth-Juncker, A. (1994). Comfort care for terminally ill patients. The appropriate use of nutrition and hydration. *The Journal of the American Medical Association, 272*(16), 1263–6.

19 Bruera, E., Belzile, M., Watanabe, S. & Fainsinger, R.L. (1996). Volume of hydration in terminal cancer patients. *Supportive Care in Cancer, 4*(2), 147–50.

20 Chadfield-Mohr, S.M. & Byatt, C.M. (1997). Dehydration in the terminally ill-iatrogenic insult or natural process? *Postgraduate Medical Journal, 73*(862), 476–80.

21 Fox, E.T. (1996). IV hydration in the terminally ill: Ritual or therapy? *British Journal of Nursing, 5*(1), 41–5.

22 Parkash, R. & Burge, F. (1997). The family's perspective on issues of hydration in terminal care. *Journal of Palliative Care, 13*(4), 23–7.

23 Steiner, M.J., DeWalt, D.A. & Byerley, J.S. (2004). Is this child dehydrated? *The Journal of the American Medical Association, 291*, 2746–54.

24 Parkash, R. & Burge, F. (1997). The family's perspective on issues of hydration in terminal care. *Journal of Palliative Care, 13*(4), 23–7.

25 Steiner, N. & Bruera, E. (1998). Methods of hydration in palliative care patients. *Journal of Palliative Care, 14*(2), 6–13.

26 Fainsinger, R.L., Maceachern, T., Miller, M.J., et al. (1994). The use of hypodermoclysis for rehydration in terminally ill cancer patients. *Journal of Pain and Symptom Management, 9*, 298–302.

27 Bruera, E., Neumann, C.M., Pituskin, E., Calder, K. & Hanson, J. (1999). A randomized controlled trial of local injections of hyaluronidase versus placebo in cancer patients receiving subcutaneous hydration. *Annals of Oncology, 10*(10), 1255–8.

28 Regnard, C.F.B. (1996). Comparison of concentrations of hyaluronidase. *Journal of Pain and Symptom Management, 12*, 147.

29 Bruera, E. (1996). Comparison of concentrations of hyaluronidase: Author's response. *Journal of Pain and Symptom Management, 12*, 148.

Chapter 8

Gastrointestinal symptoms

Justin Amery, Michelle Meiring and Caroline Rose

Key points

- Children with HIV/AIDS or cancer are very prone to mouth problems, particularly those who are malnourished.
- One of the most common causes of vomiting in children's palliative care is doctors' prescribing
- GI bleeding is very frightening for all concerned: *Anticipate* and *prepare* for it, but *don't panic* (it is quite rare for a child to bleed to death from a GI bleed).
- Diarrhoea is very common in children with HIV/AIDS and is the most common cause of illness and death during the first year of life.

8.1 Mouth care

8.1.1 Background

An adult mouth produces about 1.5 litres of saliva per day! It protects teeth and gums, prevents infections, helps digest food and acts as a lubricant. Most oral problems are due to a reduction in saliva and poor oral hygiene[1]. Children with HIV/AIDS or cancer are very prone to mouth problems, particularly those who are malnourished. They can easily be overlooked, but they should be taken seriously because, apart from the discomfort, they make eating, drinking and swallowing very painful, all of which impact significantly on the quality of life.

8.1.2 Causes of oral problems in children's palliative care

- Drugs:
  - Cytotoxic drugs which damage oral mucosa
  - Other drugs which dry the mouth (particularly anticholinergic drugs)
- Dehydration and reduced oral intake
- Debility
- Local lesions.

8.1.3 General oral care

- Keep the mouth as moist as possible and try to encourage the child to brush his or her teeth.
- Encourage the child to gargle and rinse regularly, ideally using saline, but with water if saline is unpalatable.

◆ Ask the child (or carer) to gently clean the tongue with a soft toothbrush.

◆ Encourage the child to chew pineapple which contains an enzyme which helps clean the mouth.

8.2 Sore mouth

Small children with sore mouths may present with difficulty or pain in swallowing or vomiting, reluctance to take food, excessive salivation or crying while feeding.

8.2.1 Causes

◆ Oral candidiasis (most common cause in children with HIV)

◆ Dental caries (present in 75% of patients)

◆ Cytotoxic therapy

◆ Aphthous stomatitis

◆ Recurrent herpes simplex.

8.2.2 Assessment and management of mouth pain

General treatment:

◆ use paracetamol before meals

◆ avoid spicy or sour foods

◆ use soothing liquids and ice-lollies (if available).

Table 8.1 Practical management of mouth pain

Condition	Problem	Management
Dental caries	Dry mouth and infections	General mouthcare Penicillin for infections
Oral candidiasis (present in 75% of patients)	Can present with ◆ Non-specific spongy red mucosa ◆ Angular stomatitis ◆ Classical white spots	Nystatin drops 1 ml qds Nystatin lozenges qds Miconazole (Daktarin®) oral gel Fluconazole orally: see Formulary, Chapter 20, p. 390. Amphotericin see Formulary, Chapter 20, p. 382.
Cytotoxic therapy	Marked stomatitis common	General mouthcare Use soft bland foods
Aphthous stomatitis	Shallow, cratered lesions with a raised, erythematous border and a grey, central pseudomembrane. Can be small or large.	Steroid creams in oralbase if available Prednisolone tabs crushed and the powder applied topically.
Recurrent herpes simplex	May start with itching/tingling sensation, followed by painful vesicles (which scab on keratinized tissue)	Aciclovir

8.3 Dysphagia

8.3.1 Background

This is very common in children with HIV/AIDS and cancers. Apart from the problems with not being able to swallow properly, children and families are often frightened that they might choke or inhale food.

8.3.2 Causes

- In the lumen:
  - Swallowed foreign body
  - Stuck food.
- In the wall:
  - Inflammation on mucosa due to infection (especially candidiasis)
  - Inflammation/ulceration due to drugs or other infections
  - Oesophageal reflux and spasm
  - Oesophageal carcinoma (very rare in children)
  - Neurological disorder (neuropathy due to cancer invasion or HIV infection).
- Outside the wall:
  - Physical obstruction (e.g. due to lymphadenopathy/tumour in the mediastinum)
  - Oesophageal candidiasis and/or ulceration (common in AIDS)
  - Drugs: particularly NSAID
  - Gastro-oesophageal reflux: drugs, persistent cough, recurrent vomiting.

8.3.3 Assessment

There may be little clinical evidence to help you differentiate the causes of dysphagia, unless you have access to facilities for chest X-ray and endoscopy.

- In children with cancer or HIV/AIDS:
  - Strongly suspect candidiasis in all cases (particularly if the dysphagia is painful, and/or the child has had steroids, chemotherapy or non-steroidals).
  - The absence of oral candidiasis does not exclude oesophageal candidiasis: consider if child refuses feeds, is drooling (unable to swallow own secretions) and has a hoarse cry from laryngeal candidiasis.
- If there is dental pain/trismus:
  - Think of dental caries and abscesses.
- If the child can swallow fluid easily, but food gets stuck:
  - Think of a stricture or compression.
  - Oesophageal cancer is rare in children but stricture secondary to ulceration can happen.
  - External compression form mediastinal lymphadenopathy is quite common.
- If the child struggles to swallow liquids:
  - Think of a motility disorder, a neurological disorder or a severely narrowed lumen.
- If the neck bulges or gurgles on drinking:
  - Think of a pharyngeal pouch (uncommon).

◆ If there is cough and recurrent chest infection with weak gag reflex:
  • Think of recurrent aspiration.

8.3.4 Management

Table 8.2 Practical management of dysphagia

Cause	Management
All children	◆ Treat the cause if possible ◆ Estimate feeding and hydration and manage as above ◆ Use feed thickeners for children with reflux
Candidiasis	◆ Nystatin is the cheapest and most widely available drug ◆ Miconazole (Daktarin®) oral gel as a second line (if available) ◆ Fluconazole daily for 21 days as 3rd line ◆ If you have nothing else, we have used clotrimazole 500 mg pessaries (sucked) with success! ◆ Gentian violet is cheap and although messy quite effective and sometimes more readily available than the above mentioned
Drug related	◆ Stop NSAIDs and anticholinergics if possible ◆ If not use gastroprotective drugs
Recurrent aspiration	◆ Consider tube feeding
Tumours	◆ Consider dexamethasone to reduce tumour bulk, but beware steroids in children (see Chapter 5 – Pain) ◆ Consider referral for radiotherapy if available ◆ Consider Celestin or Atkinson Tube or stent if available ◆ Consider gastrostomy if available
Pharmacological symptomatic treatment	◆ Consider acid suppression PPI (e.g. omeprazole) or H2 blockers (e.g. ranitidine) ◆ Consider motility stimulant (e.g. metoclopramide or domperidone) ◆ Try local anaesthetic (e.g. lidocaine) mixed with antacid formulation ◆ In terminal phase consider dexamethasone to give temporary relief in the last few days of life ◆ Treat residual pain using the WHO ladder

8.4 Nausea and vomiting

Box 8.1 Case scenario – Bernadette

Bernadette is a 7-year-old girl with HIV/AIDS. She has failed to respond to ARTs and has recurrent chest infections with persistent cough. She is taking co-trimoxazole (Septrin®) and erythromycin. She has moved from her family in the village to stay with her aunt in Kampala to be nearer treatment centres. She has started vomiting.

Questions:

◆ What is your differential diagnosis?

◆ How you would assess her to decide which are the most likely causes?

◆ How you would manage the vomiting?

8.4.1 **Background**

Children vomit very easily, but not always for the same reasons as adults. The prime difference is that children, particularly small children, have very sensitive gag reflexes, therefore any irritation to the back of the throat can trigger vomiting. We all have probably seen that children make themselves vomit from crying, gastric regurgitation, persistent coughing or from simple snottyness (leading to post-nasal drip). Furthermore, in our experience, nausea and vomiting in children is often (inadvertently) caused by drugs prescribed by health workers.

For this reason, it is easy to be tempted to trivialize childhood vomiting in children's palliative care. However, in fact children tend to be more resistant to vomiting from pharmacological or metabolic causes. So, for example, opioid-induced vomiting is less common in children than adults.

> Therefore, if you do see children with cancer or AIDS who are vomiting, you need to take it seriously

8.4.2 **Causes**

The physiology and pathology of vomiting are not well known by doctors and nurses in general, and consequently one sees some very unusual (and ineffective) drug regimes put in place for unsuspecting patients.

Firstly, we need to understand that vomiting can be triggered by stimulation of receptors in different parts of the gut and nervous system. The following diagram illustrates this well. Note that there are many possible triggers for vomiting, some of which (drugs, chemotherapy, radiotherapy, anxiety, upset, organomegaly) are very common in the children's palliative care setting.

8.4.3 **Assessment**

◆ If nausea is not a problem,
  • think of oversensitive gag reflex (cough, post-nasal drip, crying, gastric regurgitation), gastric stasis/compression or possibly raised intracranial pressure.
◆ If there is nausea and the child is on drugs or generally unwell,
  • think of drug causes (cytotoxics, antibiotics, NSAID, opioids), infections or metabolic causes (e.g. renal or hepatic failure).
◆ If the nausea is related to position/movement,
  • think of vestibular infection/tumour, or vestibule-toxic drugs.
◆ If there is nausea and with features of oesophagitis or gastritis,
  • think of drug-related causes (NSAID or steroids) or gastro-oesophageal regurgitation or candidiasis.
◆ If there is nausea and anxiety,
  • try to ascertain causes.
◆ If the child is well,
  • think of gastric stasis, gastric distension, constipation.
◆ If the child has a headache or neurological clinical features,
  • think of raised ICP and/or intracranial infection.

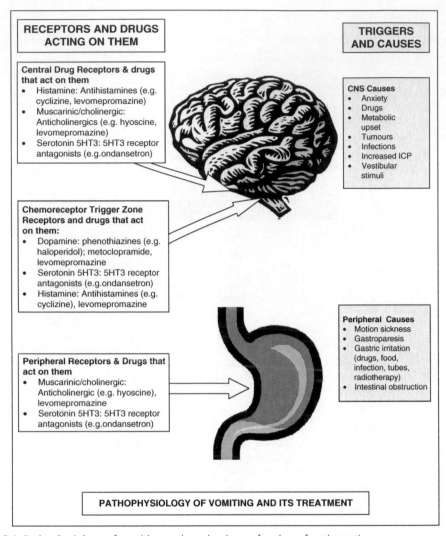

Fig. 8.1 Pathophysiology of vomiting and mechanisms of action of anti-emetics.

8.4.4 **Anti-emetic pharmacology**

If we are to prescribe rationally, it is important that we have a clear understanding of how anti-emetics work. We saw above that there are many different receptors that trigger vomiting. In the table below, we can see which antiemetics work on these different receptors.

Table 8.3 Emetic receptor activity of different drugs[2]

Drugs	Emetic receptor activity					
	Dopamine	Histamine	Muscarinic	Serotonin (5HT2)	Serotonin (5HT3)	Serotonin (5HT4)
Metoclopramide	++	0	0	0	+	+
Domperidone	++	0	0	0	0	0

Table 8.3 (continued) Emetic receptor activity of different drugs[2]

Drugs	Emetic receptor activity					
	Dopamine	Histamine	Muscarinic	Serotonin (5HT2)	Serotonin (5HT3)	Serotonin (5HT4)
Ondansetron	0	0	0	0	0	+ + +
Cyclizine	0	+ +	+ +	0	0	0
Hyoscine Hydrobromide	0	0	+ + +	0	0	0
Haloperidol	+ + +	0	0	0	0	0
Promazine	+ + +	+	0	0	0	0
Levomepromazine	+ + +	+ + +	+ +	+ + +	0	0

You can see from the table that:

◆ If available, the broadest spectrum anti-emetic is levomepromazine. It is also a sedative.

◆ Ondansetron, often thought of as an anti-emetic wonder drug, is actually very limited in its effect. It became known as a wonder drug purely within the small confines of chemotherapy units because chemotherapy hits serotonin-4 receptors, which are not well modulated by any other anti-emetics. In general children's palliative care practise however, it is not always a very effective drug.

◆ There is little point in trying promazine or metoclopramide if haloperidol isn't working.

In summary, when you are managing vomiting in children's palliative care, think rationally and systematically. Get to know the diagram and tables. Think of the most likely cause of the vomiting, guesstimate which receptors are involved and choose the appropriate anti-emetic. You will be pleasantly surprised by the results.

8.4.5 Management of nausea and vomiting

Table 8.4 Practical management of nausea and vomiting

Cause	Management
All children	◆ Explain, reassure, modify diet to ensure it is frequent, low volume, attractive foods ◆ Treat anxiety (Chapter 13 – Psychosocial and family care)
Possible iatrogenic causes?	◆ Review drug list and stop non-essential emetogenic drugs
Non-pharmacological management?	◆ Anxiety reduction (see Chapter 5 – Pain)
Features of gastritis or oesophagitis (pain, indigestion, flatulence, blood in vomit)?	◆ Stop NSAID and steroids if possible. Use omeprazole or ranitidine. If not try magnesium trisilicate (although not well tolerated in children)
Features of gastric stasis or compression (e.g. know abdominal tumour or abdominal organomegaly)?	◆ Try gastric motility stimulant (domperidone or metoclopramide)
Related to movement?	◆ Rule out iatrogenic cause ◆ Start vestibular-active drug such as cyclizine or hyoscine hydrobromide

(continued)

Table 8.4 (continued) Practical management of nausea and vomiting

Cause	Management
Related to toxic or systemic causes (e.g. infections, advanced tumours, renal or hepatic failure)?	◆ Treat underlying cause where possible ◆ Use drugs active on nervous system receptors, such as promazine, haloperidol, cyclizine
Features of raised intracranial pressure?	◆ Consider radiotherapy or shunt. If not appropriate cyclizine is drug of choice. Consider steroids but see cautions in Chapter 9 – Neurological symptoms
Above suggestions not working or is sedation indicated?	◆ Try levomepromazine (if available)

8.4.6 Pragmatic guide to management of nausea and vomiting in children's palliative care

All of this might be a bit confusing but, just like the analgesic ladder, it is important for health workers in children's palliative care to have a systematic approach to the treatment of nausea and vomiting. The following is a very brief summary of management approaches.

◆ Which drugs?
  • Cyclizine: best 1st choice all rounder with low side-effect profile (not recommended orally in children <2 years and rectally in children <6 years);
  • Domperidone: where gastric emptying is a problem (squashed or static stomach);
  • Haloperidol: next best, particularly where sedation required or opioid related;
  • Levomepromazine: very effective, but sedating. Good in terminal phase.
◆ Which conditions?
  • Raised ICP: cyclizine, ondansetron;
  • Drugs, metabolic, infective or biochemical upset: haloperidol/promazine;
  • Gastrointestinal tract stimuli: domperidone, metoclopramide.

8.5 GI bleeding

8.5.1 Background

This is a very frightening event, but massive life-threatening GI bleeding is not common in children's palliative care (except in biliary atresia and veno-occlusive disease – often a result of herbal medicine). Low grade GI bleeding is common when NSAIDs or NG tubes are used and in oesophagitis.

8.5.2 Causes

◆ From upper GI tract
  • Oesophagus: e.g. drugs, candidiasis, reflux, varices
  • Stomach and duodenum: e.g. infections, ulceration (often secondary to drugs or tubes).
◆ From tumour anywhere in GI tract
◆ Clotting disorders: e.g. leukaemia
◆ Swallowed blood: from nosebleeds or bleeding in mouth or pharynx
◆ Rarer causes in children: intussusception (<2 years), volvulus, Meckel diverticulum, arterio-venous malformation, oesophageal varices.[3]

8.5.3 Assessment

- Is the child vomiting frank blood, coffee grounds or just some blood mixed with the vomit?
  - Large volume frank red blood: think oesophageal causes
  - Large volume 'coffee grounds': think gastric bleeding, probably ulceration
  - Small amount blood staining in vomit: think swallowed blood (look for bleeding in nose, mouth and pharynx).
- Does the child have retrosternal pain and/or dysphagia?
  - Think oesophagitis.
- Does the child have epigastric pain?
  - Think of gastritis/duodenitis or ulceration.
- Is there a known bleeding disorder, or signs of bleeding elsewhere?
  - Think clotting abnormalities.
- Is the child getting central colicky abdominal pain?
  - Think small or large bowel causes such as Meckels diverticulum, volvulus or AV malformation.

8.5.4 Management

Table 8.5 Practical management of GI bleeding

Cause	Management
All children	<ul><li>*Don't panic*: Keep calm, reassure the child and family that it is unlikely to be life threatening</li><li>Position child so that blood/vomit drains easily</li><li>Provide receptacles and dark towels to collect blood</li><li>Consider siting an IV cannula for drugs and/or blood if appropriate and available</li><li>Check FBC and clotting screen if available</li><li>Start PPI (e.g. omeprazole)</li><li>Somatostatin</li><li>Consider referral for surgery/endoscopy (if available and appropriate)</li></ul>
Drugs?	<ul><li>Stop NSAIDs, steroids, warfarin, etc.</li></ul>
Tumour?	<ul><li>Consider radiotherapy referral</li><li>Consider the use of tranexamic acid (if available)</li></ul>
Massive life-threatening bleed?	<ul><li>Follow general management as above</li><li>Consider rapid and complete sedation using morphine and benzodiazepine parenterally</li></ul>

8.6 Intestinal obstruction

8.6.1 Background

This is quite a common condition in adults' palliative care, but less so in children's palliative care as pelvic malignancies are not so prevalent.

8.6.2 Causes

- Adhesions: commonest cause[4]
- Pelvic or abdominal malignancies

- Dysmotility, e.g. due to sepsis, cord compression, recent surgery, drugs (anticholinergics, antidiarrhoeals)
- Constipation mimicking obstruction.

8.6.3 **Assessment**

Bowel obstruction causes colicky abdominal pain, absolute constipation and nausea and vomiting with increased bowel sounds.

- Absent bowel sounds?
  - Consider peristalsis failure/ileus.
- Rectum full?
  - Clear rectum and review symptoms.
- Known abdominal or pelvic tumour?
  - Likely to be due to tumour itself or adhesions secondary to tumour.

8.6.4 **Management**

Simple 'drip and suck' (IV hydration and NG tube) will fail to control symptoms 90% of the time[5] but, with additional medical management, most patients will be comfortable enough to be cared for at home[6].

Table 8.6 Practical management of GI obstruction

Cause	Management
All patients	- Attend to mouth care
	- Stop feeding until cause found, and then can restart cautiously if child is hungry ('a little of what he fancies')
	- Use NG tube with suction if vomiting present
	- IV hydration if risk of dehydration and still appropriate
	- Stop laxatives
	- Consider surgery (if localized blockage, prognosis fair and child in good shape)
Constipation?	- Treat (see Section 8.7)
Peristaltic failure?	- Treat cause
	- Stop causative drugs
	- Start domperidone rectally
	- Consider stimulant laxative
Nausea and vomiting	- Avoid motility stimulant like domperidone or metoclopramide
	- Use cyclizine (sc) or haloperidol (sc)
	- Add 2nd agent if no better (e.g. levomepromazine)
Abdominal pain	- Colic: hyoscine butylbromide (sc or rectally)
	- Distension: paracetamol (rectal) or morphine (buccal or rectal or sc) – can aggravate abdominal pain in cases of intestinal obstruction
Tumour obstruction likely	- Consider dexamethasone short course

8.7 **Constipation**

8.7.1 **Assessment**

In adult medicine, it is normally taught that a rectal examination is necessary to assess constipation thoroughly. In children's palliative care this is arguable. To start with, children tend not to suffer with rectal or anal tumours which rectal examination is partly intended to pick up, and secondly rectal examination is quite traumatic for children. It is also often relatively easy to discover a sigmoid colon loaded with hard stools on simple abdominal examination. If the sigmoid is not palpable, then serious impaction is unlikely.

The following assessment algorithm will help isolate a cause in the majority of cases:

- Is the child dehydrated?
  - Think of reduced intake, or increased output (sweating, vomiting, etc.).
- What is the diet like?
  - Is it simply reduced intake, or is the child eating easy-to-eat carbohydrate-based foods that are not high in fibre or stimulants?
- Is the child immobile?
  - If possible, encourage the child to be as active as possible.
- Is there nausea and vomiting with colicky pains?
  - Think of possible obstruction.
- Is there anal pain on defaecation[7]?
  - Anal fissures are common in children and frequently lead to faecal withholding resulting in ever-larger and ever-harder stools, exacerbating the problem and setting off a vicious cycle.
- Are constipating drugs being used?
  - Especially opioids (the commonest cause in adult palliative care[8]), tricyclic antidepressants (e.g. amitriptyline), anticholinergic drugs (e.g. older antihistamines).
- Are there neurological features?
  - Neurological conditions often cause constipation[9], e.g. HIV encephalopathy, spinal cord compression.
- Are there features of metabolic conditions?
  - e.g. renal failure, hypercalcaemia.

8.7.2 **Classification of laxatives**

There are four main classes of laxatives. Availability might vary from country to country, but it should be possible to find at least one of each in most resource-poor settings:

(1) Bulk forming laxatives including bran, isphagula, psyllum, methylcellulose.

(2) Osmotic laxatives including magnesium salts, lactulose, sugar alcohols (sorbitol, mannitol, lactitol), small volume enemas (citrates, phosphates), polyethylene glycol.

(3) Stimulant laxatives including surface-active substances (docusates), bisacodyl, cascara, aloe, sodium picosulfate, castor oil, anthraquinones (senna, dantron). Senna coffee is often a locally available herbal product, as are paw-paw seeds (1–5 teaspoons daily)[10].

(4) Faecal softeners and lubricants including oils (ground-nut oil, blue-band margarines), dioctyl sodium, a plug of petroleum jelly inserted on the tip of a little finger or use a glycerin suppository (rectally).

8.7.3 **Management of constipation**

Table 8.7 Practical management of constipation

Cause	Management
Is there an obvious cause (see above)?	Treat cause: diet, rehydrate, improve mobility, alter medications, etc.
Signs of obstruction (e.g. vomiting, severe colicky abdominal pain, no flatus)	Refer for immediate surgical opinion or, at end of life, stop feed, insert NG tube, consider IV fluid and use antispasmodic
Pain on defaecation?	Check anus for fissures or candidiasis and treat with laxatives and local anaesthetic or glyceryl trinitrate cream prior to defaecation
Hard stool?	Treat with both stimulant and either an osmotic or a softening laxative. Oral preparations are best, but rectal ground-nut oil retained overnight with oral stimulants may work well. Rectal stimulants may be necessary, particularly in neurological causes. In severe cases, manual evacuation may be necessary
Is the stool soft?	Treat primarily with a stimulant, but add an osmotic laxative if necessary

8.7.4 **Manual evacuation**[11]

Manual removal of hard faeces may be necessary, particularly with neurological causes of constipation. The procedure is as follows:

(1) Explain to the child and family what is going to happen.

(2) Use distraction techniques as described in Chapter 5 – Pain.

(3) Swaddle the child if young and it is acceptable.

(4) Prepare newspaper or other receptacle for the faeces.

(5) Apply KY jelly to gloved little finger.

(6) Stroke outside of anus to relax the sphincter, then gently insert finger, stopping if spasm occurs *giving time for muscles to relax*. NB: muscles do not relax instantly. Allow 5–10 minutes of gentle, firm pressure. Do *not* push hard against a closed sphincter. Be patient.

(7) Remove small pieces of faeces piece by piece. Break up large pieces with finger before removal.

(8) Talk to child throughout procedure and stop if discomfort is too much. You can always continue another day. This procedure may need to be repeated alternate mornings by a nurse or by a relative who can be shown the procedure.

(9) Once the 'plug' has been removed, a laxative at night can be commenced.

Box 8.2 Case study – Mugisha

Mugisha is a 5-year-old boy who has been in hospital for 3 weeks for chemotherapy for his lymphoma. He was on paracetamol and codeine from the ward staff for facial pain. He was anxious in the ward and hated the toilet facilities. He had not opened his bowels for 1 week and then became incontinent with liquid faeces. He was assessed and found to have a palpable

Box 8.2 Case study (continued)

colon per abdomen with hard impacted stools on gentle rectal examination. He was diagnosed with constipation with overflow as a result of several factors. He was relatively immobile and had changed diet since being on the ward. The codeine was constipating and his fear of using the toilet facilities led to him withholding his faeces. All of these factors led to his constipation. Treatment involved providing him with more fibre in his diet; encouraging him to drink plenty; and making sure he was accompanied and reassured when going to the toilet. He required glycerin suppositories and senna syrup to enable him to start passing stool successfully again.

8.8 Diarrhoea

Diarrhoea is very common in children with HIV/AIDS and is the most common cause of illness and death during the first year of life. It is often prolonged and complicated, often with dehydration and malnutrition. AIDS-related diarrhoea can produce up to 20 stools per day with severe dehydration. Persistent diarrhoea is associated with an 11-fold increase in risk for death in HIV-infected children when compared to uninfected children. Up to 70% of diarrhoeal deaths in HIV-infected children result from persistent diarrhoea[12].

8.8.1 Causes (all children including HIV-infected children)

- Infectious causes – all children (including HIV-infected children):
  - Rotavirus (most common)
  - Bacterial (e.g. *enterobacter*, *Escherischia coli*, *Shigella*, *Salmonella species*, *Camphylobacter*, *Giardia*, *Entamoeba histolytica* and *Candida*).
- Drugs:
  - Antibiotics.
- Constipation with overflow
- Neurological: particularly paraplegia or autonomic dysfunction
- Lactose intolerance: inherited or post-inflammatory
- Ano-rectal irritation: due to faecal incontinence, candidiasis, post-radiotherapy.

8.8.2 Causes (HIV-infected children only)

- Other infectious causes:
  - Cryptosporidiosis, isosporiasis, CMV, atypical mycobacteria, strongyloides stercoralis, tricuris tricuria, cryptosporidiosis.
- HIV enteropathy
- Antiretrovirals (especially protease inhibitors).

8.8.3 Assessment

- Are there signs of acute infection? (offensive or blood-stained stool, pus in stool, fevers, abdominal pain)
  - Think retrovirus or other common infectious causes outlined above.

- ◆ Is the diarrhoea chronic[13] in an HIV-positive child?
  - • Think rarer causes of infections (see above), lactose intolerance, medications (e.g. ARTs) and HIV enteropathy.
- ◆ Are there signs of faecal impaction (previous constipation and palpable faeces per abdomen)?
  - • Consider overflow.
- ◆ Could it be due to drugs?
  - • Think antibiotics, ARTs, excess laxatives.
- ◆ Are there neurological features?
  - • Think about paraplegia or autonomic dysfunction.
- ◆ Is it related to diet and are there sugars or acid pH in stool?
  - • Think about lactose intolerance or milk protein hypersensitivity.
- ◆ Are there signs of ano-rectal irritation?
  - • Consider faecal incontinence, candidiasis, post-radiotherapy.

8.8.4 Management

Table 8.8 Practical management of diarrhoea

Causes	Management
All children	◆ Use waterproof plastic under sheet covered with cotton sheet or absorbent material ◆ Counsel carers regarding cross-infection risks ◆ Counsel family regarding nutrition ◆ Counsel family regarding household hygiene (especially handling baby's water and food) ◆ Bowies regime*
Diarrhoea – all children[14]	◆ Assess for malnutrition and use National IMCI Guidelines if present (see Chapter 7 – Feeding and hydration problems) ◆ Begin home fluids immediately ◆ Treat dehydration with oral rehydration salts (or IV fluids if severe) ◆ Emphasize continued feeding and increased feeding during and after the diarrhoeal episode ◆ Abstain from administering anti-diarrhoeal drugs in acute diarrhoea. ◆ Provide children with zinc supplementation for 10–14 days

Diarrhoea with blood in the stool	◆ If stool tests are not available, treat presumptively according to national guidelines or as follows:
	  • co-trimoxazole/nalidixic acid and metronidazole (if in an area where amoebiasis is a possibility) for children <8 years
	  • ciprofloxacin and metronidazole for children ≥8 years

Faecal impaction	◆ See Section 8.7 constipation
Possible drug causes	◆ Stop causative drugs if possible
Colic?	◆ Try antispasmodic, e.g. hyoscine butylbromide

Table 8.8 (continued) Practical management of diarrhoea

Causes	Management
Proctitis or anal irritation?	◆ Local toilet
	◆ Barrier cream
	◆ Treat for candidiasis
	◆ Metronidazole rectally if there is an offensive discharge
	◆ Consider steroid suppositories or retention enema
Diarrhoea still persisting and troublesome?	◆ Consider anti-diarrhoeal, e.g. loperamide, low-dose morphine or codeine phosphate

*Bowies regimen[15]

- ◆ Lactose-free milk (e.g. soya-based milk)
- ◆ Colestyramine see Formulary, Chapter 20, p. 386
- ◆ Gentamicin given orally to reduce bacterial overgrowth seen in chronic diarrhoea see Formulary, Chapter 20, p. 392
- ◆ Metronidazole
- ◆ In addition Vitamin A and Zinc can be added.

8.9 Questions for you

(1) You probably know how to prescribe analgesics rationally (the WHO pain management ladder). But do you know how to prescribe anti-emetics rationally? Think of a case you remember where you tried to manage a child who was vomiting. Which chemoreceptors do you think were triggering the vomiting? Which drugs would work best for those receptors?

(2) Similarly, think of a child you have seen with constipation where you have used more than one laxative. You now know that different laxatives work in different ways. Did you use a rational combination or an irrational one?

Notes

1 Watson, M., Lucas, C., Hoy, A. & Back, I. (Eds) (2005). *Oxford Handbook of Palliative Care*. (p. 238). Oxford University Press, Oxford.

2 Available online at www.Palliativedrugs.Com

3 Renee, Hsia. (2006). Pediatrics, gastrointestinal bleeding', *E-Medicine,* Available online at www. Emedicine.Com/Emerg/Topic381

4 Miller, G., Bowman, J. & Shrier, I. (2000). Aetiology of small bowel obstruction. *American Journal of Surgery, 180*(1), 33–6.

5 Regnard, C. & Hockley, J. (2003). *A Guide to Symptom Relief in Advanced Disease*. (5th edition). (p. 71). *Radcliffe Medical Press.*

6 Platt, V. (2001). Malignant bowel obstruction so much more than symptom control. *International Journal of Palliative Nursing, 7*(11), 547.

7 Clayden, G.S. (1992). Management of chronic constipation. *Archives of disease in childhood, 67*, 340–4.

8 Meuser, T., Pietruck, C., Radbruch, L., Stute, P., Lehmann, K.A. & Grond, S. (2001). Symptoms during cancer pain treatment following WHO-guidelines: A longitudinal follow-up study of symptom prevalence, severity and etiology. *Pain, 93*(3), 247–57.

9 Sullivan, P.B. (1997). Gastrointestinal problems in the neurologically impaired child. *Bailliere's Clinical Gastroenterology, 11*(3), 529–46.

10 Merriman, A. (2006). *Pain and Symptom Control in the Cancer and/or Aids Patient in Uganda and Other African Countries.* (4th edition). Hospice Africa Uganda. ISBN 9970-830-01-0.

11 Merriman, A. (2006). *Pain and Symptom Control in the Cancer and/or Aids Patient in Uganda and Other African Countries.* (4th edition). Hospice Africa Uganda. ISBN 9970-830-01-0.

12 Tindyebwa, D., Kayita, J., Musoke, P., et al. (Eds) *African Network for Care of Children Affected by HIV/ AIDS (ANECCA) Handbook on Paediatric AIDS in Africa.* (p. 95). (Revised Edition 2006). Available online at www.Anecca.Org.

13 Gwyther, L., Merriman, A., Mpanga Sebuyira L. & Schietinger H. (Eds) (2006). *A Clinical Guide to Supportive and Palliatuve Care for HIV/AIDS in Sub-Saharan Africa.* Foundation for Hospices in Sub-Saharan Africa. Available online at http:// www.Fhssa.Org.

14 WHO/UNICEF. (2004). *Joint Statement on Clinical Management of Acute Diarrhoea.*

15 Bowie, M.D. (1998). Management of persistent diarrhoea in infants. *Indian Journal of Pediatrics, 54,* 475–480.

Chapter 9

Neurological symptoms

Justin Amery, Susie Lapwood and Michelle Meiring

Key points

- Neurological problems are relatively common in children's palliative care.

- Delirium is a common problem in childhood and extremely common in children towards the end of life.

- *Don't panic*: Seizures are extremely frightening to child, family and health professionals, all of whom may see them as a herald of impending death *but* most seizures are harmless and self-limiting and you usually do not need to intervene.

- HIV encephalopathy may be at least partly reversible, but only by ART. Unless the child is close to death, ART should be started as soon as possible (if available), irrespective of CD4 counts. Delay risks further irreversible neurological destruction.

- Dystonia is extremely painful (which is why torturers use electric shocks) but often over-looked as it is usually present in children with global neurological impairment, who cannot easily communicate their pain.

- Dystonia is difficult to treat and usually requires a full range of non-pharmacological, pharmacological and even surgical interventions.

9.1 Overview

Neurological problems are relatively common in children's palliative care, and yet health professionals consistently say that this area is the clinical area they feel least confident in. This is probably not surprising as neurology is a complex area, and there are many, many symptoms, signs, syndromes and diagnoses to confuse and befuddle the health worker.

However, all is not lost. In the African children's palliative care context, relatively few neurological syndromes make up the vast majority of neurological presentations. Furthermore, these common syndromes present with obvious and characteristic symptoms and signs, which any health professional should be able to pick up with ease.

The trick is to be systematic and not to panic. This chapter hopefully helps you with both.

9.2 Neurological problems in HIV/AIDS and cancers

HIV invades the central nervous system by infecting monocytes, which cross the blood-brain barrier and establish HIV infection in macrophages and microglial cells. It is estimated that 40–70% of HIV-infected persons develop symptomatic neurological disturbances, but the brain is most commonly affected in children[1].

HIV can cause progressive encephalopathies, developmental delay, dementia and peripheral neuropathies. Children with HIV are prone to opportunistic infections of the CNS, especially meningitis. These problems are often compounded by malnutrition, lack of stimulation from ill parents, repeated absences from school resulting from their illnesses or the effects of social stigma[2]. While ART might, in mild cases where destruction is not yet severe, reverse the effects of HIV infection on the CNS, ART itself can also have neurological side effects, the most common of which is peripheral neuropathy[3].

While head and neck cancers are rare in children, as a proportion of childhood cancers they occur fairly frequently. In the West, lymphoma is the most common type of paediatric head and neck cancer, followed by neural tumours (especially retinoblastoma), thyroid malignancies and soft tissue sarcomas[4]. In Africa, where Burkitt's lymphoma is far more common than in the West, it is likely that its incidence is even greater than reported. Head and neck tumours can be difficult to manage in children's palliative care because neurological symptoms such as dystonia and neuropathic pain do not always respond to drug treatment, and because neurological destruction is irreversible, so permanent loss of important functions such as vision, hearing and mobility are common.

Other causes of chronic neurological diseases whether congenital (for example cerebral palsy or genetic conditions) or acquired (such as post-infective neurological destruction) are also common in Africa. However, these conditions do not often present in a palliative care context in Africa.

9.3 Neurological assessment in children's palliative care

The most common causes of neurological problems in African children's palliative care are as follows:

(1) CNS infections (especially malaria, OI's in HIV/AIDS and TB)

(2) CNS tumours (primary or secondary)

(3) CNS degeneration (especially HIV encephalopathy)

(4) Idiopathic (especially ART related neuropathy).

In the same way, there are relatively few neurological presentations in African children's palliative care. The most common are as follows:

◆ headache

◆ confusion

◆ seizures

◆ painful hands or feet

◆ loss of skills or dementia

◆ weakness

◆ spinal cord compression.

9.3.1 Taking a neurological history

Everyone thinks that, to be a good neurologist, you have to be able to pick up and interpret a huge range of obscure and subtle physical signs. In fact, this is not the case. The trick with neurological diagnosis is to spend time on the history, as the history will give you 95% of your diagnosis. Indeed, by the time you start examining you should have a pretty good idea of what the problem is, and should ideally have no more than two or three differential diagnoses in your mind. If you have more, the chances are the examination will end up confusing rather than clarifying matters.

The key items you need to explore in the history are as follows:

◆ Nature of the complaint?

◆ Onset: sudden, rapid or gradual?

◆ Static, deteriorating or exacerbations /remissions?

◆ Walking and fine skills?

◆ How it affects the patient's life?

◆ Associated conditions (especially HIV)?

◆ Drugs, alcohol and family conditions?

◆ Systematic enquiry for associated conditions?

The trick is to recognize certain *symptom clusters*. Once you have a good idea of these, you will find that neurology comes a lot more easily.

9.3.2 Main presenting symptom clusters in children's palliative care

In our experience, there are only seven commonly presenting symptom clusters in the African children's palliative care context, and every health worker working in African children's palliative care should at least be able to interpret these. They are listed below.

Table 9.1 Main neurological symptom clusters

Headache (If none of these accompanying features are present, the chances are that the headache is benign)	
Change in consciousness	Think of drugs, fever or raised intracranial pressure
Fever	Think of CNS infection or malignancy
Rash	Think of meningitis
Focal neurological signs	Think of destruction (e.g. tumour, bleeding, infarct, local infection)
Confusion	
With fever?	Think infections or possible tumour (esp. lymphoma)
With change to conscious level?	Think infection or increased ICP
With localizing signs?	Think of destruction (e.g. tumour, bleeding, infarct, local infection)
Seizures	
Fever?	Think infections
Known cancer?	Think tumours
Other generalized signs?	Think metabolic disorders
Always …	Think drugs (prescribed or illicit)
Painful hands or feet	
Can be caused by	Opportunistic infections (OIs)
	HIV itself
	ARTs
	Alcohol use
	Vitamin deficiencies

(continued)

Table 9.1 (continued) Main neurological symptom clusters

Loss of skills or dementia	
Acute?	Think infections, infarct, drugs, metabolic causes
Chronic: HIV negative?	Think alcohol, drugs, tumour
Chronic: HIV positive?	Think ART side effects or HIV encephalopathy
Weakness	
Acute: HIV negative?	Metabolic disorders, drugs
Acute: HIV positive?	Demyelinating polyneuropathy
Chronic: HIV Negative?	Systemic effect of most cancers and metabolic disorders. Also neurosyphilis, lymphoma encephalopathy
Chronic: HIV positive?	Demyelinating polyneuropathy, progressive polyradiculopathy, cerebral toxoplasmosis, neurosyphilis, lymphoma encephalopathy (PML)
Spinal cord compression	
No signs above the neck	If there are signs above the neck, there is an intracranial lesion
Known or likely disease	There is usually a fairly obvious underlying pathology (e.g. cancer, TB)
Paraparesis or monoparesis	Suggests lesion at or above the level of lumbar cord or lumbar nerves
Bladder or bowel impairment	Suggests lesion at or above cauda equina level. Always check perianal sensation
Pinprick level on the trunk	This helps work out the exact level of the lesion but is not helpful in practice as it does little to change the management. If radiotherapy is an option, the patient will need imaging anyway.

9.3.3 Neurological examination in children's palliative care

This is perhaps the most feared of all examinations by health workers around the world, not just in palliative care. However, recently, neurologists have pointed out that in fact, in general medical practice (such as family medicine and palliative care), a short focused neurological examination should pick up most of the key signs that are important (i.e. they will pick up any major pathologies of the type likely to cause symptoms in a children's palliative care context). The authors have slightly adapted this and presented it below.

Table 9.2 Quick neurological examination

Examination	Notes
Cognition: From your history, does he appear to have been clear and coherent with no subjective memory loss?	Y = unlikely cognitive defect N = think of organic CNS problem
Watch the child walk in	Normal gait = unlikely significant widespread pathology
	Suggestive gait = underlying pathology (e.g. spastic gait suggests upper motor neurone damage)
	In a wheelchair = paraparesis?, generalized weakness?, pain?

Table 9.2 (continued) Quick neurological examination

Examination	Notes
Ask him to walk on his heels and toes and then hop on each foot (older children only)	Y = normal motor and coordination (legs)
Can he pick up small items (e.g. small beads) with both hands?	Y = unlikely significant acuity problem or fine motor problem N = possibly abnormal, get eye check
Romberg's test and pyramidal tract test combined: get him to stand with feet together and arms out in front, palms up, eyes open then closed	(1) If trunk and arms stay steady: suggests normal sensory, vestibular and cerebellar systems (2) If trunk drifts or wobbles: suggests joint position problems of the trunk (dorsal column disorder) (3) If the arms drift: suggests problems with pyramidal tract (arms)
With his eyes still closed, you touch 1 finger on the child's outstretched right hand and ask him to touch the tip of his nose with it. Repeat on the left	OK = normal comprehension, attention, motor and coordination (arms)
Ask him to open his eyes and pretend to play the piano or tap each hand...faster...faster	OK = normal fine motor and coordination (arms)
Ask him to look only at your nose and point at which of your fingers is moving (do in all four quadrants of your own visual field)	If misses one finger, do again with each eye covered. If eyes wobble; check for nystagmus[A] Abnormal = visual field defect *Hallpike's test: the patient sits upright with legs extended. Ask them to look over one shoulder and then get them to lie down backwards quickly with the neck held in extension (either support the head as it hangs off the table or put a pillow under their upper back). After a 10 second latent period, you will see rotational nystagmus if the patient has benign positional vertigo. Repeat with the head looking to the other side.*
Now ask him to follow your finger with his eyes	OK = normal eye movements (cranials III, IV, VI)
Shine torch at his eyes and say 'Screw up your eyes tight, then open your eyes'. Then get him to look up, then ask him to show you his teeth and stick out his tongue	◆ If face equally tight, cranial VII = ok ◆ If there is pupil response on eye opening, cranial I = ok ◆ If he can show teeth clenched both sides, cranial V = ok ◆ If eyebrows raise equally, cranial VII = ok ◆ If tongue moves equally, cranial XII = ok

Lie on the couch	Fundoscopy: look for blurred optic disks suggesting raised intracranial pressure
	Check his reflexes:
	  ◆ Reduced/absent = neuropathy
	  ◆ Brisk = upper MN disease
	Check plantars: upgoing = pyramidal disorder

9.4 **Delirium and agitation**

9.4.1 **Background**

Delirium is a common problem in childhood. Most people who have children have seen their child become delirious with fevers. Delirium is defined as an acute alteration in alertness, cognition and perception. It is extremely common in children towards the end of life.

9.4.2 **Causes**

All children:

- ◆ Any febrile illness
- ◆ Uncontrolled pain (e.g. urinary retention or severe constipation)
- ◆ Metabolic causes: hypoglycaemia, hyponatraemia, uraemia, liver failure
- ◆ Drugs: opioids, steroids, benzodiazepines, tricyclic antidepressants
- ◆ Tumours
- ◆ Cerebral infections: especially malaria
- ◆ Hypoxia
- ◆ Malnutrition (particularly B1 deficiency).

In children with HIV/AIDS:

- ◆ HIV invasion of brain cells
- ◆ Meningitis (cryptococcal or bacterial)
- ◆ Toxoplasmosis
- ◆ ARTs, co-trimoxazole (Septrin®) high dose.

Also, delirium can be confused with acute anxiety. The difference is that anxious patients are not disoriented, although they may appear to be because they are so distracted they won't engage with your questions/assessment.

9.4.3 **Assessment**

- ◆ Take a history and examine
  - • Looking for signs of renal or liver failure, malnutrition, hypoxia or neurological abnormalities suggesting a central cause.
- ◆ Reassess medications
  - • Consider stopping potential culprits.
- ◆ If facilities available and investigation is still appropriate
  - • Check FBC, blood film, UEs, TFTs, LFTs and Glucose.

9.4.4 **Management**

Table 9.3 Practical management of delirium and agitation

Cause	Management
All children	◆ Reassure
	◆ Reduce risk of disorientation by turning lights on and reducing noise
	◆ Try to orient the child by reminding of place, time, etc.
	◆ Limit the number of staff involved

Table 9.3 (continued) Practical management of delirium and agitation

Cause	Management
Treat cause	◆ Ensure no unrecognized discomfort (especially urinary retention, constipation) ◆ Review medications, especially sedatives ◆ Treat intra-cranial infections and metabolic causes
If still no better	◆ Start antipsychotic (e.g. haloperidol or levomepromazine if available) ◆ Take care with benzodiazepines alone. They carry the risk of paradoxical agitation in children (unless there is an element of anxiety in which case they may help) ◆ Benzodiazepines can be used in conjunction with antipsychotics to sedate patients

9.5 Seizures

9.5.1 Background

Seizures can occur in HIV-infected children as a result of opportunistic infection or HIV invasion of brain cells. In cancers, seizures are commonly due to increased intracranial pressure, bleeding or invasion. They can of course also occur in idiopathic and secondary epilepsy. Seizures are extremely frightening to both child and family, both of whom may see them as a herald of impending death. They are also very frightening for health professionals, who may feel impotent in the face of them.

Don't panic. Most seizures are harmless and self-limiting. If the child is safe, you don't need to rush straight to drug treatment. Take a deep breath and concentrate on calming the family and your colleagues while the seizure takes its course. If there is no improvement after a few minutes, or if the child is turning blue, then you need to start treatment.

Also, do not fall into the trap of thinking that the only successful outcome is to abolish seizures completely. This may be impossible. In a children's palliative care setting, it may be that a situation where a child is not necessarily seizure-free, but with seizures having minimum distressing impact on the child, might be a 'good-enough' outcome.

9.5.2 Causes

◆ HIV invasion of CNS

◆ Opportunistic infections

◆ Tumour destruction of CNS

◆ Increased intracranial pressure

◆ Intracranial bleeds

◆ Biochemical disturbances (e.g. hyponatraemia)

◆ Hypoxia

◆ High fevers

◆ Underlying neurological/developmental disorder (static or progressive)

◆ Idiopathic/undiagnosed.

9.5.3 **Emergency management of seizures**

Table 9.4 Practical management of seizures

Cause	Management
All children	◆ *Don't panic*: take a long, deep breath; breathe it out slowly and check your watch
	◆ Ensure that the child is not in immediate danger (e.g. from falls, burns, drowning)
	◆ Remove tight clothing
	◆ Do not place anything in the mouth (e.g. spoons, tongue depressors)
	◆ Avoid leaping in with drug treatment but concentrate on calming family and colleagues
	◆ Place in side-lying position after the fit to prevent aspiration
	◆ Consider checking blood glucose level
After 5 minutes, or if the child is turning blue	◆ Give oxygen (if available)
	◆ Give rectal benzodiazepine (e.g. diazepam) or buccal lorazepam (midazolam if available)
	◆ Repeat the dose if the seizure continues for more than 5–10 minutes more.
Still no response	◆ Try a different route (e.g. buccal benzodiazepine)
	◆ Try a different drug (e.g. paraldehyde rectally – in an equal volume of ground-nut oil), phenytoin IV, phenobarbital IV
Still no response	◆ Sedate using the infusion of increasing doses of benzodiazepine and/or phenobarbital until acceptable control is achieved
	◆ Consider anaesthetic and intubation if still appropriate and available

9.5.4 **Status epilepticus**

Box 9.1 Case scenario – Flavia

Case scenario – Seizures

You are visiting Flavia, who is a 12-year old with known end-stage lymphoma with features suggestive of CNS disease (weakness of her right side). She has a severe chest infection and is feverish. She is at home with her mother and her 8-year-old sister. There are no acute medical facilities locally available. While you are there she suddenly screams and then starts a generalized convulsion.

◆ *What are the possible causes?*

◆ *What examination would you do?*

◆ *How would you manage this situation?*

Hints:

◆ Don't panic

◆ Sometimes the best thing to do is to do nothing

◆ What could you ask Flavia's mother and daughter to do that would help them and help you at the same time?

Occasionally status epilepticus may be a terminal event. If a seizure is not settling after 4–5 minutes (check your watch to be sure – time slows down when a child is convulsing), or the child is clearly becoming hypoxic, you will need to intervene. Control may be gained using the infusion of midazolam either on its own or combination with phenobarbital. These drugs are obviously respiratory depressants although large doses have been used without causing immediate respiratory compromise, especially in those who are not benzodiazepine naïve.

9.5.5 Ongoing management of seizures

In the children's palliative care situation most seizures will be secondary to an underlying pathology. This means that, as long as the pathology (e.g. cancer, infection, cerebral scarring) remains, the seizures are likely to recur. This means that health workers should always think about whether a child who presents with seizures should be started on ongoing preventative treatment.

It is beyond the scope of this book to give an exhaustive account of the ongoing management of seizures. However, for all children a good history should be taken in order to work out what precipitating factors might be and to search for possible underlying triggers. The following should be asked about[5]:

- events provoking attacks
- warnings of attacks
- motor features
- type of movement
- distribution of movement
- sensory features
- type
- distribution
- level of consciousness during attack
- length of attack
- presence of pallor, cyanosis or flushing
- characteristics and duration of the recovery phase
- predisposing factors
- family history of epilepsy
- head trauma or infection
- evidence of respiratory compromise.

In most African contexts, it is unlikely that EEG and/or brain imaging will be available or affordable. However, imaging is often not necessary[6], as the cause will often be fairly apparent from the history and from your knowledge of the child's underlying palliative diagnosis. In cases where there is developmental regression and HIV/AIDS, where the cause is not fairly obvious or where control of seizures is becoming a problem, the imaging (where available) might help pinpoint a diagnosis and offer specific treatment options (e.g. ART treatment, drainage of brain abscess, radiotherapy to brain tumours, etc.).

All children with epilepsy, and their families, should receive counselling on avoiding dangerous situations. Generally, families and children should be told that they can carry on their normal day-to-day lives as far as possible, but to avoid situations where they might be at risk if they convulse.

These might include tending fires, bathing alone (or bathing other children), climbing up to dangerous heights, etc.

The drug of choice depends on whether or not a child is on ART.

If a child is not on ART, the drug of choice for most seizures in the African children's palliative care context is carbamazepine (for tonic clonic seizures) or valproate[7]. If available, lamotrigine can be used as an alternative. Phenytoin is also effective but is becoming less used because of toxic effects. However, as most of these toxic effects are a result of long-term use, it may still be appropriate for it to be used in a palliative care context.

If a child is on ART, all anticonvulsants with the exception of valproate are likely to interfere with the metabolism of ARTs and so may cause the development of resistance (see Chapter 12 - HIV/AIDS). For this reason, unless you are an expert in ART treatment, seek advice before starting anti-convulsants. If advice is not available, then use valproate as a first line treatment as it does not interfere with ART metabolism

If you find that you cannot achieve control with one drug, expert advice now suggests:

◆ changing to another single agent rather than adding a second agent[8]

◆ when changing to a new drug, start at the initial dose and slowly increase until in the middle of its therapeutic range, and seizure control is good

◆ then slowly withdraw the old drug over a period of about 6 weeks.

9.6 Encephalopathies

9.6.1 Background

Encephalopathy in children in Africa is mostly due to HIV/AIDS (progressive multifocal leukoencephalopathy (PML) and HIV encephalopathy), although other genetic and metabolic causes are possible. It is particularly distressing for parents to watch as children 'go-backwards': gradually losing hard-earned and highly precious skills, regressing developmentally, losing their personalities, changing their behaviour and gradually becoming more and more dependent.

9.6.2 Assessment

Encephalopathy usually presents as developmental delay or regression. ANECCA guidelines suggest that diagnosis of HIV encephalopathy is mainly clinical and depends on the presence of at least two of the following for at least two months[9]:

◆ failure to attain, loss of developmental milestones or loss of intellectual ability

◆ impaired brain growth or acquired microcephaly

◆ acquired symmetrical motor deficit manifested by two or more of the following: paresis, pathologic reflexes, ataxia or gait disturbances

◆ normal CSF (or non-specific findings) and, if CT scan available, evidence of diffuse brain atrophy.

A full assessment of all of the child's functional abilities should be made (see Chapter 4 – Assessment and management planning).

9.6.3 Management

N.B. HIV encephalopathy may be at least partly reversible, but only by ART. Unless the child is close to death, ART should be started as soon as possible (if available), irrespective of CD4 counts. It is unacceptable to delay, thereby risking further irreversible neurological destruction.

Table 9.5 Practical management of encephalopathy

Cause	Management
All children	◆ Carry out full functional assessment
	◆ Address all physical, psychological and social needs holistically
	◆ Exclude other causes of neurological disease, e.g. birth asphyxia, CNS infections
	◆ Involve multidisciplinary team and draw up cohesive management plan
Pain and seizures	◆ Treat as per Chapter 5 – Pain
HIV encephalopathy	◆ Irrespective of CD4 counts or percentage, start ART if available

9.7 Head and neck cancers

9.7.1 Background

In the West, lymphoma is the most common type of head and neck cancer in children, followed by neural tumours (especially retinoblastoma), thyroid malignancies and soft tissue sarcomas[10]. Head and neck cancers (and their treatments) can be disfiguring, interfere with speech, feeding and breathing, may disturb vision or hearing and can carry a deep psychological impact for both the child and the family.

9.7.2 Specific children's palliative care problems in head and neck cancers

9.7.2.1 Neuropathic pain

◆ Features: This often occurs in the head and neck, often radiating to the arms. It can be severe, burning or shooting and may be associated with neurological signs.

◆ Management: See Chapter 5 – Pain for details. However, note neuropathic pain originating in the brain (usually due to damage to the thalamus) or spinal cord can be intractable. This is probably the most difficult of all pains to manage successfully. All non-pharmacological methods should be employed to the fullest extent. Opioids should be titrated to high doses. All adjuvants, such as antidepressants and anticonvulsants, should be tried. If available and pain persists, ketamine and/or methadone should be tried as alternative opioids that may be more effective than morphine in neuropathic pain. The author has had experience where the only analgesic with any effect in a girl with cervical tumour was nitrous oxide inhaled.

9.7.2.2 Trigeminal neuralgia

◆ Features: sharp, burning, severe pain across one side of the face.

◆ Causes: usually middle or posterior fossa tumours.

◆ Treatment: as for other neuropathic pains.

9.7.2.3 Orbital syndrome

◆ Features: severe retro-orbital headache.

◆ Causes: tumours or metastases in orbits, meninges or sphenoid cavity.

◆ Treatment: as per WHO pain ladder +/– surgery or radiotherapy. Steroids may ease pressure temporarily (but see cautions about use of steroids in children in Chapter 5 - Pain).

9.8 Spinal cord compression (SCC) and cauda equina syndrome (CEC)

9.8.1 Background

Spinal cord compression is caused by lesions in the spine pressing on the spinal cord. The spinal cord stops at L2 and becomes the cauda equina; so lesions below this do not cause true spinal cord compression. At this level, the correct term is cauda equina compression. However, in practise clinicians often use the term spinal cord compression for both. Also, in practise, both are emergencies and both require similar management.

9.8.2 Diagnosis

Usually, spinal cord compression occurs after a diagnosis of the underlying pathology (e.g. cancers or TB) is made. This is because it is a late complication. However, it might be the first presentation of a previously well child, particularly if the cause has rapid onset (such as an abscess). As with all neurological diagnoses, the history is far more important than the examination. Look for a history of severe back pain in the presence of increasing weakness in one or both legs, loss of bowel and bladder function or loss of sensation in the lower half of the body.

On examination, the leg weakness should be obvious. Reflexes are less helpful as they can be absent (if the lesion has disrupted lower motor neurons in the spinal nerves) or brisk (if the lesion has disrupted upper motor neurons in the spinal cord). You might find a loss of sensation in the lower trunk, limbs or peri-anal area.

9.8.3 Management of spinal cord and cauda equina compression

> Spinal cord compression is one of very few emergencies in children's palliative care. You need to recognize it and act on it immediately.

- ◆ Treat pain: spinal cord and cauda equina compression are usually very painful indeed; so the first step is to achieve pain control using pharmacological and non-pharmacological approaches. You will normally need WHO step 3 analgesia.

- ◆ Minimize pressure on the cord: the next step is to minimize the pressure on the cord. This reduces the chance of damage becoming permanent. It is very important as, even in a child who is dying, mobility and bowel/bladder control significantly improve the quality of life. Furthermore, being immobile will also significantly reduce the child's life expectancy. If you treat while a child is ambulant, 70% will regain function. If you wait until a child becomes non-ambulant, only 5% regain function.

- ◆ Refer for treatment of the cause: ideally, all children with SCC should be referred for radiotherapy (and/or sometimes surgery) to decompress the lesion. Where these options are available, you should give high-dose dexamethasone immediately. This will often reduce oedema around the tumour or abscess for a few days until radiotherapy or surgery is performed.

> Referral for radiotherapy should be on the same day as diagnosis. Do not 'wait and see'.

Where radiotherapy or surgical options are not available, it is less clear whether or not you should give steroids. On one hand, steroids may give some pain relief by decompressing the nerve. On the other, it might be very difficult to stop the steroids again once they are started. If the child survives for a long time after SCC/CEC is diagnosed, this means that you may leave an immobile, incontinent child on long-term, high-dose steroids, with the consequent hazards of Cushing's syndrome, diabetes, reduced immunity and probable skin breakdown. Perhaps a more sensible option would be to use a very short course until pain control is achieved using opioids and adjuvants, and then stop the steroids as soon as possible.

Box 9.2 Case scenario – Jane

Case scenario: Spinal cord compression

Jane is an 8-year-old girl with disseminated sarcoma, and known bony metastases.

She complains that, since she woke, she has bad back pain. Her mother says she seems to be unable to get out of bed. She has also wet the bed, although Jane does not appear to be aware of this.

You examine her and find that she is paralyzed in both legs and has lost sensation in her peri-anal area.

You give her 4 mg morphine and 8 mg dexamethasone and call the local hospital, where radiotherapy is available. She is admitted and found to have a lesion at L2, compressing the cord. She receives radiotherapy the same day. At your next visit you are delighted to find that she is back on her feet and able to use the toilet. Although Jane dies three months later, she maintains her mobility and independence for most of the rest of her life, and dies peacefully from a chest infection at home.

9.9 Meningitis

9.9.1 Causes

In all children

- Bacterial: especially meningococcal, haemophilus influenza type B and pneumococcal.

In children with HIV/AIDS

- TB: often presenting with sub-acute and chronic symptoms
- Viral: HIV itself as well as others
- Fungal: cryptococcal (rarely seen in young children but more common in older children and adolescents)
- Protozoal: toxoplasmosis.

9.9.2 Assessment

Suspect meningitis if the child has vomiting, headache, neck stiffness (often absent in cryptococcal meningitis), pain (worse on coughing), photophobia, irritability, confusion or convulsions. The child may have a stiff neck or rigid posture. You may see a classical non-blanching rash or a bulging fontanelle. Look for signs of raised intracranial pressure (papilloedema, unequal pupils, raised BP, low pulse and focal neurological signs). Take a blood smear to check for cerebral malaria, either as a differential diagnosis or co-existing condition. If possible, obtain a lumbar puncture unless there are signs of raised intracranial pressure. In children with HIV, differential diagnoses include tuberculous, bacterial and fungal infections (WHO, 2004)[11].

9.9.3 **Management**

Table 9.6 Practical management of meningitis

Cause	Management
All children	<ul><li>This is an emergency and needs to be treated as such unless the child is in the terminal stages.</li><li>Educate caregiver how to maintain clear airway.</li><li>Nurse the child on his/her side to avoid aspiration of fluids.</li><li>May require naso-gastic feeds especially if the level of consciousness is impaired.</li><li>Turn every 2 hours.</li><li>Change bedding when wet.</li><li>Pay attention to pressure points[12].</li></ul>
Bacterial meningitis	<ul><li>Ideally should be managed in hospital if possible.</li><li>1st line: 3rd-generation cephalosporin (e.g. ceftriaxone) if available (it is safer in children). Otherwise chloramphenicol IV.</li></ul>
Cryptococcal meningitis	<ul><li>Treat pain using WHO ladder.</li><li>Amphotericin followed by fluconazole see Formulary, Chapter 20.</li><li>Or fluconazole (requires an induction dose especially in children) see Formulary, Chapter 20.</li><li>Maintain prophylaxis with fluconazole unless the child is on ART and with sustained immune recovery see Formulary, Chapter 20.[13]</li></ul>
Tuberculous meningitis	<ul><li>12 months of rifampicin and isoniazid plus pyrazinamide and a third drug (ethambutol, ethionamide or streptomycin) for the first two months.</li><li>Some authors routinely add steroids[14].</li></ul>
Other symptoms	<ul><li>See sections on pain, delirium, convulsions.</li></ul>

9.10 **Other opportunistic infections of CNS**

These opportunistic infections tend to be seen only in cases of severe immunosuppression and even then usually only in older children and adolescents.

The following table is adapted from the ANECCA guide[15]

Table 9.7 Practical management of neurological opportunistic infections

Cause	Features	Management
CMV infection: Most common OI in children	<ul><li>Encephalitis, retinitis, radiculomylitis, neuritis</li></ul>	<ul><li>IV ganciclovir 10 mg/kg per day in two divided doses for 2–3 weeks.</li><li>or foscarnet 180 mg/kg/day in three divided doses for 14–21 days. May be used when there is sight-threatening CMV retinitis.</li></ul>

Table 9.7 (continued) Practical management of neurological opportunistic infections

Cause	Features	Management
Cryptococcus	◆ Fever, headache, seizures, change in mental status. ◆ Focal neurological signs uncommon ◆ CSF-Indian ink positive ◆ Cryptococcal antigen test, MRI, if available	◆ Induction with amphotericin followed by fluconazole see Formulary, Chapter 20.
Toxoplasmosis	◆ Encephalitis, mental changes, fever, headache, confusion. ◆ Do not do lumbar puncture if there is mass lesion.	◆ Pyrimethamine see Formulary, Chapter 20, p. 405. ◆ Plus sulfadiazine see Formulary, Chapter 20, p. 406. ◆ Plus folinic acid see Formulary, Chapter 20, p. 391. ◆ Treat until 1–2 weeks beyond resolution of signs and symptoms.
Herpes simplex	◆ Fever, altered consciousness, personality changes, convulsions and usually focal neurological signs particularly temporal lobe signs	◆ IV aciclovir 20 mg/kg given three times a day for 21 days.

9.11 Dystonia

Box 9.3 Case scenario – Jonas

Jonas is a 7-year-old boy with severe HIV encephalopathy. He has severe communication difficulties and is regressing developmentally. His mother reports he is getting increasingly distressed. You examine him and find his legs are fixed in extension, his arms in flexion and his back arches every few minutes.

Questions

1. How would you assess him?
2. How would you manage him?

9.11.1 Background

Dystonia (or muscle spasm) is a common but often overlooked feature of neurodegenerative disorders such as HIV encephalopathy and metabolic disorders. Muscle spasm is extremely painful. If you doubt that, remind yourself of how it feels when you wake with a bad cramp, or ask yourself why electric shocks are used by torturers. If you are still in doubt, remind yourself that contractures are so bad they can cause subluxations and dislocations of joints (even major joints such as the hip).

Unfortunately, because children who suffer with severe dystonias often have global neurological impairment, they cannot easily communicate their pain so it gets overlooked.

Apart from pain, dystonia has other profound impacts on the life of a child including reduced or absent mobility (or even control over movements), profound fatigue, muscle contractures leading to bone and joint deformity and reduced/asymmetrical bone growth leading to small and/ or deformed stature, excessive secretions and drooling (due to difficulty in swallowing).

Dystonia is not the same as epilepsy, but there is an overlap between the two (both are due to disturbances in nervous system electrical activity). In children with global neurological damage, epilepsy and dystonia frequently co-exist and are very difficult to differentiate. Persistent, chronic, low grade and focal seizures may mimic muscle spasms, and tonic or clonic spasms may appear as focal epilepsy. Furthermore, EEGs are rarely helpful to differentiate dystonia from epilepsy as, by the time a child has reached such an advanced stage, the EEG is usually so grossly abnormal that little sense can be made of it.

9.11.2 **Pathophysiology**

Dystonia is not fully understood, but a simple explanation is this. Remember that our muscles have to have just the right amount of tone. If they are too floppy, we cannot hold our position or mobilize/speak/swallow. If they are too tight, our position becomes locked, muscles become ischaemic and again we cannot mobilize/speak/swallow. Tone varies all the time even in healthy people. We all know what it is like to have stiff neck and shoulders when we are stressed, or for our voice to crack when we are anxious or emotional or how relaxed and supple we feel after massage or stretching.

Dystonia means that our muscle tone goes wrong. It is either too tight (in which case muscles become ischaemic and liable to tearing) or too floppy (in which case we become weak or even paralyzed).

The basal ganglia, thalamus, cerebellum and cortex work together to generate the right amount of tone, by sending the right amount of electrical activity through the upper and lower motor neurons to the muscles. When any of these structures are damaged, our muscle tone either increases or decreases to levels which interfere with daily living and may cause distressing symptoms.

9.11.3 **Causes**

- ◆ Spasticity (upper motor neuron lesions such as spinal cord damage)
- ◆ Damage to the brain, particularly basal ganglia, thalamus and cerebellum (e.g. encephalopathy, post-infection, birth hypoxia, cerebral bleeding)
- ◆ Drugs (e.g. metoclopramide, haloperidol)
- ◆ Idiopathic

Once it has set in, muscle spasm can be triggered by any number of stimuli: *pain, constipation, full bladder, noise, fear, unexpected touch*. The horrible thing about it is that it can both be triggered by pain and can also trigger pain. This leads to a vicious circle where the spasm causes pain which intensifies and prolongs the spasm, and so on.

9.11.4 **Assessment**

Assessing children with global neurological damage is very difficult. You need to re-read the chapter on assessment (Chapter 4) and remind yourself how to assess children by taking 3rd party histories and also by using physiological clues. However, there is no substitute for spending time with the child and family and really getting to know the child and his or her 'normal' level of activity and muscle tone. You may have to listen very carefully to the parents, who usually have a good idea of what is painful and what is not painful.

9.11.5 **Management**

Table 9.8 Practical management of dystonia

Cause	Management
All patients	◆ Perform a full functional assessment and address problems with mobility, position, feeding, bathing, etc. ◆ Gentle handling by familiar people ◆ Teach the caregiver how to perform regular physiotherapy ◆ If water is accessible, warm bathing can be very helpful in unlocking spasms ◆ Massage can also be very helpful
Treat causes	◆ Stop causative drugs ◆ Check that constipation or urinary retention is not an issue ◆ Ensure familiar, comfortable quiet environments ◆ Remove and treat all causes of pain as far as possible ◆ Try and control any epileptic activity
Drugs	◆ Drugs for dystonia are only effective in about 50% of cases ◆ Drugs for dystonia may improve muscle tone but overall may make things worse (e.g. spasm may be the only thing that allows a child to sit or stand) ◆ Drugs for dystonia may cause sedation and other adverse effects such as severe drooling ◆ Try baclofen and/or diazepam first line and titrate to effective dose ◆ Note that baclofen may make epilepsy worse ◆ Dantrolene and tizanidine are not licensed in children but can be useful if available ◆ Consider analgesia to treat the pain of the dystonia

Notes

1 Tindyebwa, D., Kayita, J., Musoke, P., et al. (Eds.). *African Network for Care of Children Affected by HIV/AIDS (ANECCA) Handbook on Paediatric AIDS in Africa*. (Revised Edition 2006). Available online at www.Anecca.Org.

2 Gwyther, L., Merriman, A., Mpanga Sebuyira L. & Schietinger H. (Eds.) (2006). Management of clinical conditions in children. *A Clinical Guide to Supportive and Palliative Care for HIV/AIDS in Sub-Saharan Africa*. Foundation for Hospices in Sub-Saharan Africa. Available online at http:// www.Fhssa.Org.

3 Tindyebwa, D., Kayita, J., Musoke, P., et al. (Eds.). *African Network for Care of Children Affected by HIV/AIDS (ANECCA) Handbook on Paediatric AIDS in Africa*. (Revised Edition 2006). Available online at www.Anecca.Org. Neurological Manifestations, p. 102.

4 Albright, J.T., Topham, A.K. & Reilly, J.S. (2002). Pediatric Head and Neck Malignancies: US Incidence and Trends over 20 years. *Archives of Otolaryngology-Head and Neck Surgery, 128*(220), 655–9.

5 'History Taking In Epilepsy'; *GP Notebook* Available online at www.Gpnotebook.Co.Uk

6 ILAE Neuroimaging Commission. (1997). ILAE Neuroimaging Commission Recommendations for Neuroimaging of Patients with Epilepsy. *Epilepsia, 38*(10), 1–2.

7 National Institute for Health and Clinical Excellence (NICE). (2004). Newer Drugs for Epilepsy in Children. Available online at http://www.nice.org.uk/guidance/index.jsp?action=byID&o=11532 NICE.

8 Drug and Therapeutics Bulletin. (2001), *39*(2), 12–16.

9 Tindyebwa, D., Kayita, J., Musoke, P., et al. (Eds.). *African Network for Care of Children Affected by HIV/AIDS (ANECCA) Handbook on Paediatric AIDS in Africa*. (Revised Edition 2006). Available online at www.Anecca.Org.

10 Albright, J.T., Topham, A.K. & Reilly, J.S. (2002). Pediatric Head and Neck Malignancies: US Incidence and Trends over 20 years. *Archives of Otolaryngology-Head and Neck Surgery, 128*(220), 655–9.

11 World Health Organization. (2004). *Palliative Care: Symptom Management and End-of-Life Care Module. Integrated Management of Adolescent and Adult Illness.*, WHO, Geneva.

12 World Health Organization. (2004). *Palliative Care: Symptom Management and End-of-Life Care Module. Integrated Management of Adolescent and Adult Illness.* WHO, Geneva.

13 Gwyther, L., Merriman, A., Mpanga Sebuyira L. & Schietinger H. (Eds.) (2006). Management of clinical conditions in children. *A Clinical Guide to Supportive and Palliative Care for HIV/AIDS in Sub-Saharan Africa.* Foundation for Hospices in Sub-Saharan Africa. Available online at www.Fhssa.Org.

14 Gwyther, L., Merriman, A., Mpanga Sebuyira L. & Schietinger H. (Eds.) (2006). Management of clinical conditions in children. *A Clinical Guide to Supportive and Palliative Care for HIV/AIDS in Sub-Saharan Africa.* Foundation for Hospices in Sub-Saharan Africa. Available online at www.Fhssa.Org.

15 Tindyebwa, D., Kayita, J., Musoke, P., et al. (Eds.). *African Network for Care of Children Affected by HIV/ AIDS (ANECCA) Handbook on Paediatric AIDS in Africa.* (Revised Edition 2006). Available online at www.Anecca.Org. Neurological Manifestations, p. 106.

Chapter 10

Skin problems

Justin Amery and Michelle Meiring

Key points

- Skin problems are very common in children's palliative care in Africa.
- Skin problems are very distressing, but may be overlooked or not taken seriously by health workers.
- Most skin problems benefit from simple skin care advice.
- There are simple and systematic ways of approaching management of skin problems, even if you do not know exactly what the underlying cause is.

10.1 Introduction

Skin problems are very common in children's palliative care, and particularly in children with HIV/AIDS. It is estimated that 92% of patients with HIV will experience skin problems during the course of the illness[1]. The commonest causes of skin problems in HIV/AIDS infected children are bacterial infections, fungal infections, viral infections (especially herpes) and infestations (especially scabies). Children with cancers can also suffer with fungating tumours, sores and hyperhidrosis (especially in lymphomas). As HIV/AIDS progresses, skin problems become more severe and problems such as candidiasis, oral hairy leukoplakia, folliculitis, herpes simplex and molluscum develop[2].

> It is always better to look at pictures rather than read about rashes and spots. We cannot provide an atlas of rashes in this book, but you can find an excellent and free online resource (at the time of print) at http://www.dermatlas.org/derm

10.2 General skin care

Remember that most patients with skin conditions carry fear and stigma. This applies also to children. Many people fear that skin conditions are catching, whereas most are not. Also, many skin conditions are disfiguring. So showing compassion, touching and cuddling the child and providing clear explanations to the child and family are very important.

Table 10.1 Simple management of all skin conditions

Intervention	Rationale
◆ Avoid thorough washing, bathing or showering more than once a day.	Prevents drying of skin and removal of skin's natural moisture. Dry skin fissures and is therefore more vulnerable to infections and allergens.
◆ Don't use soap or baby bath, but substitute aqueous cream or emulsifying ointment or bath oil.	
◆ Use a thick moisturizer after bathing (e.g. aqueous cream, emulsifying ointment).	
◆ Moisturize the whole body using thick moisturizer at least three times a day.	
◆ Humidify the air by boiling water.	
◆ Use soft, non-abrasive sponges, wash-clothes and towels.	Prevents mechanical irritation.
◆ Pat rather than rub dry.	
◆ Keep fingernails short and smooth.	
◆ Encourage the child not to scratch but to use finger tips to rub itchy areas.	
◆ Put mittens on small children to prevent damage from nails.	
◆ Use lactic acid, urea (10% urea cream), or sodium lactate moisturizers for itching.	Adds or helps to retain moisture.
◆ Keep topical creams and ointments cool or refrigerated.	The cooling sensation has an antipruritic effect.
◆ Avoid restrictive or non-absorbent clothing.	Guards against mechanical irritation.
◆ Use fragrance-free products rather than scented products.	Scented products may contain fragrance masking which elicit allergic responses in some patients.
◆ Avoid lanolin-based creams.	Produces a high rate of allergic response.

Children with HIV and AIDS, or skin problems due to cancer, should receive the following general skin care advice. Most skin conditions will feel better and probably improve[3]. Remember, prevention is better than cure!

10.3 Algorithm for assessing skin problems in children's palliative care

10.3.1 Steroid creams

Steroid creams are used so frequently in skin problems that some (more lazy) health professionals simply differentiate skin lesions into two classes: 'steroid positive' (i.e. respond to steroids) and 'steroid negative' (i.e. don't respond to steroids)! You should aim to be more professional than

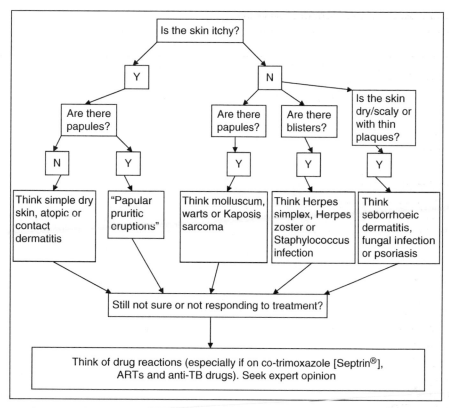

Fig. 10.1 Flow chart for skin problems in African children's palliative care.

that and try to narrow down the diagnosis as much as you can. You should be able to say what the rash is *not*, even if you cannot be exactly sure what it *is*.

You also need to be aware that overuse of topical steroids can cause significant side effects locally (e.g. striae, scarring, thinning of skin) and systemically (e.g. adrenal suppression, cushingoid symptoms). On the other hand, when used correctly, they can be very effective. Therefore, you need to strike a careful balance when using them. As my old dermatology consultant used to say, 'there is only one thing worse than using too much steroid, and that's not using enough'. The right amount/strength is the right amount/strength needed to completely clear the lesion.

'Finger tip units' are a useful measure to determine the amount of topical steroid you need to use. One fingertip unit (FTU) is the amount of topical steroid that is squeezed out from a standard tube along an adult's fingertip. This assumes that the tube has a standard 5 mm nozzle. A finger tip is from the very end of the finger to the first crease in the finger. An FTU of cream or ointment is measured on an adult index finger before being rubbed onto a child. One FTU is used to treat an area of skin on a child equivalent to twice the size of the flat of an adult's hand with the fingers together. You can gauge the amount of topical steroid to use by using your (adult) hand to measure the amount of skin affected on the child. From this you can work out the amount of topical steroid to use.

10.3.1.1 **Classes of steroids**

There are four classes of steroids, and you should get used to dealing with at least one from each group. These are as follows:

Class 1: Very Potent

- Clobetasol propionate 0.05%
- Diflucortolone valerate 0.3%.

Class 2: Potent

- Triamcinolone acetonide 0.1%
- Betamethasone valerate 0.1%
- Betamethasone dipropionate 0.05%
- Mometasone furoate 0.1%
- Fluocinonide 0.05%
- Diflucortolone valerate 0.1%.

Class 3: Moderate

- Betamethasone valerate 0.025%
- Hydrocortisone 1%
- Clobetasone butyrate 0.05%
- Alclometasone dipropionate 0.05%
- Fluocinolone acetonide 0.00625%.

Class 4: Mild

- Hydrocortisone 0.5% - 2%
- Fluocinolone acetonide 0.0025%.

Class 2: Potent (50–100 times as potent as hydrocortisone)

- Betamethasone valerate
- Betamethasone dipropionate
- Diflucortolone valerate
- Fluticasone valerate
- Hydrocortisone 17-butyrate
- Mometasone furoate
- Methylprednisolone aceponate.

Class 3: Moderate (2–25 times as potent as hydrocortisone)

- Aclometasone dipropionate
- Clobetasone butyrate
- Fluocinolone acetonide
- Triamcinolone acetonide.

Class 4: Mild

- Hydrocortisone 0.5–2.5%.

10.3.1.2 Skin absorption of topical steroids

Children's skin is much thinner than adult skin, and so you should always 'step down' at least one class compared to the recommended adult potency. Also, steroids are absorbed at different rates from different parts of the body. A steroid that works on the face may not work on the palm. But a potent steroid may cause side effects on the face. For example[4]:

- Forearm absorbs 1%
- Armpit absorbs 4%
- Face absorbs 7%
- Eyelids and genitals absorb 30%
- Palm absorbs 0.1%
- Sole absorbs 0.05%.

10.4 Itchy skin

10.4.1 Causes

The commonest causes in children's palliative care are:

- simple dry skin (Xerosis)
- atopic dermatitis
- contact dermatitis
- scabies
- chicken pox
- obstructive jaundice.

10.4.2 Assessment

Dry skin

- very common in debilitated children (e.g. cancers, HIV/AIDS)
- especially where malnutrition or malabsorption are present
- associated with eosinophilia
- prone to secondary infection so needs to be taken seriously
- may cause simple dryness, or later scaling and fissuring, eventually serous oozing and crusting.

Atopic dermatitis

- usually on face and flexures
- very itchy, red lesions, initially vesicles, then red, weeping fissures
- when chronic may develop thickened lichenified lesions
- often co-infection with staphylococcus.

Contact dermatitis

- any area where contact with allergen or irritant
- most frequently due to being left in wet nappies or clothes
- appears similar to atopic dermatitis.

10.4.3 **Management**

Table 10.2 Practical management of itch

Cause	Management
All patients	◆ All of these causes will respond well to basic general skin care (see above)
	◆ Try to identify and remove allergens and irritants
	◆ Use loads of emollients to trap moisture in the skin
	◆ Use barrier creams (e.g. zinc oxide) where contact is inevitable (e.g. in the nappy area)
	◆ Urea containing creams may help
	◆ Slightly sedating antihistamines may also help (e.g. chlorphenamine)
Itching	◆ Try wet wraps: damp cotton material soaked in potassium permanganate, water or saline
	◆ Apply these over steroid ointment (for itch) and/or povidone-iodine (for infection)
Skin lesions	◆ Use adequate amounts of steroid cream (class 4 to the face or flexures, class 3 or 2 to thicker skin)
	◆ Use 'one step down' in infants and babies (start with hydrocortisone 0.5%)
	◆ If infection suspected add cloxacin
Seborrhoeic dermatitis	◆ Selenium sulphide shampoo
	◆ Or antifungal creams
	◆ Also topical steroids

10.5 **Papular pruritic eruptions**

10.5.1 **Causes**

- insect bites and infestations (e.g. scabies, fleas, bed-bugs)
- allergies (e.g. papular urticaria)
- infections
- folliculitis
- fungal infections.

10.5.2 **Assessment**

PPE's are recurrent and persistent papules, which are itchy and which cause hyperpigmentation or hypopigmentation as they heal.

10.5.2.1 **Scabies**

- Look for reddish, pruritic papules with evidence of burrows in finger webs, wrists and umbilical region.
- In babies, look also in palms, soles and scalp.
- Often associated with impetigo.
- Can get severe diffuse disseminated scabies in HIV-positive children: 'Norwegian scabies'.

10.5.2.2 **Folliculitis**

- Inflammation of the hair follicle (may be inflammatory or infectious or both).
- Often associated with staphylococcus aureus infection.
- May be triggered by other organisms such as pityrosporum yeasts or demodex mites (D. folliculorum) which cause eosinophilic inflammation.
- Causes erythematous papules and pustules *located around hair roots*.

◆ Pustules and crusts suggest bacterial infective element.

◆ May develop into painful furuncles or boils.

10.5.3 Management

Table 10.3 Practical management of papular pruritic eruptions

Cause	Management
General treatment	◆ As for itchy dry skin above
	◆ Topical steroids (start with hydrocortisone 1% and increase potency as needed)
	◆ Topical antipruritics such as UEA with 1% menthol or calamine lotion or
	◆ Consider sedating antihistamine such as promethazine or chlorphenamine
Scabies	◆ Treat the whole family
	◆ Wash all clothes and bedclothes
	◆ Benzyl benzoate 25% apply and wash off after 24 hours (younger children dilute 1:2 in water)
	◆ Lindane (Gamma benzene hexachloride) 1% lotion: apply and wash off after 24 hours
	◆ Sulphur 5–10% ointment: apply daily for 3 days (better choice in young babies)
	◆ Add flucloxacillin as staphylococcus co-infection is common
Folliculitis	◆ Treat empirically using agents active against fungal, bacterial and demodex mites as well as an anti-inflammatory agent
	◆ E.g. clotrimazole or ketoconazole; erythromycin (topical or oral) and metronidazole 0.75% lotion or solution plus steroid (mid potency)
	◆ Treat boils and furuncles with oral antibiotics (e.g. cloxacillin or erythromycin)
	◆ If extensive or recalcitrant try oral antifungals
Fungal and yeast infections	◆ Treat with topical anti-fungals if localized
	◆ If extensive consider using systemic anti-fungals

10.6 Scaly patches and plaques

10.6.1 Seborrhoeic dermatitis

Assessment:

◆ Usually in scalp, axillae, groin and neck.

◆ Greasy, scaling or crusting, slightly itchy or non-itchy patches or thin plaques.

◆ Usually on scalp, nasolabial folds, ears, eyebrows, forehead.

◆ Can be very severe and widespread in AIDS and may involve the presternal area, axillae, groin, genitals and buttocks.

◆ Probably triggered by follicular yeast pityrosporum ovale.

Management:

◆ Simple skin care (as given above).

◆ Inflammatory lesions on the face can be treated with low-potency topical corticosteroid (e.g. hydrocortisone 1%).

◆ Antifungal agents such as selenium sulphide shampoos, clotrimazole or ketoconazole topical cream can be very effective.

◆ Dry, scaly skin can be managed with tar or salicylic acid-based shampoos.

◆ Improves with anti-retroviral treatment in HIV-infected children.

10.6.2 **Psoriasis**

Assessment:

- Can occur in one of two forms: localized lesions or generalized.
- Lesions are well-circumscribed, erythematous plaques with thick, 'silvery' scales that can be easily scraped off leaving a reddish base.
- Usually on areas of pressure/trauma, e.g. extensor surfaces, sacrum, hands, feet and scalp.
- In AIDS patients often presents as generalized plaques or atypical forms.
- Atypical forms include 'erythrodermic' and 'pustular' psoriasis.

Management:

- Generalized skin care.
- Emollients.
- Topical mid-potency steroids (Classes I, II or III) reduce inflamation.
- Topical keratolytic agents such as tar and salicylic acid to reduce scaling.
- Vitamin D derivatives (e.g. calcipotriol if available) reduce cell turnover.
- Generalized disease may require systemic therapy which can cause problems with immuno-suppression (e.g. methotrexate).

10.6.3 **Fungal and yeast infections**

Assessment:

- Look for erythematous patches or plaques with sharply defined advancing edges.
- In the scalp may present with patches of alopecia.
- If in body folds and nappy area it is often due to candida.
- May be extensive in HIV/AIDS patients.
- May resemble any of the eczemas or even psoriasis.
- If possible scrape edge of the lesion onto a microscope slide, add a drop of 10% potassium hydroxide, add coverslip and warm over a flame for 3–5 seconds and examine for hyphae[5].

Management:

- Keep body folds clean and dry and dust with cornflour or talc.
- Initially try topical antifungal preparations for 2–3 weeks, e.g. gentian violet 0.5% aqueous solution or Whitfield's ointment or imidazole creams (such as 1% clotrimazole).
- Use oral antifungal agents if no response or widespread (e.g. griseofulvin, fluconazole, ketoconazole, itraconazole or terbinafine).
- Beware of potential drug interactions in patients on ARTs. You may need to monitor LFT's more frequently.
- Tinea corporis or capitis usually requires 6 weeks or more of griseofulvin, nail infections take several months to resolve.

10.7 **Non-itchy papules and nodules**

10.7.1 **Molluscum contagiosum**

Assessment:

- Skin-coloured smooth papules with central umbilication.

Management:

♦ Local destructive methods are often used but of questionable benefit, and may even spread lesions further.

♦ Therefore simple reassurance that the lesions will disappear of their own accord within a year or two should suffice.

10.7.2 **Viral warts**

Assessment:

♦ Warty, skin coloured, painless papules, often flat on plantar surfaces.

Management:

♦ Topical 25% podophyllin or 50% trichloracetic acid, or local destructive methods if causing distress (but of questionable benefit).

♦ Condylomata accuminata (severe warty lesions in children with HIV/AIDS): usually improves with ART's and topical treatments as above, but may require destructive methods and sometimes even radiotherapy.

10.7.3 **Kaposi's sarcoma**

Assessment:

♦ Single or multiple painless, purplish lesions often associated with lymphoedema, often on face, oral mucosa and legs.

♦ May progress from flat, smooth patches to nodules or plaques.

Management:

♦ ART often results in tumour regression.

♦ Radiotherapy for local lesions.

♦ Palliative chemotherapy is often very helpful.

10.8 **Blistering lesions**

10.8.1 **Herpes zoster**

Assessment:

♦ Often preceded by pain, tingling and numbness in a dermatome.

♦ Followed by an eruption of vesicles which burst open to form sores, eventually scabbing.

♦ May be very painful.

♦ In advanced HIV may disseminate.

Management:

♦ Frangipani milk (the sap from cut frangipani leaves or stalks) helps reduce pain by paralyzing the nerve endings and helping healing with minimal scarring.

♦ Consider hospitalizing in AIDS especially if disseminated, systemic or patient unable to take oral meds.

♦ Aciclovir. See Formulary, Chapter 20, p. 380.

♦ Give prophylaxis to immunocompromised contacts with varicella-zoster immune globulin (VZIG) 125U per 10 kg (max 625U) within 48–96 hours of exposure.

♦ Use analgesia as per WHO ladder (see Chapter 5 – Pain) with adjuvants (e.g. amitryptyline).

10.8.2 **Herpes simplex**

Assessment:

- Often preceded by pain, tingling and numbness.
- Often starts in or around the mouth.
- Followed by an eruption of vesicles which burst open to form sores, eventually scabbing.
- May be very painful.
- In advanced HIV may disseminate.

Management:

- Aciclovir if extensive, if the eye is involved or if there is persistent ulceration.
- Treat secondary bacterial infection.
- Miracle Paint[6].

10.8.3 **Impetigo and ecthyma**

Assessment:

- Red, crusting, sometimes blistering lesions, with yellowish tinge in exudates.
- Can form large ulcers called ecthyma.
- Often suprainfection of other skin lesions.

Management:

- If mild, use topical antibacterial.
- If severe or persistent, use oral antibiotics: flucloxacillin/cloxacillin and phenoxymethylpenicillin or erythromycin.
- Advise regular washing with soap or povidone-iodine solution.
- Advise contacts that it is contagious so use own towels, bed-linen, etc.

Box 10.1 Case study – Mohammed

Mohammed is a 2-year old with HIV/AIDS Stage 3. He is generally doing well and his CD4 count remains high. He has not started ART yet. His mother brings him to you as he has developed a widespread, slightly itchy rash, predominantly over his face, scalp and trunk. When you examine you see that the rash is quite scaly and greasy, but you cannot see any plaques, fissures, papules or nodules.

- What are the most likely causes?
- How could you differentiate?
- How would you manage Mohammed?

10.9 **Fungating tumours**

Causes:

- In children, most commonly due to Kaposi's sarcoma and lymphoma.

Assessment:

- Painful, ulcerated enlarging growths with unpleasant odour and secondary infections.

Management:

◆ Consider debridement or palliative radiotherapy (if available).

◆ Cleanse regularly with salt water or antibacterial solution (e.g. metronidazole solution – 2 litres saline + 13 crushed 400 mg metronidazole tablets).

◆ Use ripe paw-paw for sloughing, crushed and applied twice daily for 5 days[7] or charcoal, live yoghurt or honey.

◆ Apply metronidazole tablets crushed into a powder.

◆ In South Africa, a local 'recipe' that has been found to be useful is as follows: 1 tub of aqueous cream, 40 × 400 mg crushed metronidazole tablets and 10 mg of morphine powder (highly concentrated).

10.10 Causes of changes in skin colour

Table 10.4 Causes of changes in skin colour[8]

Colour/clinical	Diagnosis	Site/s	Likely cause	Treatment
Purple; ↑ or ↓ pigmentation	Photosensitive drug reaction	Face, arms, neck	TB drug, thiazide	Stop drug Topical steroid Sun screen
Purple patches, plaques, nodules	Kaposi's sarcoma	Legs, arms, trunk, face, mouth	Human Herpes virus type 8 (HHV8)	See section on Kaposi's sarcoma
Purple and red areas; lips may be painful	Toxic epidermal necrolysis	Whole body, skin and mucosae	Co-trimoxazole, TB drug, anticonvulsant, nevirapine, EFV	Stop drug See section on cutaneous drug reactions
Purple-red patches with blisters	Fixed drug eruption	Anywhere on skin or mucosae	Laxatives, co-trimoxazole, analgesics	Avoid drug
Purple/blue nails	Blue nails of HIV	Nails	Unknown	None
Red, with scaling over whole body	Erythroderma (eczema, psoriasis, drug reaction)	Whole body	Anticonvulsant, co-trimoxazole, TB drug, allopurinol	Stop drug Topical steroid
Round red patches with central necrosis	Stevens–Johnson syndrome	Skin lesions anywhere, red eyes, erosions of mucosae	Co-trimoxazole, TB drug, anticonvulsant, analgesic	Stop drug See section on cutaneous drug reactions
Red defined area with fever and pain	Cellulitis	Leg, face most common	Streptococcus pyogenes	Penicillin by injection

10.11 Hyperhidrosis (excessive sweating)

Causes in children's palliative care:

◆ Infections

◆ Lymphomas

◆ High-dose morphine

◆ TB in older children.

Management:

◆ Explanation and reassurance that there is nothing more sinister going on is often all that is required.

◆ Use frequent sponging advise about absorbent clothing and bedding.

◆ Treat the cause if possible.

◆ If available use aluminium chloride hexahydrate to sweaty areas: noting it may take several weeks to reach maximum effectiveness.

◆ Drugs are not that effective but ones that might help include:

  • anti-muscurinics such as amitriptyline, propantheline, imipramine, etc.

  • cimetidine (note interactions with ART)

  • propranolol.

10.12 **Questions for you**

◆ Without looking back, try and write down the following:

  • The simple skin care advice you should give to all children who have skin problems.

  • What are the most common causes of popular pruritic eruptions?

  • The best treatments for herpes simplex and herpes zoster.

◆ Now check back and remind yourself.

Notes

1 Gwyther, L., Merriman, A., Mpanga Sebuyira L. & Schietinger H. (Eds.) (2006). *A Clinical Guide to Supportive and Palliative Care for HIV/AIDS in Sub-Saharan Africa.* (p. 125). Foundation for Hospices in Sub-Saharan Africa. Available online at http:// www.Fhssa.Org.

2 Hartshorne, ST. (2000). Common dermatological problems among HIV/AIDS patients. *CME. YOURSA Journal of CPD,* *18,* 321–6.

3 Tuthill, J. & Garnier, S. (2003). Prevention of skin breakdown. In Gwyther, L., Merriman, A., Mpanga Sebuyira L. & Schietinger H. (Eds.) (2006). *A Clinical Guide to Supportive and Palliative Care for HIV/AIDS in Sub-Saharan Africa.* Foundation for Hospices in Sub-Saharan Africa. Available online at http:// www.Fhssa.Org.

4 Dermnet New Zealand: Available online at http://dermnetnz.org/treatments/topical-steroids.html.

5 Gwyther, L., Merriman, A., Mpanga Sebuyira L. & Schietinger H. (Eds.) (2006). Dermatologic Problems. *A Clinical Guide to Supportive and Palliative Care for HIV/AIDS in Sub-Saharan Africa.* Foundation for Hospices in Sub-Saharan Africa. Available online at http:// www.Fhssa.Org.

6 Merriman, A. (2006). *Pain and Symptom Control in the Cancer and/or AIDS Patient in Uganda and Other African Countries.* (4th Edition). Hospice Africa Uganda. ISBN 9970-830-01-0.

7 Merriman, A. (2006). *Pain and Symptom Control in the Cancer and/or AIDS Patient in Uganda and Other African Countries.* (4th Edition). Hospice Africa Uganda. ISBN 9970-830-01-0.

8 Gwyther, L., Merriman, A., Mpanga Sebuyira L. & Schietinger H. (Eds.) (2006). *A Clinical Guide to Supportive and Palliative Care for HIV/AIDS in Sub-Saharan Africa.* Foundation for Hospices in Sub-Saharan Africa. Available online at http:// www.Fhssa.Org.

Chapter 11

Urinary symptoms

Justin Amery and Michelle Meiring

Key points

- Urinary symptoms tend to come together in groups.
- Diagnosis is usually made on history alone.
- Most urinary symptoms are exacerbated and can be caused by anxiety.
- Catheterization may be necessary, but can be traumatic. The use of special techniques and drugs can reduce this trauma.

11.1 Assessment of the urinary system

Urinary symptoms tend to come in 'clusters'. Clinical examination tends to reveal little of use, except where the bladder or kidney is palpable, so your diagnosis will mostly be based on the history. Urinary dip-sticks, if available, can be very useful in looking for blood, sugar, white cells and so on. Common clusters of urinary symptoms in children's palliative care include:

- **Frequency alone** might be due to infection, anxiety, diabetes mellitus or obstruction with overflow.
- **Frequency with dysuria** (pain on urinating) suggests lower urinary tract infection (UTI), i.e. bladder and urethra.
- **Simple loin pain** suggests kidney infection or stone or tumour.
- **Loin pain radiating to groin** suggests higher UTI (i.e. kidney and ureter) or stone or both.
- **Poor stream, frequency and continuous lower abdominal pain** with a palpable smooth mass arising from the pelvis suggests urinary retention.
- **Change in colour** suggests blood (or possibly drugs such as rifampicin, senna, bile, etc.).
- **Haematuria** suggests infection or stone or glomerular damage (e.g. inflammation, tumour).
- **Incontinence** is often normal in children and can be a symptom of regression (secondary to the upset of their illness and treatment) in children who were previously dry.
  - If there is a palpable bladder, think of retention with overflow due to local tumour.
  - If there are other neurological features think of neurological damage (e.g. spinal cord compression or neurodegenerative conditions such as HIV).

11.2 **Urinary retention**

11.2.1 **Causes**

- Opioids
- Drugs: Anti-cholinergic drugs, tricyclic antidepressants, opioids
- Neurological: Spinal cord compression
- Physical: Faecal impaction, pelvic tumour (e.g. lymphoma)
- Infective: UTI.

11.2.2 **Management**

Table 11.1 Practical management of urinary retention

Cause	Management
All patients	◆ Stop offending drug if possible ◆ Try gentle bladder massage and warm baths ◆ Consider catheterization
Drugs	◆ If due to morphine bethanechol or carbachol may help, but the problem usually settles after a few days
Urinary tract infection (UTI)	◆ Ensure good fluid intake ◆ If catheter in place, consider changing (but don't treat asymptomatic bacteriuria) ◆ Start antibiotics after considering local antibiotic sensitivities ◆ If unsure, in the community setting, the 1st line antibiotic is usually amoxycillin, although this may vary from place to place. In hospital settings, use local guidelines.
Physical obstruction	◆ Catheterize ◆ If due to tumour, consider radiotherapy referral if available and appropriate
Spinal cord compression	◆ Catheterize ◆ If radiotherapy is available and appropriate, start high-dose steroids and refer immediately

Box 11.1 Case study – Thomas

Thomas is an 8-year-old boy with leukaemia with widespread marrow infiltration. He has been getting severe back and nerve root pain, so last week you started him on morphine and amitriptyline. Today he presents in distress saying he has not passed urine for nearly 24 hours. When you examine him you find his bladder is palpable up to the umbilicus

- What is the diagnosis?
- What could be the causes?
- How would you manage this situation?

11.3 Catheterization in children

11.3.1 Tips for urinary catheterization in children[1]

- Catheterization is painful and traumatic.
- Always use distraction techniques (see Chapter 5 – Pain).
- Consider incident (procedural) analgesia such as morphine or anxiolytic/sedative (e.g. benzodiazepine) in young or anxious children.
- Always use anaesthetic gel if available, or lubricating jelly if not.
- Catheterize the child as upright as possible to ensure drainage.
- Choose the catheter size according to age and gender.
- Girls can accommodate larger catheters as the female urethra is more flexible than the male urethra.
- The larger the catheter diameter, the quicker the urine will drain.
- Use the shortest length possible to avoid knotting, tangling or kinking.
- When inserting a catheter
  - Into a female urethra, angle the catheter in a downward fashion.
  - Into a male urethra, resistance is very likely to be met at the external sphincter. By holding firm steady pressure against the sphincter, the muscle will eventually fatigue, and you will feel a release of pressure. When this happens, continue pushing the catheter into the bladder. Never force a catheter against resistance. If you do not feel a release of pressure (entering into the bladder) the catheter may be doubling back on itself. In this case, remove the catheter and choose a bigger size in order to exert enough pressure on the sphincter to push through.
- When urine appears into the catheter, insert the catheter a little further (1–2 cm) in order to assure that the catheter tip is fully within the bladder (you can push a Foley catheter right up to the hilt to be certain).
- After balloon inflation, gently tug on the catheter to bring the balloon down to the bladder neck before taping the tube in place.
- If you are unable to catheterize after above, stop and seek specialist advice.

11.3.2 Guidance for gauge and length of catheters in children[2]

Table 11.2 Catheter length guide

Age	Male	Female
Gauge		
Newborn	5, 6 or 8 Fr	5, 6 or 8 Fr
1–2 years	8 Fr	8 Fr
3–5 years	8 or 10 Fr	8 or 10 Fr
6–10 years	8 or 10 Fr	8 or 10 Fr
11–12 years	10 or 12 Fr	12 Fr
13 years and older	12 or 14 Fr	12 or 14 Fr

(continued)

Table 11.2 (continued) Catheter length guide

Age	Male	Female
Length		
Newborn	6 cm (+/−2 cm)	1.5–2 cm
2 years	8 cm (+/−2 cm)	1.5 –3 cm
5 years	10 cm (+/−2 cm)	1.5 –3 cm (+/−2 cm)
10 years	12 cm (+/−2 cm)	1.5 –3 cm (+/−2 cm)
12 years	16–20 cm (+/−2 cm)	4–6 cm (+/−2 cm)

NB: If paediatric catheters are hard to come by, sometimes the authors have used sterile feeding tubes (especially if you are just going to empty the bladder and withdraw).

11.4 **Irritable bladder**

11.4.1 **Causes**

♦ Infection
♦ Neurological damage (e.g. spinal cord compression, sacral plexus damage or neurodegenerative conditions)
♦ Anxiety
♦ Catheter.

11.4.2 **Features**

♦ Urge to pass urine frequently
♦ Maybe with actual incontinence.

11.4.3 **Management**

Table 11.3 Practical management of irritable bladder

Cause	Management
Non-pharmacological	♦ Reassurance ♦ Warm bathing ♦ Distraction
Infection	♦ See above
Neurological causes	♦ Trial of oxybutynin in children >5 years or tricyclic antidepressants in all children

11.5 **Haematuria**

11.5.1 **Causes**

In a children's palliative care setting, the most likely cause in a child is infective. Other causes include:

• Bilharzia
• Glomerular inflammation or injury (e.g. glomerulonephritis, nephritic syndrome)

- Clotting disorders
- Vasculitic disorders
- Disorders of renal vasculature
- Tumours in the renal tracts
- Developmental anomalies.

11.5.2 **Management**

Table 11.4 Practical management of haematuria

Cause	Management
All children	◆ Explain and reassure the child and family that it looks worse than it is due to the dilution effect of urine ◆ Manage cause
Severe bleeding	◆ Consider sedation with opioid and/or benzodiazepine (see Chapter 18 – Caring for children at the end of life) ◆ Catheterize if still appropriate ◆ Bladder washout using saline initially (to remove clots) and then silver nitrate 1 in 10,000 (if available) for 30 minutes (or continuous infusion for 24–48 hours) ◆ Refer to hospital if available/appropriate
UTI	◆ See above
Tumour	◆ Consider tranexamic acid if available

11.6 **Question for you**

(1) Have you ever been unable to pass urine when you are desperate? Remember how uncomfortable that was and imagine that this continued and worsened for 24 hours. Prompt diagnosis and management of urinary retention is very important.

Notes

1 Cinnati Childrens Hospital Policy On Urinary Catheterization/Bladder Irrigation. Available online at www.cincinnatichildrens.org/NR/Rdonlyres/104DECEF-6231-4B0C-B8F8-16CB8A72FD47/0/Catheterization.Pdf
2 Cinnati Childrens Hospital Policy On Urinary Catheterization/Bladder Irrigation. Available online at www.cincinnatichildrens.org/NR/Rdonlyres/104DECEF-6231-4B0C-B8F8-16CB8A72FD47/0/Catheterization.Pdf

Chapter 12

HIV/AIDS*

Justin Amery, Jenny Sengooba, Ivy Kasiyre
and Michelle Meiring

Key points

+ AIDS is by far the biggest and the main non-acute cause of childhood death in Africa.

+ Even in the era of ARTs, palliative care remains a crucial part of HIV/AIDS care because treatment sometimes fails, and, more often, is not available or affordable.

+ Palliative care also has an enormous role to play in the relief of distressing symptoms (some which may be as a result of side effects to ARTs) and immune reconstitution illnesses.

+ HIV/AIDS brings a huge physical, psychological and social burden to infected children and their families.

+ HIV/AIDS is a multi-system, multi-organ disease, not just a disease of the immune system.

+ Most symptoms caused by HIV/AIDS can be managed successfully, using the same principles as with symptoms due to other pathologies.

+ It is not necessary to be an HIV/AIDS expert to provide good children's palliative care, but you do need to know about side effects and interactions of ARTs, which can be significant in palliative care settings.

+ Providing palliative care to children with HIV/AIDS generates some very difficult ethical dilemmas.

12.1 **Background**

In many ways this chapter does not belong to a textbook of Children's Palliative Care. Usually, palliative care does not focus on diseases. Instead, it usually focuses on children's problems and symptoms. There are no chapters in the book on other conditions – even cancer. However, AIDS is not like any other condition. It is unique in children's palliative care in Africa. It carries particular challenges and requires particular approaches. In fact, it is difficult to grasp the magnitude and depth of the impact of AIDS on children's health. To help us understand why children's palliative care is so important in Africa, it might be useful to be aware of the following background and facts.

---

* The authors of this chapter are particularly indebted to the following sources: the ANNECA handbook[1], A Clinical Guide to Supportive and Palliative Care for HIV/AIDS in Sub-Saharan Africa[2], the Hospice Africa Uganda 'Blue Book', the WHO World Health report 2003 – Shaping the Future[3] and the UK DFID 'Child Mortality Factsheet'[4].

All evidence and figures quoted below are derived from these sources (see foot note):

◆ Most infections in African children are caused by mother-to-child transmission (MTCT). These result from a variety of factors: the high HIV infection rate in women of childbearing age, the high birth rates/fertility rates and low uptake and coverage of PMTCT.

◆ Of close to 40 million people living with HIV at the end of 2003, 70% lived in Africa, and 60% of those infected in Africa were women.

◆ Of the 2.1 million children under the age of 15 years living with HIV worldwide, at least 90% live in Africa. UNAIDS estimated that in 2003 there were 630,000 new paediatric HIV infections. It is currently estimated that in developing countries 1,600 children are infected daily by their HIV-infected mothers.

12.2 The effects of HIV/AIDS on children in Africa

HIV/AIDS affects African children in many ways:

◆ In Africa, more than 400,000 children under 15 died of AIDS in 2003 alone.

◆ Africa is already burdened with high morbidity and mortality rates due to infectious diseases and malnutrition in children and HIV/AIDS complicates this picture further.

◆ Maternal ill health, especially HIV-related, has a negative effect on infant survival irrespective of the child's HIV status.

◆ Infant and early childhood mortality among children of HIV-infected mothers (HIV exposed) is 2–5 times higher than that among children of HIV-negative mothers (HIV unexposed).

◆ There are over 13 million orphans worldwide who have lost one or both parents due to AIDS. It is projected that by 2010 the number of children orphaned by AIDS will increase to more than 25 million.

◆ In 2001, 10 countries in Africa had orphan rates higher than 15%, with at least half of the orphans resulting from AIDS (see Figure 2.3).

◆ The impact of AIDS on families and communities also affects non-orphaned children. With the deepening poverty that results from sick and dying parents, children are the first to suffer. They suffer mental, psychological and social distress and increasing material hardships. The children may be the only caregivers for their sick or dying parents/guardians, may drop out of or interrupt school, and are at risk of discrimination and abuse, both physical and sexual.

◆ Children with HIV/AIDS in resource-constrained countries experience high rates of morbidity and mortality relatively early in their lives, with up to 75% mortality by 5 years of age.

◆ Improvements in basic HIV care, and more recently antiretroviral therapy, have improved survival among HIV-infected children in developed countries. On the other hand, HIV-infected children in resource-limited settings continue to have little access to even basic HIV and supportive care.

◆ Globally, but particularly in resource-constrained settings, the terminal care needs and services for children with life-threatening illnesses are poorly understood and poorly developed.

◆ Delivering basic HIV/AIDS care, antiretroviral treatment and children's palliative care to HIV-infected children and their families requires continuity, good record keeping, significant planning, resources and infrastructure, all of which are scarce in resource poor settings.

◆ Children with HIV/AIDS have a variety of clinical care and psychosocial and socioeconomic needs, as well as the need to enjoy their rights as children.

12.3 Challenges facing palliative care for children with AIDS in Africa

All of the challenges facing children's palliative care which were outlined in Chapter 1 apply with AIDS. In fact, AIDS is by far the main non-acute cause of childhood death in Africa, and therefore the condition which children's palliative care practitioners need to focus on very carefully.

There are particular reasons why children's palliative care in AIDS is a challenge, however. These include:

- The very high prevalence of multiple symptoms in children with AIDS.
- Inadequate knowledge and skills in children's palliative care and management of childhood HIV/AIDS among care providers.
- Lack of prioritization by governments, health systems and education systems.
- The fact that the symptoms and manifestations of the disease change rapidly with disease progression.
- The variability of access to vital treatments such as ART.
- Frequency of ART treatment failure (often due to poor adherence).
- Significant morbidity due to side effects of ART treatment.
- Families refusing to engage in HIV treatment services for a variety of social and cultural reasons.
- Lack of resources for identification, monitoring, treatment and follow up.
- Severe infrastructural weaknesses limiting access to health facilities, drugs, support and other treatment.
- Prolongation of the chronic disease phase resulting in more complex and expensive management.
- Wide range of drug toxicities of ART.
- Competing effectiveness and toxicity of different drugs leading to complex decisions about sustaining or withdrawing treatments.
- Emergence of co-morbid conditions (e.g. hepatitis, chronic psychiatric illness).
- Development of immune reconstitution illnesses in children started on ARTs – especially in late stages of HIV.
- Stigmatization of AIDS resulting in failure to engage with health care services.
- Guilt associated with mother-to-child transmission.
- Possibility/likelihood that more family members are infected, sick or dying.
- Many family members affected resulting in multiple bereavement and overstretched carers.
- Breadwinners in families are often the most affected by AIDS.

12.4 Relevant information about HIV and its pathology

HIV attacks the immune system of the individual leading to the decline in CD4 cell counts. CD4 cells are a group of T-lymphocytes vital in fighting infections and immunosurveillance. HIV infection may be asymptomatic for a number of years whilst the virus insidiously damages the immune system. As the level of immunity falls children become susceptible to specific types of infections.

In children immunosuppression is defined according to the age group since children usually have higher cell counts in all blood lines than adults[5]. In children in the developed world, the median time from the onset of severe immunosuppression to an AIDS defining illness is

12–18 months in children not receiving antiretroviral drugs. HIV-infected infants frequently present with clinical symptoms in the first year of life, and by one year of age an estimated one-third of infected infants will have died, and about half by 2 years of age. There is thus a critical need to provide antiretroviral therapy (ART) for infants and children who become infected.

It is important to look for opportunistic infections as a cause of pain and symptoms in HIV-positive children. Treating them may enable a patient to stop analgesics and improve their quality of life greatly, even returning to school and normal activities. Many of these infections can be treated with inexpensive medications (e.g. candida, toxoplasmosis, tuberculosis and pneumonia), although some treatments are more expensive, such as treatment of cryptococcal meningitis.

12.4.1 Pathophysiology of HIV/AIDS

It is important to understand that the HIV virus causes pathology in two ways:

1. By suppressing the immune system

2. By directly infecting and damaging organs and systems

Organs and systems that can be directly infected and damaged include:

- The central nervous system: The HIV virus damages the central and peripheral nervous system, causing HIV encephalopathy and both central and peripheral neuropathies. These can cause a range of problems from subtle developmental and cognitive delay through to global neuro-degeneration with severe disability and ultimately death. Other less common problems include vascular myelopathy of the spinal cord and a sensory polyneuropathy affecting the hands and feet which can cause severe pain.

- The gastrointestinal system: HIV enteropathy is used to describe a syndrome of diarrhoea, mal-absorption and weight loss for which no other explanation is found. Villous atrophy is a common histological finding and small bowel permeability is increased.

- The heart: Causing HIV-related cardiomyopathy.

- The kidneys: Causing HIV-related nephropathy.

- The respiratory system: Causing lymphocytic interstitial pneumonitis (LIP) and debilitating chronic lung disease often complicated by cor pulmonale.

12.5 Psychosocial issues

Children with HIV/AIDS are liable to suffer with all of the psychosocial problems of children with any other life-limiting condition. A full discussion of these can be found in Chapter 13 – Psychosocial and family care. However, the additional issues that HIV-infected children face are arguably even greater. This is because of the nature of the HIV virus: its infectivity, its long latent period, its tendency to decimate whole families and the fact that it is still highly stigmatizing. As an example, some particular challenges that children with HIV/AIDS face would include:

- Psychological distress at illness and at the prospect of death and dying (as described in Chapter 13)
- High risk of being orphaned leading to:
  - lack of parental nurturing
  - lack of basic needs
  - loss of inheritance
  - need to work
  - less educational skills.

- ◆ Social isolation due to
  - stigma
  - effects of the condition (e.g. chronic coughs, disfiguring skin conditions).

12.6 **Prevalence of symptoms in AIDS**

12.6.1 **Incidence of different symptoms**

HIV-related conditions that are observed to cause pain particularly in children include[6]:

- ◆ meningitis and sinusitis (headaches)
- ◆ pneumonia and chest pain
- ◆ otitis media
- ◆ shingles
- ◆ cellulitis and abscesses
- ◆ severe candida dermatitis
- ◆ very painful oral lesions such as herpes, acute necrotizing gingivitis and severe dental caries
- ◆ intestinal infections, such as mycobacterium avium intracellulare (MAI) and cryptosporidium
- ◆ hepatosplenomegaly
- ◆ oral and esophageal candidiasis
- ◆ disseminated Kaposi's Sarcoma
- ◆ dystonic pain secondary to encephalopathy.

12.6.2 **Pain**

Pain in AIDS can be caused by:

1. The effects of specific opportunistic infections (e.g. headache with cryptococcal meningitis, visceral abdominal pain with disseminated mycobacterium avium complex).
2. The effects of HIV itself or the body's immune response to it (e.g. distal sensory polyneuropathy, HIV-related myelopathy).
3. The effects of medications used to treat HIV disease (e.g. dideoxynucleoside-related peripheral neuropathy, zidovudine-related headache, protease inhibitor-related gastrointestinal distress).
4. The non-specific effects of chronic debilitating illness.
5. Procedural pain due to repeated procedures such as venesection, tube feeding, lumbar punctures and so on.

Table 12.1 AIDS pain syndromes and most common pain diagnoses in AIDS[7]

Pain type	N	%
Somatic pain	107	71
Neuropathic pain	69	46
Visceral pain	44	29
Headache	69	46

(continued)

Table 12.1 (continued) AIDS pain syndromes and most common pain diagnoses in AIDS[7]

Pain type	N	%
Pain site		
Joint	47	31
Polyneuropathy	42	28
Muscle	40	27
Skin	23	15
Bone	31	20
Abdominal	25	17
Chest	19	13
Radiculopathy	18	12

It should be noted that in some instances the incidence and/or prevalence of pain may have actually increased with the advent of ART. As is often the case with AIDS, the irony of decreased mortality rates is that by surviving longer some children may thus be vulnerable to new complications and pain, as in the observed increasing prevalence of peripheral neuropathy which occurred with longer survival according to the Multi-Center AIDS Cohort Study[8].

Despite the high prevalence of pain in AIDS, several studies have also demonstrated that pain in children with AIDS is likely to be under-diagnosed and under-treated (see Chapter 5). This failure to diagnose and treat pain may reflect both the general under-recognition of pain by most physicians and/or the additional reluctance to consider seriously any self-report of pain in children.

In addition to pain, children with AIDS have been found to have a high prevalence of other symptoms, particularly but not exclusively in the advanced stages of the disease[9–12]. Moreover, one recent study suggested that physicians frequently also fail to identify and under-treat common non-pain symptoms reported by children with AIDS[13]. Symptoms include a mixture of physical and psychological conditions, such as fatigue, anorexia, weight loss, depression, agitation and anxiety, nausea and vomiting, diarrhoea, cough, dyspnoea, fever, sweats and pruritus.

12.6.3 Other symptoms

The prevalence of the 10 most common symptoms for children with HIV/AIDS in Africa has been reported as follows[14]:

- fever, sweats or chills (51%)
- diarrhoea (51%)
- nausea or anorexia (50%)
- numbness, tingling or pain in hands/feet (49%)
- headache (39%)
- weight loss (37%)
- vaginal discharge, pain or irritation (36%)
- sinus infection or pain (35%)
- visual problems (32%)
- cough or dyspnoea (30%).

12.7 **Management of symptoms in children with AIDS**

Individual symptom management advice is covered more fully in the relevant chapters of this book. However, to demonstrate the overlap between disease-specific treatment and palliative treatment that is a feature of AIDS, the following table will give an overview.

Box 12.1 **Case study – Miriam**

Miriam is a 4-year-old with HIV/AIDS complicated by abdominal lymphoma. She was started on ARTs 3 months ago. Her mother says she is crying a lot, complaining of abdominal pain, has gone off her food and is not gaining weight as you had hoped. Her father died 6 months ago of HIV/AIDS.

- What do you think could be some of the causes of her symptoms?
- Write a holistic problem list.
- Write a management plan for each of the problems.

Table 12.2 Practical management of symptoms in HIV/AIDS

Symptom	Causes	Disease-specific therapy	Palliative therapy
Fatigue, weight loss, anorexia	HIV infection Opportunistic infections Malignancy Anaemia	ART Treat infections Transfusions Nutritional support	Explanation and reassurance Lifestyle modifications Steroids
Pain	See above	ART Treat specific diseases using antibacterials/ antifungals/antivirals	Treat underlying cause Remember non-pharmacological approaches Consider ART Use WHO pain ladder
Nausea and vomiting	Drugs, gastrointestinal, infections	Stop drugs Treat infections using antifungals, antiparasitics, antivirals and antibiotics	Anti-emetics Prokinetics H2 blockers (e.g. rantidine) or PPI (e.g. omeprazole). Small frequent feeds, fluids between meals, offer cold foods, eat before taking medications, dry foods, avoid sweet, fatty, salty or spicy foods.
Dysphagia	Candidal oesophagitis	Antifungals	If severe, reduce inflammation by giving steroids initially (may need IV initially). The ideal treatment is fluconazole which may need to be given intravenously. If this is not available, we have had some success using clotrimazole pessaries 500 mg to be sucked daily for 5 days. Use analgesic ladder for pain.

(continued)

Table 12.2 (continued) Practical management of symptoms in HIV/AIDS

Symptom	Causes	Disease-specific therapy	Palliative therapy
Sore mouth	Herpes simplex, apthous ulcers, thrush, gingivitis	Aciclovir	Keep mouth clean; clean with soft cloth or gauze in clean salt water. Give clear water after each feed. Avoid acidic drinks and hot food. Give sour milk or porridge, soft and mashed. Ice cubes, ice cream or yoghurt may help, if available and affordable.
Chronic diarrhoea	Infections (gastroenteritis, parasites, MAC, cryptosporidium, CMV) malabsorption, malignancies, drug-related	Antibiotics/antivirals/ antiparasitics	Rehydration (Bowie's regimen), vitamin A and zinc, diet modification (e.g. yoghurt rather than fresh milk if lactose intolerance is a possibility), micronutrient supplements. Kaolin (cosmetic only) or bismuth. Oral morphine can alleviate intractable diarrhoea as can loperamide if available.
Constipation	Dehydration Tumours Drugs	Rehydrate Treat tumours with DXT or chemo if appropriate Adjust medication	Activity Diet modification Laxatives
Ano-genital ulceration	Commonly due to herpes simplex virus Candidiasis	Herpes: aciclovir (oral) or an emulsion mixture of nystatin 5 ml, metronidazole powder 400 mg and aciclovir 200 mg Antifungals	Crush a tablet of prednisolone and apply the powder to the affected part.
Breathlessness	Pneumonia Anaemia Tumour Effusion Weakened respiratory muscles	Treat cause Antibiotics Iron or transfusion if severe Treatment of tumour (if appropriate) Drainage (if appropriate)	Fan and maximize airflow Counselling Distraction Relaxation Guided imagery Opioids Benzodiazepines
Persistent cough	Infections, LIP, bronchiectasis, TB, effusion, tumour	Antibiotics PCP treatment Anti-TB treatment Treatment of tumour (if appropriate) Drainage	Nebulization with physiotherapy Suppressant (e.g. low-dose morphine) Phsyiotherapy Humidification Steroids (LIP)

Table 12.2 (continued) Practical management of symptoms in HIV/AIDS

Symptom	Causes	Disease-specific therapy	Palliative therapy
Severe dermatitis	Seborrhoeic dermatitis Infestations Folliculitis Fungal infection Hypersensitivity Renal and liver disease	Antibacterials/antifungals/ antiparasitics Hydration Steroids	Emollients, antihistamines, antiseptics, topical steroids. Antimuscarinic antidepressants (e.g. amitriptyline) Anxiolytics Keep nails short to minimize trauma and secondary infection from scratching
Shingles and post-herpetic neuralgia	Herpes zoster	Aciclovir if caught early	Liquid from frangipani tree when applied to the vesicles (before they break) causes paralysis of nerves for up to 8 hours. Break off a small branch and collect the white fluid into a clean jar. Paint this onto the area. (This fluid can be kept up to 24 hours). Post-herpetic neuralgia – use amitriptyline, valproate, phenytoin or carbamazepine for shooting pain (but beware of interactions with ARTs). Add morphine if necessary
Convulsions	Infections and infestations, encephalopathy, malignancies, PMLE		Diazepam or phenobarbital or paraldehyde for acute control, then convert to longer term therapy. Beware of interactions between anticonvulsants and ARTs
Metabolic disorders	Anticonvulsants, glucose, mannitol, steroids		Rehydrate. Ensure good oxygenation. Give high energy, low protein feeds until disorder resolves. Treat individual cause
Fevers, sweats	HIV MAC CMV Lymphoma	ART Azithromycin Aciclovir Chemotherapy	NSAIDS Steroids Hyoscine Cimetidine
Pressure sores	Malnutrition Reduced mobility	Nutrition Mobilization	Wound dressing, metronidazole powder to control odour, honey applications on clean, debridement if necessary
Delirium/ agitation	Electrolytes disturbances Toxoplasmosis Cryptococcal meningitis IC sepsis	Correct imbalances and rehydrate antifungals and antibiotics	Assist orientation Haloperidol or promazine Benzodiazepines
Depression	Reactive Chronic illness	Play therapy Counselling Distraction (role of antidepressants in children still uncertain)	Counselling Distraction

12.8 **Antiretroviral therapy in children's palliative care**

12.8.1 **Introduction**

A significant proportion of children receiving children's palliative care in the African context will be on ARTs, usually including nucleoside reverse transcriptase inhibitors, non-reverse transcriptase inhibitors and a few on protease inhibitors. It is very important to understand that significant drug interactions can occur in children receiving palliative care drugs who are also on ARTs. Furthermore, most of these medications may need to be administered in the presence of other co-morbid conditions such as hepatitis, pancreatitis, gastritis, hypertriglyceridemia, hyperglycemia, lipodystrophies, HIV-associated nephropathies and opportunistic infections. These can increase the risk and the effects of interactions and adverse effects of drugs.

12.8.2 **Important pharmacology in children's palliative care and HIV/AIDS treatment**

It is beyond the boundaries of this book to deal with the whole pharmacology of ARTs. If you are regularly prescribing and managing ARTs, or if you do not have ready access to advice and support from professional ART providers, you should familiarize yourself with the relevant pharmacology using other more detailed sources. The aim of this chapter is to highlight at least the major risks.

The key system to understand is the cytochrome P450 (CYP) enzyme system. This group of enzymes is largely located in the liver, but also in the kidneys, lungs, brain, small intestine and placenta. The CYP system is responsible for the metabolism of almost all clinically useful medications, most importantly the antiretroviral agents (PIs and NNRTIs), several drugs used in the management of opportunistic infections in advancing HIV disease, many of the newer serotonin-specific reuptake inhibitors (SSRIs) and other psychotropic agents, endogenous substances such as steroids and prostaglandins, environmental toxins, anti-malarials and dietary components.

The primary role of the CYP system is to make the drugs more water-soluble and less fat-soluble, so that biliary excretion of the drugs can take place. As a result, these enzymes can affect the amount of active drug in the body at any given time. Such changes can be positive, enhancing efficacy, or negative, worsening toxicity and adverse events.

12.8.3 **How to recognize significant interactions and adverse effects in children's palliative care**

Any child with seemingly exaggerated toxicities on usual doses of medications or manifesting treatment failure in the absence of factors such as resistance or poor adherence/compliance should be considered to be suffering from an unidentified drug–drug interaction until proven otherwise. In such cases, careful review of the child's medication profile is necessary. Fortunately, the majority of drug–drug interactions are minor in nature and do not require extensive changes to the child's drug regimen. However, the minority of drug interactions that can be clinically important can reduce the effectiveness of both HIV/AIDS treatment and palliative care treatment, and so need to be addressed.

12.8.4 **Common effects of children's palliative care drugs on ARTs**

Certain drugs commonly used in children's palliative care can induce or inhibit the CYP system.

- ♦ Those that induce CYP can reduce the amount of available ARTs in the system, thereby making treatment failure more likely.
- ♦ Those that inhibit CYP can increase the amount of available ARTs in the system, thereby making ART toxicity more likely.

> Unless you are a specialist in HIV/AIDS, if you wish to use CYP inducers or inhibitors in children who are on ARTs, you should liaise with your local ART providers to discuss whether ART doses need to be altered.

12.8.4.1 Known CYP inducers

- Carbamazepine (Tegretol®)
- Rifampicin (Rifadin®)
- Phenobarbital
- Phenytoin
- Prednisolone
- Cigarette smoke
- Omeprazole
- Isoniazid.

12.8.4.2 Known CYP inhibitors

- Ketoconazole
- Itraconazole
- Erythromycin
- Fluoxetine
- Diltiazem
- Verapamil
- Clarithromycin
- Omeprazole
- Ciprofloxacin
- Fluconazole
- Metronidazole
- Co-trimoxazole (Septrin®)
- Haloperidol
- Cimetidine.

12.8.5 Common effects of ARTs on children's palliative care drugs

Some PIs and NRTIs can induce or inhibit the CYP, thereby increasing or reducing the effects of certain drugs commonly used in children's palliative care. Different PIs and NRTIs have different effects on the CYP system – some are more powerful inducers or inhibitors than others. The most potent inhibitor is ritonavir.

Where the child is taking CYP inducers or inhibitors, you may find you need to use different starting and continuation doses than would otherwise be the case. As a general rule, drugs that inhibit the CYP system cause the most dangerous interactions as they increase the level of toxic drugs thereby making dangerous toxic effects more likely.

Some of these interactions are potentially very harmful. These are outlined below.

12.8.5.1 Highest risk drugs when used with CYP inhibitors

- Tricyclic antidepressants (e.g. amitriptyline): risk of prolonged QT interval and sudden cardiac deaths.
- Macrolides (e.g. erythromycin): risk of prolonged QT interval and sudden cardiac deaths.
- Newer antihistamines (e.g. loratadine): risk of prolonged QT interval and sudden cardiac deaths.
- Cisapride: risk of prolonged QT interval and sudden infant death syndrome.
- Quinine and chloroquine: risk of prolonged QT interval and sudden cardiac deaths.
- Chloral hydrate: risk of prolonged sedation and respiratory depression.
- Benzodiazepines: risk of prolonged sedation and respiratory depression.
- Methadone: risk of prolonged sedation and respiratory depression
- Rifabutin (Mycobutin®): Ritonavir increases the risk of rifabutin-induced hematological toxicity by decreasing its metabolism.
- Co-trimoxazole (Septrin®): risk of increase in allergic reactions, especially rash.
- Beta blockers: risk of significant falls in blood pressure and heart rate.
- Haloperidol: risk of increased dystonic side effects and drowsiness.

Box 12.2 Case scenario – Samuel

Samuel is a 12-year-old boy with HIV/AIDS who is on ART. You start him on the normal recommended dose of haloperidol as he has unexplained vomiting. He starts making grimacing movements and complaining of pain and stiffness in his muscles. What do you think has happened?

12.8.5.2 Tips for counselling children and families about potential cardiac interactions

While children are generally less prone to cardiotoxicity than adults, this is not always the case, particularly where there are co-morbid cardiac conditions. All children using these drug combinations should be counselled to:

- Immediately report tachycardia, lightheadedness, palpitations, vomiting or diarrhoea.
- Avoid use of street drugs, substances of abuse or excessive use of alcohol.

12.9 Ethics and communication

Fuller discussion of ethics can be found in Chapter 17. However, there are particular issues that apply in children's palliative care in children with HIV/AIDS. These arise partly because ARTs are so effective, even in children who are apparently moribund (the so-called 'Lazarus effect') and partly because ARTs can be quite toxic, burdensome and expensive.

1. Balancing risks versus harms at the end of life: For example, should a child with very advanced HIV neuropathy causing global neurological and functional loss be given ARTs, thereby potentially extending lifespan when the quality of life could be argued to be overly burdensome to the child?

2. Benefits versus harms of treatment: For example, deciding whether to treat severe side effects of ARTs with more drugs, such as anti-emetic therapy for protease inhibitor-induced nausea and vomiting or alternatively to stop/change ARTs.

3. Deciding when or whether to withdraw drugs such as PCP prophylaxis or ARTs when a child is clearly at the end of life.

4. The question of the justice of life sustaining treatments such as ARTs being limited either to children whose families can afford them or, where ARTs are available, on a rationing system.

5. The cost to society of widespread ART treatment in children versus the benefits to society.

12.9.1 Continuation versus discontinuation of ART

One issue that frequently arises involves the question as to whether or not to stop ARTs in a child who is either not responding or who is felt to be unlikely to respond to them. The issue is this:

ARTs can be life saving and also can relieve symptoms (even though this takes time) but there are situations where the child's prognosis is so poor that the burden to the child of starting or continuing ARTs is greater than the potential benefits. For example, a child with AIDS who also has advanced resistant lymphoma or severe encephalopathy is not likely to recover with (or despite) the ARTs, even if they can be tolerated. As ARTs have significant side effects, and can interact with some palliative medication; and as ARTs can add to the confusion of 'poly-pharmacy', it is reasonable to consider withholding or withdrawing them. On the other hand, in some cases, the child and family may have such a strong emotional investment in continuing ARTs that withholding or withdrawing may prove very difficult.

The key to all this is 'informed consent'. The child and family need to be given all the information about possible benefits and burdens of treatment, in a way that they can understand. There are two problems with this. Firstly, without a 'futuroscope' it is very difficult to assess the outlook of the child in trying to come to a reasonable recommendation for the child and family (further discussion of prognostication can be found in Chapter 18 – Caring for children at the end of life). Secondly, the issues involved are complex and technical, and so getting the information across to the child and family in a way they can understand is a skilled counselling task that may require considerable time.

We have tried to deal with the issue of communicating difficult topics in Chapter 2 – Communicating with children and their families. Prognostication requires a very good understanding of both the evidence and the specifics of the individual child (his or her nature, history, investigations, previous management and so on). Even then, prognostication is little more than educated guesswork, but the guess is often crucial to a decision which literally has life and death consequences. To help you, here are some indicators of a poor prognosis in HIV/AIDS[15]:

Laboratory markers:

◆ CD4 + T-lymphocyte count < 25 cells/mm³

◆ Cd4 < 15%

◆ serum albumin < 2.5 gm/dl.

Clinical conditions:

◆ CNS lymphoma

◆ PML

◆ cryptosporidiosis

◆ severe wasting

◆ visceral Kaposi's sarcoma

- advanced AIDS dementia (more in adults)
- toxoplasmosis
- severe cardiomyopathy
- chronic severe diarrhoea
- life-threatening malignancies
- advanced end-organ failure (e.g. liver failure, congestive heart failure, COPD, renal failure, chronic lung disease).

Note: All of these factors may potentially be over-ridden in the setting of effective antiretroviral therapy

Ultimately, it is almost certain that you will be called upon by a child's family to give your opinion as to the child's likely prognosis, because it is very stressful and exhausting not to know when death is going to occur. This stress and exhaustion can be complicated by guilt and anxiety triggered by wishing that everything could be all over with. In the author's experience, as long as you explain that you cannot be certain, it is usually possible to talk in terms of hours, days, weeks or months, but not more specifically than that.

12.10 **Prescribing for opportunistic infections in children with HIV/AIDS**

12.10.1 **Chest infections**

Bacterial pneumonia (non-severe)	- Follow national or IMCI guidelines If no guidelines - Oral amoxicillin or penicillin see Formulary, Chapter 20 - Or co-trimoxazole see Formulary, Chapter 20 - Plus paracetamol or ibuprofen. See Formulary, Chapter 20 - If recurrent (>3x/y) investigate for TB, foreign body or chronic lung disease.
Severe pneumonia	Admit if possible. Supportive care - Supplemental oxygen - Correct severe anaemia (Hb <5 g/dL) by transfusion - Oral or IV hydration - Monitor fluid input/output - Analgesic/antipyretic - Vitamin A supplementation Specific therapy - Unknown organism: Amoxicillin 3rd-generation cephalosporin (e.g. ceftriaxone) or ampicillin *plus* cloxacillin *plus* gentamicin. See Formulary, Chapter 20 - If <1 year: consider PCP (see below) - If staphylococcal skin lesions or bullae on CXR or postmeasles, or with poor response to 1st line add cloxacillin or vancomycin - If repeated pneumonia, poor response, bronchiectasis or chronic lung disease; suspect gram negatives and add gentamicin or ceftazidime

Pneumocystis pneumonia:	*Pneumocystis carinii* pneumonia (PCP) (Also know as *Pneumocystis jiroveci*): If PCP is suspected, continue to treat for bacterial pneumonia, but also treat for PCP:
Major cause of severe pneumonia (15–30%) and death (30–50%) in HIV-infected infants, peaking at 3–6 months of age	Supportive management ◆ See section on cough and dyspnoea ◆ Hydration ◆ Vitamin A supplementation ◆ Correct severe anaemia by transfusion ◆ Oxygen ◆ Prednisolone. See Formulary, Chapter 20 Specific care ◆ High-dose co-trimoxazole ◆ or sulfamethoxazole. See Formulary, Chapter 20
TB	NB Treatment for TB should be started 2 months (2 weeks to one month) prior to starting ART to avoid the immune reactivation syndrome ◆ Treat as recommended by national guidelines. ◆ Take care with possible interactions between antiretroviral, antifungal and antituberculous drugs
Lymphocytic interstitial pneumonitis	◆ Oxygen ◆ Steroid, e.g. prednisolone. See Formulary, Chapter 20 ◆ Bronchodilators (e.g. nebulized salbutamol). See Formulary, Chapter 20 ◆ Start ART if available ◆ Physiotherapy ◆ Treat associated cor pulmonale with diuretics (e.g. furosemide) and potassium supplementation

12.10.2 Skin infections

Scabies	Children <1yr ◆ 25% benzyl benzoate for 12 hours or lindane (gamma benzene hexachloride) ◆ 2.5% sulphur ointment ◆ Screen and treat other household contacts where appropriate ◆ Wash and iron bedding and clothing or hang it out in the sun
Ringworm	◆ Whitfield's ointment (benzoic acid with salicylic acid) ◆ 2% miconazole cream ◆ For scalp lesions give oral ketoconazole if available. If not use griseofulvin, but beware of side effects. See Formulary, Chapter 20
Herpes zoster	◆ Analgesia (e.g. paracetamol or ibuprofen and add adjuvant, e.g. carbamazepine or amitriptyline if necessary) ◆ IV aciclovir. See Formulary, Chapter 20 ◆ Prevention in exposed child: varicella-zoster immune globulin within 48–96 hours of exposure. See Formulary, Chapter 20
Impetigo treatment	◆ Hygiene ◆ 10% iodine solution 3x daily or zinc oxide cream ◆ If pyrexial or resistant: cloxacillin or flucloxacillin or erythromycin for 7–10 days

(continued)

Chickenpox	◆ Topical calamine lotion
	◆ If available all HIV-infected children should receive aciclovir. Where supplies are limited, it should be used for disseminated chicken pox with complications
Herpes simplex	◆ Local antiseptic (e.g. gentian violet)
	◆ Analgesia: paracetamol or ibuprofen and add adjuvant e.g. amitriptyline if necessary
	◆ If disseminated: aciclovir. See Formulary, Chapter 20

12.10.3 Mouth infections

Oral candidiasis	◆ Nystatin drops 5 ml qds
(present in 75% of patients)	◆ Nystatin lozenges qds
	◆ Fluconazole
	◆ Amphotericin. See Formulary, Chapter 20
Recurrent herpes simplex	◆ Aciclovir

12.10.4 CNS infections

Bacterial meningitis	◆ 1st line: chloramphenicol or 3rd-generation cephalosporin (e.g. ceftriaxone). See Formulary, Chapter 20
Cryptococcal meningitis	◆ Treat pain using WHO ladder
	◆ Amphotericin followed by fluconazole. Fluconazole requires an induction dose especially in children. See Formulary, Chapter 20
	◆ Maintain prophylaxis with fluconazole unless the child is on ART and with sustained immune recovery[16].
Tuberculous meningitis:	◆ 12 months of rifampicin and isoniazid plus pyrazinamide and a fourth drug (ethambutol, ethionamide or streptomycin) for the first 2 months[17]
	◆ Corticosteroids as adjunctive therapy in more serious cases
CMV infection:	◆ IV ganciclovir.
	◆ Foscarnet may be used when there is sight threatening CMV retinitis.
Cryptococcus	◆ Induction with amphotericin followed by fluconazole
Toxoplasmosis	◆ Pyrimethamine plus sulfadiazine and folinic acid. See Formulary, Chapter 20
	◆ Treat until 1–2 weeks beyond resolution of signs and symptoms.

12.11 Questions for you

- ◆ Think of the last few children you have seen with HIV/AIDS. What symptoms were they suffering from (either as a result of the condition or as a result of the treatment)? What would you do differently having read this chapter?
- ◆ What psychosocial problems did these children face?
- ◆ Have you ever been part of a decision as to whether or not to stop ARTs? What were the two sides to the decision? What did you decide and why?

Notes

1 Tindyebwa, D., Kayita, J., Musoke, P., et al. (Eds.). *African Network for Care of Children Affected by HIV/AIDS (ANECCA) Handbook on Paediatric AIDS in Africa.* (Revised Edition 2006). Available online at www.Anecca.Org.

2 Gwyther, L., Merriman, A., Mpanga Sebuyira L. & Schietinger H. (Eds.) (2006). *A Clinical Guide to Supportive and Palliative Care for HIV/AIDS in Sub-Saharan Africa.* Foundation for Hospices in Sub-Saharan Africa. Available online at http:// www.Fhssa.Org.

3 WHO World Health Report. (2003). Shaping the Future. WHO, Geneva. Available online at www.Who.Int/Whr/2003/Chapter1/En/Index2.Html. Department For International Development (DFID).

4 Department For International Development (DFID). Available online at www.Dfid.Gov.Uk/Mdg/Childmortalityfactsheet.

5 WHO: *Antiretroviral therapy of HIV infection in infants and children: towards universal access.* WHO Guidelines 2006. Available online at http://www.who.int/hiv/pub/guidelines/art/en/index.html

6 Strafford, M., Cahill, C., Schwartz, T., et al. (1991). Recognition and treatment of pain in pediatric children with AIDS. *Journal of Pain and Symptom Management, 6,* 146.

7 Reprinted With Permission From Hewitt D, Mcdonald M, Portenoy R, et al. (1997). Pain syndromes and etiologies in ambulatory AIDS children. *Pain, 70,* 117–23.

8 The Multicenter AIDS Cohort Study (MACS) is an ongoing prospective study of the natural and treated histories of HIV-1 infection in homosexual and bisexual men conducted since 1984 by sites located in Baltimore, Chicago, Pittsburgh and Los Angeles. Data from the MACS have been the basis of more than 780 publications in peer reviewed journals. Available online at http://www.statepi.jhsph.edu/macs/history.html.

9 Larue, F., Brasseur, L., Musseault, P., et al. (1994). Pain and symptoms in HIV disease: A national survey in France. Third congress of The European Association For Palliative Care [Abstract]. *Journal of Palliative Care, 10,* 95.

10 Foley, F. (1994). 'AIDS Palliative Care'. Abstract: 10th International Congress on the care of the terminally ill. *Journal of Palliative Care, 10,* 132.

11 Moss V. (1990). Palliative care in advanced HIV disease: Presentation, problems, and palliation. *AIDS, 4*(S), S235–42.

12 Fontaine, A., Larue, F. & Lassauniere, J.M. (1999). Physicians recognition of the symptoms experienced by HIV children: How reliable? *Journal of Pain and Symptom Management, 18,* 263–70.

13 Breitbart, W., Mcdonald, M.V., Rosenfeld, B., Monkman, N.D. & Passik, S. (1998). Fatigue in ambulatory AIDS children. *Journal of Pain and Symptom Management, 15,* 159–67.

14 Mathews, W., Mccutcheon, J.A., Asch, S., et al. (2000). National estimates of HIV-related symptom prevalence from the HIV cost and services utilization study. *Medical Care, 38,* 762.

15 Republic of South Africa Department of Health (2001) Conditions Suggestive of Less than Six Months Prognosis in Children with AIDS. *Recommendations for Managing HIV Infection in Children.*

16 Gwyther, L., Merriman, A., Mpanga Sebuyira L. & Schietinger H. (Eds.) (2006). Management of clinical conditions in children. *A Clinical Guide to Supportive and Palliative Care for HIV/AIDS in Sub-Saharan Africa.* Foundation for Hospices in Sub-Saharan Africa. Available online at http:// www.Fhssa.Org.

17 Gwyther, L., Merriman, A., Mpanga Sebuyira L. & Schietinger H. (Eds.) (2006). Management of clinical conditions in children. *A Clinical Guide to Supportive and Palliative Care for HIV/AIDS in Sub-Saharan Africa.* Foundation for Hospices in Sub-Saharan Africa. Available online at http:// www.Fhssa.Org.

Section 3

Holistic care

We decided to put the symptom control chapters before the other chapters as our research suggests that these areas are what health workers think they need to know about children's palliative care.

However, our research also shows that in practise, health workers run into difficulty with interpersonal and intrapersonal skills far more often than they do with technical symptom control skills. Such skills include communication, assessment, awareness of culture and spirituality, self-awareness and ethical issues.

In many ways, this section is probably more important than Section 2. You can think of the symptom control section as a worm on the hook. You are here, so you must have been hooked. Now that you are here, please read on. We are pretty sure that the contents of the next section will get you out of more scrapes than anything you have read so far.

Chapter 13

Psychosocial and family care

Justin Amery, Nkosazana Ngidi, Caroline Rose, Collette Cunningham, Carla Horne and Linda Ganca

Key points

- Children are members of numerous social groups: families, clans, tribes, schools and communities.
- To understand the effects of life-limiting illnesses on children, you need to understand the interplay of all of these.
- In early childhood, a child has little concept of himself or herself as separate from the mother or family.
- The story of childhood can be seen as a story of separation from family and integration into a wider society.
- Children and their families coping with life-threatening illnesses and the end-of-life have to withstand extreme pressure and stress.
- Children can express this psychological stress in different ways and can be helped to manage it in different ways.
- Families are systems and individual children are parts of those systems: you cannot manage one without the other.
- Families are usually resilient and have unique (if idiosyncratic) systems for coping with stresses. Your job is less about finding solutions and more about helping them find the ones that are already there.
- In a similar way, communities have personalities, strengths and weaknesses: you need to understand yours if you are to help children and families find the support they need.

13.1 Introduction

This is a large subject area with the potential to include a very wide range of issues. In practise each child and family are likely to present very different challenges and viewpoints particularly in regard to psychosocial and family care. This chapter will attempt to present an overview of these issues and to explore in detail further those that are particularly pertinent to children's palliative care in Africa.

'Psychosocial' means the dynamic relationship between the social and psychological experiences where the effects of one continually influence the other[1]. The health status of children is interconnected with their social status and can have psychological consequences. For example, a child who is orphaned, HIV positive and living with relatives may or may not be treated well by the extended family; this can influence both the health of the child but more importantly their psychological status (see the case study below).

Box 13.1 Case study – Philip

Philip is a 6-year-old boy who is very sick from HIV/AIDS, which he contracted from his mother during pregnancy. She died and Philip has moved to live with his aunt. He has no known father. His aunt (a peasant farmer) has five other children. She is uneducated and knows little about HIV/AIDS.

Philip is seen in an HIV treatment centre after his uncle eventually brings him. He is very withdrawn, uncommunicative and tearful. After assessment he is started on ARTs and improves physically, but remains withdrawn. Eventually, he is seen by a counselor, who builds trust and confidence by playing with him over a few sessions. Eventually, while playing a game with some household implements, he confides in the counselor that he is kept apart from everyone at home; has his own spoon and bowl; and is not allowed to eat, wash or play with the other children. He sleeps in a small hut outside the main house. The counselor visits the aunt at home and counsels her on HIV. With support, Philip is allowed to join the rest of the family, sleeping, eating and playing with the others. He starts at school. He becomes much happier and more open. He also begins to start taking responsibility for his own ARTs.

The important thing to realize is that a child is a member of a number of social groups: the family (immediate and extended), the school, the local community, the clan and tribe and the wider community. These can be illustrated quite nicely as a series of concentric circles (see Box 13.2) with the child in the middle, then the family, then the local community and then the wider community.

One circle merges into the next; so there is no clear point at which one ends and the next begins. In other words, the child is at the centre of a highly complex and interactive *system*, which reacts and responds to the pressures and stresses of life-limiting illnesses.

The aim of this chapter is to describe how these various rings interact. We will start with the outer ring that of the community, before moving inwards to describe the family and then the child himself.

13.2 **Community aspects**

A community may be defined as a social group of people sharing a common environment that has similar intent, belief, resources, preferences and needs, which affects the identity of individuals living within. Learning about the community in which the child lives and the role that the family plays in that community can help us to assess the type of support the family may or may not need. 'Community' is likely to mean different things to different families. For example, to some it may mean their community or groups in their area, to others their church, mosque or school. For the purposes of this chapter, local community is defined in reference to the social environment of the child, wherever that may be (church, school, home, village, institution and refugee camp).

The local community may be able to help the child and family with their many needs, whether emotional, financial, childcare, transport or spiritual. Practical examples include a Pastor being able to drive a child to hospital, a local charity providing material resources such as a radio or books for a bed-bound child or a community volunteer spending time with a child in hospital so that the mother can have a break and attend to other issues. Families who are not well integrated

Box 13.2 Community circles of support

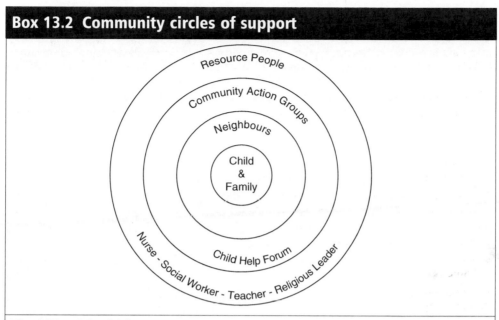

The child and the child's immediate family are at the centre of the concentric rings. Each child is depicted as being at the centre of his or her own family. Surrounding the child and family are the neighbours who are in turn surrounded by their community. Finally, all communities form part of a larger social system that incorporates government and civil structures. The people involved in each concentric 'ring' can provide some form of assistance to the child and the child's family that culminate in 'Circles of Care'.

in their community are likely to need more input of practical and emotional support from the palliative care team.

13.2.1 Community assessment

Whenever a child is assessed, it is important to assess the community resources (see Chapter 4). For example, it is important to assess whether the child can go to school easily and if not to try and find an alternative solution. Similarly, one should assess if the child and family are reachable by phone either through a contact in the community or directly with the family.

A community assessment will also reveal how much support can be given by community groups working in the area. It is important not to presume that a family who appear to have a lot of support or a prominent position in the community will not need the help of the palliative care team. For example, a prominent local leader, who has always been the person in the community to whom people come for advice and support, may find it very difficult being the one in need of help.

If you plan to refer to a community group, ensure that you provide clear and written details of the case and instructions for ongoing care, with details of how you can be contacted should the need arise. Continuity of care for the child and family is crucial, and poor communication between professionals and carers is a common cause of failure of continuity. Considering all these issues will result in the development of a satisfactory 'care plan' that meets all the needs of the child and their family.

13.2.2 **Housing**

For obvious reasons it is important for the palliative care team to know and understand about the child's living conditions. Again, assessment is important and a carefully developed care plan for the child should reveal all issues pertaining to the child's living environment. For example, if a child lives under unsanitary conditions with poor water availability, this will adversely influence his/her health. Similarly, if the area is malaria endemic and the child does not have a mosquito net, this is a potential risk to the child, given that children with HIV, cancer and other illnesses are susceptible to malaria.

The role of the palliative care team is not to fix everything. However, much can be done to improve the quality of life of the child and family by making small and affordable changes. There is no right and wrong way for a child or family to be living; what is important is that the child is comfortable. In meeting the basic needs of the child and the family, linkages with others outside the palliative care team are important; these can be linkages with local government structures, community programmes, local NGO programmes, local faith-based organizations and others.

13.2.3 **Transport**

In Africa, we have observed that one of the biggest reasons for a child not accessing health care or adhering to management plans is the expense or the lack of availability of transport. Early assessment of the family's access to transport means that interventions and planning can take place to meet this need and ensure compliance with any prescribed treatment. The role of the palliative care team is to evaluate possible interventions to resolve the problem and this will include assessing available community resources. In addition, assessment needs to look at the possibility of a more accessible local health facility for the family.

Where appropriate and available, Home Based Care (HBC) programmes can be utilized for follow-up care in the community, thus reducing the number of times the child and family have to travel to the health facility. They can also help to arrange for shared lifts or seeing if there is anyone in the community who is able to bring them to the hospital. Many HBC programmes also have their own available transport that allows for transferring clients to hospital and other facilities.

If and when a child is at the latter stages of their illness, the palliative care team will assist the family in deciding the best place for the child to be nursed. Often, children and families prefer to be at home in the final stages of illness. It is also important to note that the cost of transporting a dead body can be prohibitively expensive for families so do not delay in getting a child home if that is their wish.

Sometimes the family chooses the hospital, hospice or other health facility. In these cases, transport will be required and appropriate plans will need to be made for the transfer of the child. However, it is important for the palliative care team to reassure the family that the child can be nursed in their home environment.

13.2.4 **Finance**

Having a sick child can be extremely expensive for any family. Costs may include hospital stays, transport, medication, special food and investigations. Lack of money can be a major distress for many families, particularly if it means that the child is going without medications or food. Assessment of a family's financial situation can highlight areas where the palliative care team or others may be able to help. All efforts should be made to ensure that prescribed medication is only essential and cost-effective. Above all, families should be given support to plan for costs ahead, to seek alternative sources of income and to look to family, friends or organizations that may be able to help them. It is also important to keep in mind that a child's illness may require the main breadwinner to be away from work and therefore this negatively impacts on their financial income.

13.2.5 Education

In children the continuation of normality and normal routines, despite illness, is extremely important. Many of the children we look after speak of missing school, friends and classmates as one of their biggest distresses. Children should be encouraged to attend school for as long as they are able to. This may mean attending on a part-time basis or attending with an adult carer.

For the school-going child, teachers should be included in the care of the child as part of the multidisciplinary palliative care team and to ensure the holistic needs of the child are being met. In an ideal situation someone from the palliative care team should visit the school (with permission of the child and family) to talk to the teachers and children about the child's illness.

Teachers can organize age appropriate education to children either on a one-to-one bedside basis or in a communal space, put aside in the hospital or hospice for teaching. Community volunteers, with appropriate experience and training, can also work with the team to ensure teaching input for the children.

For some children it may not be possible to attend school because they are too sick or because they are spending long periods of time in a hospital or other health care facility. For these children steps should be taken to attempt to maintain links between them and their school (and friends) and to continue their education to as great an extent as possible. Parents can go to school to collect work from the child's teacher, children can write to their school friends and where possible the child can be visited at home or in hospital, by their teacher and classmates. Teachers can encourage classmates to reply to the sick child so that they feel they are still part of their class. This can have the added benefit of enabling classmates and other children to learn to talk openly about death and dying, and hence erode some of the cultural taboos which often impede good children's palliative care.

13.2.6 Sources of support in the community

Most African countries do not have statutory social security programmes to protect and care for the underprivileged. If they do, these programmes are often not functioning fully and are rarely easily accessible to vulnerable children. However, most communities have developed some support systems, formal and informal, and an important role of the children's palliative care health worker is to become aware of circles of support within the local community, so as to be able to access them easily when needed for a particular child or family. These might include individual people (friends, neighbours and professionals); community groups (such as churches and other CBOs); and government/statutory agencies (like social welfare organizations, children's homes, etc).

Question: Do you have a written or computer database of local people, groups or organizations you can turn to find support for your patients? If not, should you have one?

13.3 **Family aspects**

13.3.1 **Basic family theory**

In early childhood, a child has little concept of him or herself as being separate from the mother or immediate family. The story of childhood is, in many ways, a story of increasing understanding of – and movement towards – oneself as an individual separate from parents and family. However, full independence (if it comes at all) does not come until well into adulthood.

Therefore, it is essential that all health workers realize that you cannot assess a child without assessing his or her place and role within the family. Family psychologists refer to the family as a 'system' rather than as a group of individuals. Like a child's mobile hanging from the ceiling, or like a set of wind-chimes, when you move one part, the others all move too. Each member of the system is thereby affected by what happens to any other member of the system.

Another way you can think of a family is as a large budding amoeba or as a tree with fruit. Each bud/fruit is a child: some are fully attached and some are nearly separated. However, in no sense can you say that the child is fully independent of the whole.

When you realize that families are systems, and that individual children are parts of those systems, it becomes clear that:

+ caring for children means caring for the whole family (and vice versa)
+ problems with the child are problems with the family (and vice versa)
+ solutions for the child have to be solutions for the whole family (and vice versa).

13.3.1.1 **Types of families**

In traditional western approaches, families are described as nuclear, single-parent, extended and reconstituted. The nuclear family comprises a mother, father and children. In single-parent families there is either a mother only or a father only. An extended family refers to nuclear families which share daily lifestyles closely with other blood relations, and these can be grandparents, uncles, aunts and cousins. Reconstituted families are those where one or both of the marital couple have been previously married and have children from their previous marriages.

Health care professionals practising within an African context should be aware that some families do not all fit so neatly in the categories above. According to Fine[2], boundaries between family units in South Africa are often indistinct, in that sometimes it is not clear who belongs to whom. For an example, a person when asked who his or her mother is can identify any one of a number of aunts or his or her grandmother. If the person grew up in a small rural village he or she may identify all adult women who had played a 'mother role' in his or her upbringing.

Families that the children's palliative care team works with may vary in many ways, one being that they come from different demographic backgrounds, ranging from urban and peri-urban areas to traditional rural areas. Knowledge of who constitutes the child's family and who the child calls is important.

Knowing what type of family a child comes from assists in future decision-making processes. Within the African traditional family setting for an example, the biological parents could be the main caregivers of the child yet not be the ones who make final critical decisions like whether to go ahead or not with procedures or treatments. This role could belong to a senior member of the family who may not even be staying with the family. Knowledge of the type of family a child comes from may be helpful for the team in anticipating emotions and feelings that may be projected along the trajectory of the illness.

In a reconstructed family, where one of the ill child's parent is divorced, and there is still tension between the divorced parents, the team could anticipate projection of feelings when dealing with those involved. Awareness of such issues helps to prepare the palliative care team members to be objective and not to take things personal.

13.3.1.2 Roles within a family

The onset of HIV and AIDS has resulted in a dramatic change in traditional family roles as we know them. Grandparents and children have assumed the role of primary caregivers for their grandparents and siblings, respectively. Declining economic conditions also have resulted in a shift in traditional gender roles where men go to work and women stay at home and look after children. Being aware of the different roles that family members play is vital as the team needs it to identify how this impacts on the care of the child.

Finding out family support systems ensures that the palliative care team works with individuals that the child or family have identified/selected. The child should always be included in the discussions, according to his/her developmental stage.

13.3.1.3 Family bonds and sub-groups

Families are held together by attachments and bonds which develop early in life amongst family members and these are maintained right through life. Depending on the family dynamics these can be strengthened or severed over a period of time resulting in the formation of subgroups within families. For example a child may develop closer bonds with maternal relatives rather than paternal relatives. These attachments or bonds tend to be more prevalent or more defined during a family crisis and these influence the decision-making process of family members.

The ongoing support that extended family members give to the ill child and their family is invaluable. It continues even after the death of the child. Health care professionals involved in children's palliative care should be sensitive to these support systems and bonds. The team can be a motivating factor in such situations by verbally acknowledging practical and emotional support provided by the extended family members, like visits and taking shifts to assist in giving feeds. As health care professionals embark on the journey of accompanying each child they care for and their family, it is imperative to consider the unique bonds and dynamics of each family. Such considerations may result in the formation of positive relationships and collaboration between families and health care teams, which will result in the improvement of the child's quality of life and provision of dignity in death.

13.3.1.4 Family trees or genograms

The first step in helping a family is to get to know them and this is facilitated by drawing a genogram. A genogram is a useful technique when working with families. It is a simple yet very useful tool that is used to take a three generational family history, record the patient's support system and promote discussion with individuals and their families. At a glance when looking at a genogram one is able to determine whether the child comes from an extended family, a nuclear family, a reconstituted family or a single parent family. The parent or guardian of the child can tell you of her previous losses and how depressed she was afterwards and she felt like killing herself; when drawing a genogram as a health care professional this gives you clues of how the mother might react in the event of the child dying.

The genogram may help to clarify areas of strength and vulnerability and such information helps to explain and or predict the family's current style of coping adaptation and creation of meaning of the child's illness. From a systems viewpoint, it is important for health care professionals from the time of diagnosis of the child's illness to know the family life cycle and the stage of development of each family member and not just the patient.

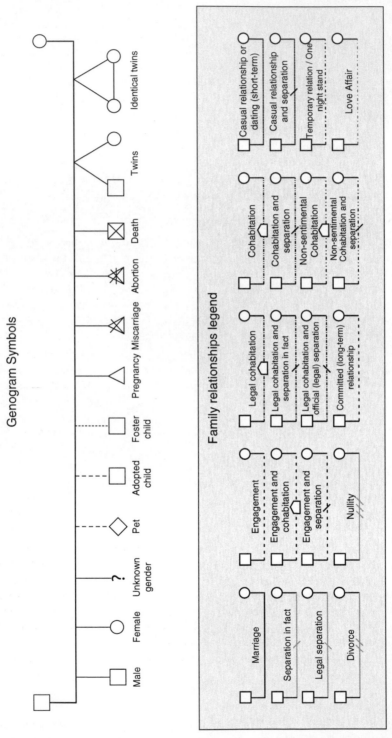

Fig. 13.1 Genogram symbols and relationships[3].

13.3.2 Family assessment

It follows therefore that assessment of a child must include a comprehensive assessment of the family. There are many ways to assess families, and it is beyond the bounds of this book to capture them all. However, one suggestion would be that, in the children's palliative care context, at least the following should be assessed[4].

Box 13.3 The main elements of a family

The main elements of a family assessment should include the following:

- Child and family's knowledge and reactions to the disease.
- Beliefs, attitudes and expectations regarding treatment and outcome.
- Coping ability during previous crises.
- History of depression and/or non-prescribed drug and alcohol use.
- Nature and stability of residential and occupational arrangements.
- Quality of relationships between family members and extended family members.
- Who is aware of the diagnosis and what was their reaction?
- Socioeconomic status of the family.
- Sociocultural factors or religious beliefs that might affect treatment decisions and adaptation.
- History of previous losses.
- Sources of emotional and financial support and availability of medical insurance.
- Health status of all family members.

13.3.2.1 The family conference

It is a good idea to arrange regular 'family conferences'. The aim of family conferences is to assist the family with identifying problems that they are facing. The following steps are a suggestion for how you might go about running the conference:

1. Allow the family to describe the problem the way they see it and how it is affecting them.
Listening is very crucial at this stage as it allows the family to tell their own story at their own pace without interference from the health care professional. Deep listening involves being fully present with the other without distraction and making comments whilst the client is still talking. Deep listening is not only about not asking questions but also about not making noises or exclamations which might be viewed by the client as judgemental and inhibit the communication process, making them to think that perhaps they are not supposed to say what they are saying. When appropriate make gentle open ended enquiries to reassure them about your interest. This type of listening is not aimed at making a therapeutic judgement as most practitioners are used to. By doing this, the health care practitioner gets a true picture of the family's problems and the simple act of telling a story and being listened to is in itself therapeutic.

2. Ask them what they have done in the past when they were faced with similar problems.
This helps you as a health care professional to identify their previous coping strategies, identifying those that you can maximize to help them deal with their current situation.

3. What was the outcome?
This is important for the health care professional and the family to focus on strategies that have yielded positive results and learn from those that didn't, analysing what it is that made others not yield the results that the family aspired to achieve.

4. Ask them if a miracle could happen what would they like to see happen.

Asking the 'miracle question' comes from the notion that when people are faced with problems already in their mind they have a picture of what they would like to see happen. It is therefore important for them to identify this for themselves rather than you as a health care professional advising them on what the ideal situation could be. When they are able to identify their own scenario it is therefore much easier for them to work through processes and co-create what they need to put in place to achieve the ideal situation.

5. What would they have to do to make this happen to make their current situation better?

This enables family members to tap into their own internal resources shifting the locus of control from external to internal.

6. Help them to identify strengths that they already have which could help them to achieve this.

The health care professional should encourage the family to identify their strengths also helping them to identify their previous strengths which they have used before and that they might have mentioned in step 2.

7. Ask them how they would implement this in their daily lives to help them cope now and in future.

The art of successful problem solving using the strengths perspective is the ability of each family member to take what they have learned and take it forward and apply it in their daily life. When dealing with a sick child families might be presented with different problems and challenges everyday but how they react to them depends on how they have reacted in the past to similar problems, what they learned from that and how they use the same coping skills to apply to other problems in their lives.

13.3.3 The problems families face[5]

In addition to feelings of sadness and loss, the fact that one of the children has a life-limiting illness places additional strains on families, such as guilt at failing to protect the child, recriminations within the family and removal of attention and affection for siblings of the sick child. The financial strains of caring for a seriously ill child can be very difficult, for example from travelling to hospital in the city, buying medications and so on. If the parent and/or child are away in hospital it can involve periods of separation from the rest of the family and difficulty in the home situation. This can compound financial problems if the breadwinner is away. Particularly with HIV/AIDS, parents and siblings may well already have had to cope with multiple losses. Stigma, especially if the illness is HIV/AIDS, is a big problem, as stigmas are negative emotions around the existence of the child's illness. It is common for parents in particular to feel anger, blame, guilt and regret around the illness in the family and about the loss of parental roles. Often, families have to cope with role reversals or role changes with children looking after sick adults or grandparents caring for orphans. Parents may be upset in their own grief and be unavailable to support each other or their other children. Siblings often have to 'step up' to take a caring role, often becoming the primary source of information and support for the sick child. Finally, after a child has died, any surviving children may serve as a painful reminder of the dead/dying child. Feelings of hostility may be displaced onto the surviving children, which can lead to further guilt.

13.3.4 Family support

The main role of the health worker is to try and help the family restore good communication. In most cases, families are naturally resilient and have systems and strategies for dealing with problems and threats. It is very common for health workers to come in with 'solutions' for families which do not fit the family's history, dynamics or systems – and therefore don't work! Most families can find their own solutions most of the time. Therefore, try to act as an intermediary in the family so that everyone understands each other's feelings and concerns, and allow them to find their own way forward.

Specifically, this usually means giving everyone in the family a chance to talk about their feelings, and listening with understanding and trying to help with issues confronting them.

Some questions that might help get you started include:

♦ What do you think X already knows about his/her illness or about what might happen to him/her?

♦ What kinds of questions has X been asking you and how did you answer?

♦ What have you told X about his/her illness or treatment?

When you meet parents for the first time to discuss concerns about their child, it can be very difficult to get started. It is easy to start 'lecturing', particularly if you are feeling nervous. A better way to begin is to get them to start talking while you listen. As they talk (and as you are seen to be listening) they will relax and trust you more.

Remember they are probably feeling overwhelmed and dealing with their own stress and depression. There may be times when you have to challenge parents, but (particularly until you have built up trust) it is usually better to act as an adviser and supporter, walking alongside the family through their difficult times. Try to avoid giving concrete advice, but rather turn questions around: 'I'm not sure. What do *you* think?'

There are however, some practical things that you might be able to do to help. These include the following:

♦ Asking if it is possible to involve extended family members to help.

♦ Looking for sources of basic needs support: financial, food, bedding, etc.

♦ Helping the family identify community support groups that they may not have been aware of, e.g. church groups, NGOs or government agencies.

♦ Advise them about supporting remaining children.

Box 13.4 Role plays – supporting parents and families

Supporting parents and families[6]: Group work activity

Bring together a group of parents and carers of children under your programme. Divide participants into small groups and give each group a copy of one of the scenarios outlined below. Each group should present a short role-play (10 minutes) showing the carers' situations and ways of offering them support and relieving the stress. Ask the group to be creative, to think of how they and others can provide practical help as well as ideas which will permanently improve their situation and allow them to cope in your absence. Discuss the ideas that came out of the role-plays. Go on to discuss other difficult situations that are common for carers, and the ways that the carers can be supported and helped.

> **Box 13.4 Role plays – supporting parents and families** *(continued)*
>
> *Role-play scenario 1:*
> *Samukelisiwe is an elderly woman who is looking after her sick HIV-positive daughter and her daughter's 5 children. Samukelisiwe is poor and is finding it hard to feed the children who are aged 1 year to 7 years. None of the children go to school. Samukelisiwe's son-in-law died last year from AIDS. Samukelisiwe is not as physically strong as she was when she was younger and she is finding it difficult to care for her daughter, who needs help to walk and who has frequent diarrhoea.*
>
> *Role-play scenario 2:*
> *Tafara is a 15-year-old boy who is caring for his HIV-positive mother. His mother can still walk but is unable to cultivate their garden or do any heavy work. Tafara has had to stop going to school to look after his mother. He often has to wash his mother's soiled clothing because she is too weak to do it. They have little money for food and no money to buy any medicines.*

13.3.5 Working with siblings

Siblings also face emotional difficulties during the terminal phase of illness. Most attention is on the sick child and brothers/sisters may feel unloved. They also often have to set up to a caring, supportive role for both parents and sick child. The siblings may also have misconceptions about the nature of the illness or have fears about developing the same illness[7].

Not surprisingly, siblings will often face emotional difficulties during the terminal phase of illness. Siblings may face all of the psychological problems outlined in this chapter. They may become irritable, anxious, withdraw socially and underachieve academically.

Again, the best thing a health worker can do is to facilitate good communication in the family, and to allow the families to use their own systems and strategies for managing problems. If you have to offer any recommendations, they should be along the lines of:

- Treat the children equally, taking into account the special needs of the dying child.
- Spend periods of time alone with the siblings.
- Keep in contact with the siblings if you are in hospital with the sick child.
- Permit and encourage the siblings to continue living their lives as normally as possible.
- Provide the siblings with a clear concept of the child's illness.
- Be honest and truthful with the sibling, otherwise they may blame parents.

13.4 Psychological aspects

13.4.1 Definition

Psychological care deals with the mind of the individual child. It includes unique feelings, emotions, thoughts, attitudes and beliefs of the child and the family.

Children and their families coping with life-threatening illness and the end-of-life are exposed to a range of factors that may affect their psychological health. These include traumatic experiences of sickness, physical disability, loss of home, rejection, domestic violence, physical or sexual abuse and loss of loved ones. They have to adjust to a huge amount of change, which demands a certain amount of emotional maturity and strength. Some of the aforementioned events can be the most stressful faced in one's life and it is important to have support from others at this time.

When a child is receiving palliative care, the support comes from their family, friends, community and the palliative care team.

Psychological care of the child suffering from chronic illness can be divided into three main levels. These are psychological issues at the:

◆ Child level

◆ Family level

◆ Community level.[8]

13.4.2 Psychological issues at the child level

A child with a life-limiting illness faces severe psychological stress form a variety of sources. The role of the palliative care team is to identify, assess and manage these problems. These problems might include[9]:

◆ actual separation and separation anxiety

◆ fears and anxieties associated with their own illness

◆ fears and anxieties regarding their upcoming death

◆ disfigurement

◆ loss of physical and cognitive capacity

◆ bereavement after the death of other loved ones

◆ poor communication due to denial or misplaced attempts to protect each other

◆ displacement to other homes

◆ stigma and rejection due to underlying illness

◆ neglect: especially where one or both parents have died

◆ physical and sexual abuse

◆ having to care for other sick family members.

13.4.3 How children deal with stress

Children tend, however, to have very good built in stress management systems, but too much stress can seriously affect a child. The role of the health worker is usually no more than to ensure

---

Box 13.5 Coping with stress – Ama's story[10]

Ama's story: You can use this story as a way of helping children identify with and then talk about their own stresses:

Ama's mother has AIDS and her father has gone away. Ama is responsible for caring for four brothers and sisters and helping her mother. She hopes to go on to secondary school. It is the farming season. The children helped her to plant and now the weeds are growing fast. The food in the granary is almost finished and the price of food is increasing. The rains have brought malaria and her little sister has fever. It is the time for exams and paying fees. If she doesn't pay her fees, she will be thrown out of school. Ama wakes in the night and thinks about all her problems, her heart beats fast and she shakes. Sometimes she has nightmares that her mother is dead and they have no food or money and the children are hungry. She finds herself shouting at the little ones and slapping them. They are shocked. Why is their sister behaving like this? Ama is suffering from stress. She feels afraid because she cannot see how she can cope with all the family problems.

that these stress-management systems are not inhibited or blocked by the health professionals or the home environment.

Play is probably the most useful coping mechanism that children have (see Chapter 3 – Play and development). Talking, particularly with older children and adolescents, is also very helpful. Perhaps you can set up groups so that children with similar problems can chat or play together. Laughter is also a great therapy.

Remember, just like adults, different children are different. Some find comfort in company, others in peace and quietness. Some like talking and some like listening. Some like to dance others like to read. It doesn't matter what it is, as long as it is something they enjoy.

13.4.4 Relaxation for children

You can also help children manage their stress by teaching them how to relax. This technique, originally designed for adults, actually works remarkably well for children. Try it and see.

Box 13.6 Relaxation for children

Get the child or children sitting or lying down somewhere quiet and comfortable and give him or them the following instructions:

- Close your eyes and breathe slowly, focusing on the breath going in and out of your body.
- Make sure that you breathe out fully: don't force it, but just let all the air find its way out slowly and naturally.
- Now concentrate on your feet, relaxing it and letting it go heavy and floppy.
- Now do the same for your legs, bottom, tummy, chest, hands, arms, shoulders, neck, head, face, eyes and tongue.
- Feel how heavy your body is. Let it become heavier so it feels as if it is almost sinking.
- Try to bring to your mind something or someone beautiful, such as a flower or a candle or a piece of music or a favourite place or a special person.
- Try to empty your mind of everything else but the thing you are focusing on.
- Allow a gentle smile to break on your face.
- Gently open your eyes and slowly stretch.

13.4.5 Emotional reactions

Just like adults, when stress gets too much, children can get emotional. Commonly they cry, but they might also get angry, have tantrums, become frightened or withdraw. Emotional reactions can be alarming for the child, family and (of course) for health workers, who tend therefore to avoid them. However, remember that it is normal for children under such psychological stress to feel emotional from time to time, and being able to express emotions to a trusted person may well ease a great deal of the child's psychological pain.

Here are some tips to help you address and manage emotional reactions[11]:

- Try to create a safe, non-threatening space where feelings, fears and taboos can be discussed and explored openly.
- Allow plenty of time.

- Be aware of your own feelings and fears. This will give you confidence.
- Share your own feelings openly. This will encourage trust.
- Remember no feeling is 'wrong'.
- If strong emotions burst out, allow them to wash over you and they will gradually die away. As long as the child or other people (including you) are not in any danger, the best thing you can do is nothing. Just be there for them.
- Allow 'time-outs' if the child or family need to take a break.
- Try to use feelings constructively, such as by developing dramas, poems, role-plays and stories.

13.4.6 Stigma

Both cancer and AIDS are stigmatizing illnesses. People fear them and avoid them. This avoidance only serves to isolate the child and family even further. Even worse, both cancer and HIV/AIDS can be disfiguring or cause foul smells or difficult conditions such as incontinence of faeces and urine. All these things can cause pain and embarrassment to a child and further their social isolation, particularly if they are reacted to badly by peers or family members.

These all can have an effect on a child's body image leading to feelings of low self-esteem, depression and fear of intimacy. The effects of stigma can be far reaching for the child and lead to feelings of social isolation, low mood and anxiety. It can mean children are subjected to abuse and ill treatment, are unable to do the things they want (like playing with friends or going to school) and will impact on their quality of life both physically and emotionally.

The fear of being stigmatized creates barriers to open and honest disclosure of a child's illness. Some children may manage stigma by telling only a few chosen people about it, but the downside of this is that it creates an obstacle to honest and open communication with people in a child's life. Disclosure of illness requires the palliative care team to support the child and the family through the process by clearly helping them to understand the illness and its consequences. It is, however, important to ensure that the child is given some control over how the plans of when, how and to whom the nature of their illness is disclosed.

Children should be given opportunities to openly discuss these issues and their worries and anxieties, and attempts can be made to cover the disfigurements with bandages or scarves. With the children's permission sensitization of the family, peers and community about the nature of a child's illness can reduce difficult reactions which in turn can reduce the feelings of isolation and low self-esteem associated with disfigurement. Try to find out ways of introducing children to others with similar problems, so that they realize that they are not alone.

Stigma usually comes about through lack of understanding of illness, long-standing myths and fear. These can be tackled by careful education and sensitization, informal and formal counselling and open and honest discussion with the child, family and other significant people.

Box 13.7 Case scenario – Hamid

Hamid had a retinoblastoma which was treated by radiotherapy. The disease and treatment led to the loss of his left eye. Hamid felt disfigured and, as a result, became shy and withdrawn. A volunteer gave Hamid some smart sunglasses. Hamid is rarely seen without them and is back to his sunny and happy self. His retinoblastoma has not recurred.

13.4.7 **Abuse**

Sadly, sexual abuse and violence are very common and serious problems that transcend racial, economic, social and regional lines in SSA and in the world generally. Children are particularly likely to be victims, as they are physically weaker, less mature and usually dependent on their abusers. Abuse may take the form of emotional and physical neglect, physical violence, rape and sexual assault, sexual exploitation and/or female genital mutilation.

It is hard to get an accurate data about the prevalence of sexual abuse and violence in SSA as many people will not report it, and when people do find it is often not taken seriously and offenders not punished. However, here are a few statistics which serve to point out how common and serious it is in Africa:

- Worldwide, 40–47% of sexual assaults are perpetrated against girls of age 15 or younger[12].
- Surveys conducted in Africa reveal that 46% of Ugandan women, 60% of Tanzanian women, 42% of Kenyan women and 40% of Zambian women report regular physical abuse[13].
- In a Nigerian survey, 46% of women report being abused in the presence of their children[14].
- In Uganda, 49% of sexually active primary school girls say they had been forced to have sexual intercourse[15].
- In Kenya, 50% of adolescent girls interviewed admitted receiving gifts from older men ('sugar daddies') in exchange for sex[16].
- In Malawi, 55% of adolescent girls surveyed report that they were often forced to have sex[17].
- In Uganda, 31% of school girls and 15% of boys report having been sexually abused, mainly by teachers[18].

Studies have shown that children who witness violence may experience many of the same emotional and behavioural problems that physically abused children experience, such as depression, aggression, disobedience, nightmares, physical health complaints and poor school performance[19]. Given the high prevalence of abuse, it is likely that a significant proportion of the case loads of health workers in SSA are being abused. It is also likely that a large number of health workers are themselves victims of abuse. These are huge additional burdens for dying children to carry, and it is one health workers have a moral and ethical duty to prevent and report.

Box 13.8 Child protection – How prepared are you?

Try and answer the following questions:

- Do you know the approximate rate of child physical and sexual abuse in your country?
- Do you know who is responsible for investigating and managing allegations of child abuse in your community?
- Does your organization have a child protection policy?
- Have you ever had training in child protection?
- Do you know what to do if you suspect a case of child abuse?
- Do you know how to recognize the signs of emotional, physical and sexual abuse?
- Have you ever seen a case of child abuse in your work setting?

If the answer to any of these questions is no, and if you are working with children, perhaps you need to think if you should be doing more to protect children under your care. Speak to your bosses and set up a child protection policy and training in your work-place as a matter of urgency.

13.4.8 **Insomnia**

Insomnia may be a problem for children and their parents, particularly where anxiety is present. Non-pharmacological interventions such as gentle massage, guided imagery and relaxation exercises can be used in the first instance. Talking about the anxieties and fears causing the insomnia and developing coping strategies for these is also important. If drugs are required, diazepam can be used in older children and triclofos in younger ones (see Chapter 20 for doses). Ensuring that the child has an environment conducive to sleep, quiet, cool and comfort is also important.

13.4.9 **Depression**

Depression, low mood and anxiety can be seen in children's palliative care. Anxiety about the future, about separation from parents and about death and dying can be observed in children. Sadness about the loss of normal life, lengthy stays in hospital and depression relating to chronic pain are also factors that must be considered. There is no magic secret to treating such children and their families, what is required is care and compassion, honesty in answering questions and allaying fears and showing that you have time to talk. Some children might not want to talk to a doctor, nurse or social worker but prefer to confide in a priest, teacher or volunteer. (This is fine but it is essential that these people are, in turn, given the support they need to cope with this.) Pharmacological treatment for depression and anxiety in children is available but most anti-depressants (particularly selective serotonin reuptake inhibitors – SSRIs) are not usually recommended for children. However, where other interventions have failed, tricyclics such as amitriptyline can be trialled. Benzodiazepines can be used in extreme cases of anxiety.

In children non-pharmacological interventions can be extremely useful and effective. Formal or informal counselling is likely to benefit every child. Use of play, art and music therapy is also likely to be useful in these situations. A particularly anxious child may also benefit from breathing exercises, guided imagery, relaxing music and story telling.

Confusion and terminal agitation may be a problem for some children. Haloperidol has an important role in treating this problem.

Parents and family members may also require medical treatment for psychological conditions. Advice should be taken on this by colleagues with experience in this field.

13.4.10 **Counselling children**

Formal counselling of a child may become necessary if any of the suggestions above are not enough. In the average children's palliative care setting in SSA, it is unlikely that you will have enough time or training to manage this alone, so it is probably best to refer to local agencies if available. It is beyond the scope of this book to go into much detail and the reader is referred to other sources such as the CRS Guide[20].

However, if services are not available and/or you find yourself in the position of counselling a child, the following structure will help:

1. Find a quiet, child friendly place with toys, crayons and everyday objects that he or she can use in acting out or telling his/her story.

2. Assessing what the child already knows.

3. Assisting the child in deciding whether or not he/she would like to discuss the issues more fully.

4. Establish ground rules of safety, trust and confidentiality.

5. Help the child identify what he or she does to cope with stress (see above) and reinforce and encourage those as strengths.

6. Try and get the child to begin to tell you his/her story, either verbally or through play or stories. *Don't rush.*

7. Begin to draw up a list of the main problems and issues that might be underpinning their distress.

8. Start discussing these, offering plenty of encouragement and congratulations, for each try to help the child come up with coping strategies that work for him/her. Don't be too directive. Use the child's own inner resources and the resources of the family and community to build strategies.

9. Don't make empty promises.

10. Keep following up the child until he/she has worked through the issues.

11. If the child is at risk, take steps to involve the necessary agencies. Do not keep it to yourself.

13.4.11 Play therapy

Playing (see Chapter 3 for more details) is how children explore and make sense of their world. Play is also a safe way for children to act out concerns and fears. It is also a way that they learn to interact with others, share, socialize, feel part of a group and feel loved, appreciated and accepted. In other words, play is incredibly important for children (and probably for adults too!).

Play has been shown to help children[21]:

- make sense of the world
- think, plan and make choices
- with problem solving
- relax and build up strength
- find and give comfort
- deal with emotional issues
- develop imagination
- express feelings in a non-threatening way
- create an environment where stress, pain and anxiety are reduced
- regain confidence and self esteem
- understand treatment and illness
- learn the sensory and concrete information that they need to prepare for hospital procedures and treatment.

Play also aids health professionals in assessment and diagnosis and provides distraction from pain, painful procedures and the difficult environment of health-care settings.

Play does not have to be with expensive toys and playthings. Children love to play simple games (tag, football, ring-a-ring of roses). They like to sing, dance, play, make believe and sometimes just hold a cuddly toy such as a doll or teddy. Toys can be produced cheaply using local and waste materials (e.g. dried beans in a material bag, bead-making from paper, board games from pieces of cardboard). Paper, coloured pens and sand are also very useful for drawing materials as all children like to draw and it is an important medium for children to express their feelings (refer to Chapter 2 – Communication with children and their families). In our experience people are very keen to donate toys and books and this should be encouraged to ensure a sustainable play service. As with education, a play service within a palliative care team can be delivered extremely well by a team of appropriately trained volunteers.

Friends and siblings should be encouraged to visit and play with the child to ensure that the child remains part of their family and community. Throughout illness and if close to end-of-life it is recommended that families keep to their routines and maintain age appropriate disciplinary habits in order to preserve consistency and familiarity for the child and any siblings[22].

For all these reasons, learning to play with children is a key skill for anyone who works with children. Playing with children will help you help children. In addition, children's play helps health workers to begin to understand what type of emotions their patients experience, as their play involves imitation and acting of feeling.

Box 13.9 Play therapy in action in Uganda[23]

Four children aged 6, 8, 9 and 14, all HIV-positive, came to the clinic for medical checkups and were told to go for free play. They started acting out a situation in which someone had died in the home. One child acted as a child wailing because her mother was dying and crying out 'whom have you left me with' (ondekede ani) in Luganda. The older child among the group acted out trying to roll the body and telling others to be firm. When the Health Care Worker heard them shouting, she came close and watched what they were doing. When she asked them what they were doing, they explained and gave the reasons they were playing the game. Their play-acting helped the children cope with their own real situations and let the HCW know what they were dealing with at home.

Play therapy can include the following:

- Free play (see box above): Children don't need help to play. All you need is some space and may be a few materials such as paper, pencils, balls, sand and so on. Just let them go and watch. You will learn a lot!

- Music therapy: Music therapy is a rather grand word for allowing children to make noises joyfully. It can include singing or playing of instruments (home-made or otherwise). As well as being simple fun and a welcome distraction, music can enable children (and adults) to reflect on their lives.

- Narrative therapy: Narrative therapy is another grand word which simply means story-telling. Children love to tell and be told stories, particularly when their own stories (or stories like them) can be woven in. It can be very helpful in allowing children simply to express themselves in a non-threatening way, but also can enable children to 'rewrite' their own stories in a way which makes more sense or gives them comfort or control[24, 25].

- Drama: Drama or role-play is a very effective form of play therapy, especially for older children and teenagers. It encourages children to work together to tell their own stories, as individuals and as a group. It is a group activity, so has the added benefit of creating friendships and supportive relationships with others going through similar experiences. It can be particularly helpful for children who are neglected, or abused.

- Memory work[26]: (described in more detail in the chapter on bereavement) Creating memory boxes or books is a combination of play therapy, narrative therapy and art therapy. Apart from allowing children to express fears and concerns, it also assists with preparation for bereavement and planning for future care of children. They also give children a sense of their roots and of belonging.

13.5 **Questions for you**

1. Reflect on your own family:
   - What are the systems at play?
   - Who are the key decision-makers?
   - How do junior members of your family make their views and wishes known?
   - How does your family cope with extreme stress?
   - What emotional expression is permissible in your family?
   - What would you say are the strengths and weaknesses of the way your family deals with stress?

2. What things were you most terrified of as a child?
   - Looking back, can you think of why?
   - What gave you comfort when you were scared?

3. Do you know how to relax?
   - Try the relaxation technique suggested above on yourself.

4. Child abuse:
   - Do you know the approximate rate of child physical and sexual abuse in your country?
   - Do you know who is responsible for investigating and managing allegations of child abuse in your community?
   - Does your organization have a child protection policy?
   - Have you ever had training in child protection?
   - Do you know what to do if you suspect a case of child abuse?
   - Do you know how to recognize the signs of emotional, physical and sexual abuse?
   - Have you ever seen a case of child abuse in your work setting?

Notes

1   Tindyebwa, D., Kayita, J., Musoke, P., et al. (Eds). *African Network for Care of Children Affected by HIV/AIDS (ANECCA) Handbook on Paediatric AIDS in Africa.*(Revised Edition 2006). Available online at www.Anecca.Org.

2   Fine, D. (1995). *A Special Bond.* (p. 199). Ravan Press, Johannesburg.

3   Copied from Wikipedia article on Genograms at http://en.wikipedia.org/wiki/Genogram

4   Wiener, L. & Septimus, A. (1991). Psychosocial Consideration and Support for the Child and Family. In: Pizzo P.A. & Wilfert C.M. (Eds.) *Pediatic AIDS: The Challenges of HIV Infection in Infants and Children, and Adolescents.* Williams and Wilkins, Houston.

5   'Supporting Families' Module: Hospice Africa Uganda Distance Learning Diploma Course Notes, 2006

6   Liverpool Associates In Tropical Health (LATH), Nigeria, with support from DFID. (2003). *HIV/AIDS Care & Counselling: A Training Curriculum For Community Volunteers.* Email: Lath@Liv.Ac.Uk

7   V. Marston, J., Swartz, E. & Sephiri, K. (1990). *Identifying Children in Distress.* Research Undertaken For Save The Children, UK The St Nicholas Children's Hospice. Bloemfontein, South Africa.

8   Tindyebwa, D., Kayita, J., Musoke, P., et al. (Eds). Module 4: Psychosocial Aspects of Pediatric HIV Care. *African Network for Care of Children Affected by HIV/AIDS (ANECCA) Handbook on Paediatric AIDS in Africa.* (Revised Edition 2006).

9   Marston, J., Swartz, E. & Sephiri, K. (1990). *Identifying Children in Distress.* Research Undertaken for Save The Children, UK The St Nicholas Children's Hospice. Bloemfontein, South Africa.

10 Gordon, G. *Choices: A Guide for Young People*. MacMillan, Africa. Available online at www.Macmillan-Africa.Com.

11 Adapted From *'Understanding and Challenging Hivstigma:Toolkit For Action'*. ICRW.

12 Heise, L. (1993). Violence Against Women: The Missing Agenda. In M. Koblinsky, J. Timyan, J. Gay (Eds) *The Health of Women: A Global Perspective*. Westview Press, Boulder, CO.

13 Wood, K. & Jewkes, R. (1997). Violence, Rape, and Sexual Coercion: Everyday Love in a South African Township. *Gender and Development*. 5(2), 41–6.

14 Odunjinrin, O. (1993). Wife Battering in Nigeria. *International Journal of Gynaecology and Obstetrics*, 41, 159–64.

15 Noble J, Cover J. & Yanagishita M. (1996). *The World's Youth, 1996*. Population Reference Bureau, Washington, DC.

16 Wjau, W. & Radeny, S. (1995). *Sexuality Among Adolescents In Kenya*. Kenya Association For The Promotion Of Adolescent Health, Nairobi.

17 Njovana, E. & Watts, C. (1996). Gender Violence in Zimbabwe: A Need for Collaborative Action. *Reproductive Health Matters*, 7, 46–52.

18 Sebunya, C. (1996). Child Abusers Face Mob Justice: *Aids Analysis Africa*, 6(3), 15.

19 Heise, L.L., Pitanguy J., Germain, A. (1994). Violence Against Women: The Hidden Health Burden. World Bank Discussion Papers, No.255, World Bank, Washington, DC.

20 AIDS Relief and Catholic Relief Services: *Psychosocial Care & Counselling for HIV Infected Children and Adolescents: A Training Curriculum*. Catholic Relief Services 228 W. Lexington St. Baltimore, Maryland 21201-3413 | 888-277-7575 | info@crs.org. January 2008 (in press).

21 Provided by the Children's Rights Centre, Durban. Available at www.childrensrightscentre.co.za.

22 Bruce, P., Himelstein, M.D., Joanne, M., Hilden, M.D., Ann Morstad Boldt, M.S. & David Weissman, M.D. (2004). Pediatric Palliative Care. *New England Journal of Medicine*, 350(17), 1752–62.

23 Gwyther, Merriman, Mpanga Sebuyira & Schietinger (Eds). A Clinical Guide to Supportive and Palliative Care for HIV/AIDS in Sub-Saharan Africa. Part 5: Care of Children and Adolescents (Box 29.5).

24 Morgan, A. (1999). Once Upon a Time. . . . Narrative Therapy with Children and Their Families. Dulwich Centre Publications. Adelaide.

25 Soskolne, T. (2003). Moving Beyond the Margins: A Narrative Analysis of the Life Stories of Women Living with HIV/AIDS in Khayelitsha. CSSR Working Paper No. 33. March Centre for Social Science Research. University of Cape Town, Cape Town.

26 Denis (2003). In Gwyther, Merriman, Mpanga Sebuyira, Schietinger (Eds) A Clinical Guide to Supportive and Palliative Care for HIV/AIDS in Sub-Saharan Africa. Part 5: Care of Children and Adolescents. Foundation for Hospices in Sub-Saharan Africa. 2006. Available online at www.Fhssa.Org

Chapter 14

Pre-bereavement and bereavement

Justin Amery, Collette Cunningham,
Nkosazana Ngidi, Eunice Garanganga,
Carla Horne and Jenny Ssengooba

Key points

- There is more than one way to support children.
- Choose the things that you and the child feel most comfortable with.
- Accept that some things just can't be 'made better' in a short space of time.
- Talk to children using words they understand.
- When explaining something, ask questions to check that the child has understood you (and also to check you have understood them).
- Give information in bite-size chunks. Pieces of the 'jigsaw puzzle' can be put together over time to make the picture complete.
- Encourage children to ask questions and ensure that you keep answering them – even if it's for the 100th time.
- Answer questions honestly and simply.
- Try to find ways in which children can be involved.
- Keep talking about the person who has died/is dying.
- Be willing, if appropriate, to refer people to child bereavement services.

14.1 Introduction

In this chapter we will look at how we can help children and their families to deal with issues of loss and bereavement during illness, as death approaches, during death and after death. In children's palliative care children may be the ones that die and may also be the ones that are bereaved (as sons, daughters, siblings or other close relatives). They may also be both, particularly where the family is affected by HIV. In children's palliative care we also have to take into account the needs of parents, for whom the loss of a child is particularly traumatic, as well as for different adult family members.

However, this chapter will not deal specifically with adult bereavement alone but in the context of family. Adult bereavement information can be found in more detail elsewhere.

Instead, we will focus on children's bereavement, for those who are going to die (and have to deal with the impending loss of their own lives) and those who are left behind. Similarly, we will not differentiate between those children who are grieving at their own impending loss and those who are grieving for someone they have lost. In general terms, the principles and practise of managing both groups are similar.

14.1.1 Definitions

It is important to distinguish between grief and bereavement as people are often confused and see them as the same.

- **Bereavement** is a state of having lost someone or something dear to you.
- **Mourning** is our external expression of loss. It is a style of expressing loss. Families, communities and cultures may mourn differently. Rituals help to bring healing and closure.
- **Grief** is the emotional and social reaction to loss. In children, grief can come from the loss of parents, siblings, failure of exams, death of pets, etc.

14.1.2 Charter for bereaved children[1]

Winston's Wish, an excellent NGO working with bereaved children in the UK, has developed a 'Charter for Bereaved Children', summarized below. The principles work well in both resource-rich and resource-poor settings.

B   Bereavement support

E   Express feelings and thoughts

R   Remember the person who has died

E   Education, truthful answers and information

A   Appropriate and positive response from schools

V   Voice in important decisions

E   Everyone involved should be supported

M   Meeting other children with similar experiences

E   Established routines, including previously enjoyed activities and interests.

N   No blame: children should be helped to understand that they are not responsible

T   Tell their story and for those stories to be heard

14.2 Children and grief

Bereaved children usually experience 'deep pockets of sadness' when they have lost their parents or siblings, and when they know that they have an incurable sickness. They may not easily be able to share this sadness with family members or with their peers. Often this pain can remain inside, and as the child grows the sense of loss may remain with them and be felt differently. Adults generally underestimate the fact that a child may be affected by the loss. Yet children, like adults, experience pain and loss of their dear ones. Children who are not allowed to grieve normally are at higher risk of developing problems and complications at the time and later in life.

In the African palliative care setting, children may have to confront their own death or the death of a loved one at the same time as grieving for many other family members who have died as a result of the HIV epidemic, malaria or other causes.

14.2.1 How children grieve

Generally, children

- revisit their grief every time their developmental level gives them new insights into what happened

- grieve as part of a family: grieving for the person and environment they have lost, affecting those who remain, and in turn being affected by them[2]

- may have fluctuations in their grief between sudden sadness and equally suddenly appearing happy. This can be very confusing.

14.2.2 Myths and realities of child and adolescent grief

Table 14.1 Myths and realities of childhood grief from 'Pediatric Palliative Medicine' in the NEJM[3]

Topic	Myth	Realities
Do children and adolescents grieve?	Young children do not grieve	All children grieve
	Children do not grieve as much as adults	Children and adults express grief differently but just as intensely
	Children are lucky as they are too young to understand	Children are vulnerable in their growing
	Children should be protected from pain and suffering	Children cannot be protected in play, the media or life experiences
	Children can resolve grief quickly	Children's grief has no time limits
	Children and adolescents understand, experience and express grief identically	Children and adolescents are developmentally distinct
Should children and adolescents be exposed to a loved one who is dying?	Children will be bewildered by being with a loved one who is dying	Children need to understand and make sense of their experiences in order to help learn that dying and death are part of life
	Children will be traumatized by their last encounters with a dying person	Children value the opportunity to spend time with their loved one during that person's last days and weeks
	Happy memories will be overshadowed by watching their loved one die	Children can learn values through participating in the death of a loved one
	Children should be protected from seeing a loved one die	Children may later resent their exclusion: their involvement will assist in grieving
Should children take part in funerals and other death rituals?	Children should not be permitted to take part in such rituals	Children can benefit by helping plan and by attending funerals, including allowing them opportunities for questioning and learning from emotional responses of adults
	If they are allowed, participation should be limited and they should be protected from seeing strong emotional reactions	Children benefit from the support of others to overcome feelings of isolation

(continued)

Table 14.1 (continued) Myths and realities of childhood grief from 'Pediatric Palliative Medicine' in the NEJM[3]

Topic	Myth	Realities
	Adults know better whether or not to allow a child to participate in such rituals	Difficulties arise from forcing children to attend or excluding them from attending against their will
Are dying children and adolescents aware of their situation and how can they be helped?	Dying children <10y are not aware they are dying	Dying children know they are dying; adult denial is ineffective in the face of children's emotional perceptions
	Dying children do not experience anxiety because they are unaware they are dying	Dying children experience fear, loneliness and anxiety
	Dying children have no concerns for themselves or others	Dying children worry, may try to put their affairs in order, strive to protect their parents and fear being forgotten
	Dying children's questions should not be answered	Dying children need honest answers and unconditional love and support

Permission 10: reprinted with permission from the Massachusetts Medical Society.

14.2.3 Normal effects of grief in children

It is common for children to experience a regression[4] in their behaviour during their period of mourning. Young children may experience bed wetting, loss of appetite, tummy upsets, restlessness, disturbed sleep, nightmares, crying, attention seeking behaviour, difficulty in concentrating, increased anxiety and clinginess. These only become a cause for concern when they occur over a prolonged period of time. Older children often display changes in personality and alterations in their normal behaviour including signs of depression, anger and rage, sleep and appetite disturbances, angelic behaviour, rudeness, learning problems, lack of concentration and refusal to go to schools. School work may be affected by underachieving or overworking. They may do everything 'right', even to the extent of parenting their parents. Boys, particularly teenagers, are likely to experience difficulties at school in the early months following parental death, but bereaved children do not necessarily develop long-term learning problems.

In adolescents, bereavement can cause a regression to a younger, more dependent stage in their development. Emotions may be suppressed, resulting in a display of apparent indifference or lack of feelings. In a search for love and affection, they may change their behaviour and become vulnerable in sexual relationships. Some children exhibit exaggerated displays of power to counteract their fears, and this may take the form of super-hero manifestations or may look like what we would characterize as naughty behaviour, acting out, anger and/or belligerence. This can also be an antidote to fear, manifesting in an outward display of personal power: 'I am strong enough to control life with my force.'

The important message is that health workers should advice families to be on the lookout for changes in behaviour. For example, a child who was previously chatty and has become uncommunicative should generate more concern than one who has always been uncommunicative.

14.2.4 **Characteristics of grief in different age groups**

Table 14.2 Characteristics of grief in different age groups

Characteristics	What you can do to help
Infants	
◆ Sense something missing even if they cannot vocalize it ◆ Miss all aspects of the person: touch, feel of their body, sound of their voice, their expressions, their smell and activities experienced together ◆ Often suffer separation effects ◆ May regress, be more irritable, more clingy or more withdrawn	◆ Recognize children are strong and adaptable ◆ Create stability ◆ Hold when upset ◆ Try and gently engage if withdrawn (using interactive games such as peekaboo, water play, touch games, singing)
Young Children	
◆ Do not understand death is final ◆ May believe that dead people will return ◆ May not initially respond to hearing that someone has died ◆ Grieve at the absence and separation ◆ Are upset at moments when they feel the 'goneness' but not at other times. ◆ Miss all aspects of the person: touch, feel of their body, sound of their voice, their expressions, their smell and activities experienced together ◆ Often suffer separation effects ◆ May regress, be more irritable, more clingy or more withdrawn ◆ May use their bodies to speak their feelings: it is a physical experience	◆ Create stability ◆ Hold when upset ◆ Try and engage if withdrawn ◆ Allow and encourage active play and communication ◆ Feedback verbally what you are seeing to help them to verbalize how they feel (e.g. you are bouncing, you are shouting, your face is red because you are sad and cross that your mother is not coming back) ◆ Be ready for contradictory statements such as 'my father's dead' and 'I hope he'll be back before my birthday' or 'He's picking me up tonight' by explaining gently that he won't be coming back because dead people do not come back
Older children	
◆ May grasp the concept of death as final and irreversible ◆ May be curious about what happened to the person who died. ◆ May believe the person is still alive and functioning elsewhere ◆ May have trouble with abstract concepts such as afterlife ◆ May start to show aggressive tendencies, risky or impulsive behaviour	◆ Ensure that there is no misplaced guilt: e.g. 'You do know, don't you, that your Mother didn't die because of anything you did' ◆ Gently confront and correct magical thinking when it comes up ◆ Ensure that there is a clear and stable routine ◆ Ensure that you always have a clear plan for getting back together when you part 'I will be here at home waiting when you get back from school' ◆ Don't be upset if children become more clingy

(continued)

Table 14.2 (continued) Characteristics of grief in different age-groups

Characteristics	What you can do to help
◆ May have magical thinking (I was mean to Joseph so he died, he might come back if I am good) ◆ May start to express fears about their own future	◆ Respond if the child needs more affection ◆ Try and stimulate withdrawn children with interactive games such as drawing together, mutual storytelling and so on
Adolescence	
◆ Abstract thinking develops ◆ May show philosophic pondering about the meaning of life and death ◆ Grief may appear as withdrawn depressive symptoms ◆ May think in terms of an afterlife as well ◆ Often have powerful emotions and may be surprised by them	◆ Be prepared for long and difficult discussions ◆ Be prepared to say 'I don't know' ◆ Try and accept and explain strong emotions ◆ Ensure that they have a stable 'base' without restricting or overprotecting them

14.3 **Bereavement support**

William Worden describes a useful concept called 'bereavement work'[5]. Children who are going to die or be bereaved, and children that have been bereaved, are faced with numerous emotional, social and spiritual challenges which they will have to overcome. Different children will face different challenges and cope with these in different ways. There is no one right way for any child. However, there is always something that health workers can do to support children along their path. This section describes some of the things we can do to help. The section looks at ways you can support a child and family.

◆ Before death – pre-bereavement

◆ At the time of death

◆ After death.

But before going into details, you might find this general piece of advice useful.

> Remember four key things:
> 'Be loving, be accepting, be truthful, be consistent'.

14.3.1 **When should bereavement work start?**

Children will begin to feel grief as soon as they understand that they or their loved one is going to die. Therefore, bereavement work should start as soon as a child is diagnosed with a terminal illness. Health workers often feel lacking in confidence in this area, but you do not have to be a bereavement specialist to be able to offer effective help. There are many ways that you can help the child and family before, during and after the bereavement.

14.3.2 **The pre-bereavement stage**

It is a common misconception that bereavement starts after death. In fact, bereavement starts as soon as a person is aware of his or her impending loss. This might be the loss of a loved one, or loss of one-self. Therefore, bereavement work for health workers does not start after death; it starts at the moment of diagnosis. In the section below, we have outlined some tips on what and how to approach pre-bereavement in children's palliative care. However, as a general rule:

> Never lie to children or prevent them from talking. It is immoral, unethical and negligent. Children have as much right to ask questions and be given honest, accurate information as adults do.

14.3.2.1 **Encourage the child to talk and communicate**

◆ Families and carers often feel that children are incapable of coping with the distress and the anxiety of loss.

◆ Children are not always given information about their disease or the disease that their loved ones have. They may even be lied to by their loved ones or prevented from expressing their fears and concerns. However, denial and protectiveness by parents are not effective ways of supporting grieving children[6] or those who are sick.

◆ Communicate openly, honestly and factually, giving age appropriate information.

◆ Avoid using abstract explanations such as 'your mother has gone to sleep'.

◆ Allow the child to express anger or fear and help the child to do so without harming himself or anyone else.

◆ Do not impose expectations on the child (e.g. by saying 'you will definitely feel better in time' or 'it's time you got over it now').

◆ Encourage normality and continuity in other areas (e.g. school).

◆ Try to avoid separation from other loved ones such as siblings.

14.3.2.2 **Denial**

◆ Denial is rarely a fixed state – individuals move in and out of it, sometimes in the same conversation.

◆ Accept that it might be appropriate for the child to deny.

◆ Try to help the child work through it by gently discussing issues around death and dying.

◆ Make it easy for the child to ask questions.

◆ Try and explore things that offer reminders (e.g. photos, fond memories and the grave).

◆ Try to make the loss real for the child by including him or her in such activities as the burial ceremony and last funeral rites.

14.3.2.3 **Anticipatory grief**

◆ Children can suffer anticipatory grief when they feel that their death or the death of the loved one is near.

◆ They might project their feelings onto others (e.g. that parents may die too) and become very anxious about this.

- They may worry about what will happen to their loved ones when they are gone.
- They may also express their ideas and fears through play or art.
- They may become withdrawn, quiet and increasingly irritable.
- Try to help them communicate what they are feeling (see above and Chapter 2).
- Involve them in discussions around illness, death and dying and in decisions regarding their care.
- Try never to go against a child's choice unless you absolutely have to: the more control children feel they have, the less fearful they will be.

14.3.2.4 Stigma

- Stigma affects all aspects of caring for children and adolescents infected and affected by HIV/AIDS and cancers.
- Stigma in the pre-bereavement stage has the effect of isolating children and their families physically and psychologically.

14.3.2.5 Fear

- Children are particularly scared of pain and separation.
- They may regress, become clingy and develop nightmares or physical symptoms.
- You may get asked very difficult questions (see Chapter 2 – Communicating with children).
- Ensure regular, honest and open communication.
- Ascertain the child's fears and concerns, and talk them through.
- Give as much control as possible: once you have an idea of the child's fears and concerns, agree an action plan for how you will deal with each.

14.3.2.6 Avoidance, separation and rejection

- Death and disease may be taboo or too painful for families to mention.
- For many reasons, family members often clam up, and non-family members or distant relatives may stay away.
- The combined effect is to isolate the child and family just when they need most support.
- Try to encourage children and family members to share how they feel, and explain why it is that avoidance and separation are so tempting but so counter-productive.
- Encourage children and families to be open with each other and others, and to give permission to each other to show emotions, to not know what to say and to value just being together for comfort and support.

14.3.2.7 Telling others

- Encourage children to tell other people what they mean to them, and encourage families to tell the children.
- Everybody has some regrets in their life, including children, even if these seem trivial to adults.
- Remember young children think magically, and may attribute huge consequences (even their or their family member's death) to tiny causes (that they upset mummy that day).

- Try to encourage children to unburden themselves of their concerns and put straight any misplaced fears or concerns.
- More than any other emotion, regret can be reduced when it is shared.

14.3.2.8 Handing over

- The time will come where you begin to hand over to the child (giving responsibility back to the child for deciding how to approach the impending death).
- Perhaps the most important thing at this stage is to help the children to understand exactly what will happen to them (if they are bereaved) and what will happen to their loved ones (if they are to die). Try to look at the world through a child's eyes, or you might overlook something which seems trivial to you but might carry huge importance to them (e.g. who will take them to school, whether they will have to change where they sit or sleep at home, who will look after their favourite toy).
- You can use a number of practical techniques to make this easier. Further details can be found in Section 14.5 below.

14.3.3 At the time of death

What happens at the time of death has profound implications for surviving loved ones. A painful, traumatic death will often leave survivors feeling guilty, angry and traumatized. A 'good death' can help survivors to look back on the positives of a child's life, not tortured about the painful moments of death. Therefore, management at the time of death is crucial; yet it is precisely the time when health workers often feel least confident and most out of their depth. This section aims to help you minimize the trauma of witnessing a loved one die. Further details can be found in Chapter 18 – Caring the children at the end of Life.

14.3.3.1 Don't panic

- The best thing you can do is go through all the worst case scenarios in your head in advance and practise exactly what you will do for each.
- We repeat, the best thing you can do is go through all the worst case scenarios in your head in advance and practise exactly what you will do for each.
- Have you done it yet? If not, do it now.
- You might feel very nervous, even out of your depth.
- But however you feel, the child and family will feel much better if you look calm and in control (even if you don't feel that way inside!).
- Calm is catching, as is panic. Panic helps nobody, so try and ooze calmness. It really works.
- If you feel like panicking, make an excuse to go outside for a bit (a mock phone call is always useful) until you calm down.
- Above all, remind yourself that:
  - the child is dying and there is nothing you can do to stop it
  - it is a very sad experience for all, and you are not going to stop that either
  - it is extremely unlikely you will make things any worse
  - there are almost certainly symptoms you can control and comforting words you can say

- even if you feel that there is nothing you can do, and however useless you feel, just by being around you are helping and making the experience easier for the family, so stick at it.

14.3.3.2 Offer choices and control to the child

◆ The child may or may not be conscious and aware at the time of death.

◆ If they are aware, try to do everything you can to give them choice and control.

◆ Talk through in detail what might happen (best and worst case). For each scenario, explain and agree exactly what the plan is.

  - e.g. *'You might start to get breathless over the next few days. That is to be expected and we can easily deal with it by giving you some medicines. Do you want to ask anything about that?'*

◆ Try to involve them in any plans so that they will keep active:

  - e.g. *'If you start to feel breathless I need you to help me. Can you do that? Good. What I need you to do is to concentrate on those special breathing exercises I taught you. Shall we practise them again now?'*

14.3.3.4 Offer choices and control to the family

◆ In exactly the same way, you need to do everything you can to give the family choice and control (don't forget siblings).

◆ Talk through in detail what might happen (best and worst case). For each scenario, explain and agree exactly what the plan is.

  - e.g. *'Moses might start to get breathless over the next few days. That is to be expected and we can easily deal with it by giving him some medicines. Do you want to ask anything about that?'*

◆ Try to involve them in any plans so that they will keep active:

  - e.g. *'If Moses starts to feel breathless I need you all to help me. Mum, I need you to cuddle him so that he feels reassured, but not too tight. Try and make sure he can always see you. Dad, I want you to make a fan and gently fan Moses' face so he feels that there is plenty of air around. Esther, I want you to help Moses think about something else by doing his breathing exercises with him, and maybe singing him some songs when he gets tired. Can you do that? Good'.*

14.3.3.5 Remember

◆ Fear of the unknown is always greater than fear of the known.

◆ The whole experience will be completely new to the child, and probably to the family too.

◆ They will watch you like a hawk, constantly checking to make sure that you are able to guide them through the process with as little trauma as possible.

◆ The more they know and understand what is happening, the calmer they will be.

◆ So commentate on everything you do and think.

  - e.g. *'Ok, I am noticing that Moses is starting to get a bit breathless, but I am not concerned as we can easily manage that. Mum, Dad and Esther, remember what we agreed for you all to do? Ok, go ahead. I am just giving Moses a medicine called diazepam. It will help him feel less breathless when it starts working in about 15–20 minutes. He will probably fall asleep too. If it does not completely work, I will give him some more. While we are waiting for it to work I will stay around, so don't worry. Do you have any questions?'*

14.3.4 After death

After death, different families and cultures adopt different practises. This is covered in more detail in Chapter 15 – Spirituality. However, we will cover the key generic points below.

14.3.4.1 Seeing the body

- Seeing the body and attending the funeral is often helpful, but should always be the child's choice. No child should be denied the opportunity by an adult, nor be forced by an adult to see the body. Keep offering the option, and the opportunity to change their mind, for as long as possible.

- Seeing the body may help a bereaved child to:
  - begin to say goodbye
  - begin to accept the reality and finality of the death
  - begin to understand what has happened
  - be less scared.

- Tell them that they can change their minds – at any time.

- Give them clear and detailed information about what will happen:
  - e.g. *'Daddy is lying in the box called a coffin on a table. He doesn't look exactly the same as when he was alive. He is completely still. If you touch him he won't be warm but a bit cold. He is wearing his pale shirt and his dark grey trousers. There are quite a lot of flowers in the room and also some cards.'*

- Let them choose what they do when they enter the room: keep still by the door, touch or stroke the body, leave something like a drawing with the body.

- Give them the choice as to whether they want someone with them, or whether they would like a little private time on their own.

14.3.4.2 Attending the funeral

- According to different cultures, it may or may not be the norm for children to see the body or attend the funeral.

- If it is not possible, try and arrange an alternative 'saying goodbye' ceremony (see Section 14.5).

- If it is possible, make sure the child realizes that they will be welcome there.

- Try to ensure that they are with someone who will support them. This should not be the person closest to the dead person, who should not be asked to be supportive of a child at a time when they may be feeling their own grief most intently. A favoured aunty might be ideal.

- Give clear and detailed information about what will happen.

- Reassure them that it is *all* of the body of the person who has died that is being buried or cremated. Some younger children are confused and wonder what happens to the head, arms and legs.

- Explain that the dead person can no longer feel anything or be scared.

- Explain that there might be a 'party' after and not to be surprised or upset by that.

- Prepare them for some of the things that adults may say to them. For example, boys may be told that they are the 'man of the house now' and will appreciate reassurance that they are not.

- Create opportunities to be involved (e.g. through placing a drawing with the body or saying something or choosing some hymns.

14.3.4.3 **Alternative 'goodbyes'**

- If the child cannot or does not want to attend the funeral, try to encourage an alternative goodbye ceremony. For example:
  - Hold a memorial at home or at the grave with specially chosen music, songs, drawings and little tributes.
  - Visiting a place with special memories.
  - Create a special place of their own choosing.
  - Holding a small ceremony.
  - Releasing balloons to which special messages are attached saying something to the loved one or remembering something special.
  - Lighting a candle and sharing special memories with each other.
  - Starting a memory box.

14.4 **Problems that can arise**

It is difficult to offer sensible generalizations about how children react to death of different loved ones. Children, their temperaments, personalities and circumstances are so varied. Children and young people will have a range of reactions including not talking about the person who has died, deep sadness, rage, disturbed sleep, nightmares, lack of appetite or overeating, loneliness and a sense of abandonment, anxiety about themselves or other loved ones, a feeling that there is no point in anything, lack of interest in previous enthusiasms, or not wanting to attend school or see friends.

Their response will also vary according to their age, the cause and nature of the death (for example, whether sudden or expected, or by violence), the family circumstances (for example, whether parents lived together, whether major life changes will now be necessary), any previous experience of death or trauma within the family, the age and relationship with their siblings, their position within the family, how long they had known each other, their own resilience and the support and care they receive.

Dysfunctional bereavement may manifest itself in a number of different ways:

- Regression, e.g. sleep disturbances, food refusal
- Excessive self criticism and guilt
- Self-destructive behaviour
- Self-harm
- Taking on a parent role
- Truanting
- Petty delinquency
- Silence and withdrawal
- Overt depression.

Mostly, these changes are temporary and gradually disperse with time. However, sometimes they can persist or even become severe. It is ultimately a subjective judgement as to whether a 'normal' reaction strays into becoming an 'abnormal one'. Your judgement will depend partly on the child, partly on the reaction and partly on the family's capacity to cope. Remember though, when treating any psychological issues in childhood, you have to remember that the child's identity as an individual is heavily wrapped up in the child's identity as a member of a family (see Chapter 4 – Assessment and management planning). Therefore, what appears as a problem for an individual child is also usually a problem for and partly attributable to the whole family. What constitutes a troubling and abnormal behaviour for one family might be completely understandable and acceptable to another. So try and manage not just the child, but the whole family.

14.4.1 Risks for dysfunctional bereavement

There are a number of factors which can trigger so-called dysfunctional bereavement[7]:

♦ Features of the loss, e.g. sudden, violent, mutilating, random or prolonged deaths.

♦ Features of the child, e.g. previous emotional or behavioural problems, multiple losses, adolescence.

♦ Features of the relationship, e.g. attachment issues, complicated or abusive situations, death of father (particularly for adolescent boys) or the mother (particularly for younger children and teenage girls), unsupported or conflicted family.

14.4.2 Anger

♦ Anger is a natural reaction and children may express their anger outwardly or inwardly. Sometimes children might turn their anger on themselves.

♦ Try to decide whether the anger is causing any harm to the child (e.g. due to physical self-harm or neglect or because it is leading to ostracism at home or at school).

♦ Try to encourage the child to express his or her feelings of anger using verbal, non-verbal communication or play.

♦ Try to explain to the family where the anger is coming from and that it will pass as long as it is not reinforced by rejection from other family members.

♦ Agree with the child and family what is acceptable and when, and how to discharge anger constructively when it becomes too much.

14.4.3 Guilt and self-blame

♦ Try to explore the child's ideas and fears:

• Children might blame themselves for the sudden traumatic situation in their lives.

• Younger children often think that the death has occurred because of their bad behaviour.

• Older children might get a false reassurance from the unwarranted self-blame (i.e. that they can prevent unwanted events if only they try harder).

♦ Put right any misconceptions if you can, e.g. *'It's not your fault. You are a child and could not have stopped the germs getting into Daddy's body. Even the doctors with all of their medicines could not do that. The germs killed daddy. You did not'.*

♦ Encourage the child to focus on the future instead of things that he/she cannot change.

♦ Encourage the child and family to communicate openly with each other rather than keeping feelings of blame bottled up inside.

♦ Explore what other sources of support are available to the child.

14.4.4 Sorrow

♦ When a child feels sorrow, he or she may be ready to accept the truth of the loss without protest.

♦ Sorrow can be an expression of a child's feelings of vulnerability as he or she continues to live without the person who died.

◆ The child may grieve a loss of security.

◆ Touch is so important: loving arms suggest safety and acceptance in a world that has become more frightening and uncertain.

◆ Try to acknowledge the one who has died gently and regularly, particularly on aspects of his/her life or personality that were good.

14.4.5 Sleeping difficulties

◆ Sleeping is a form of parting, and perhaps even a form of mini-death, so it is not surprising that bereaved children often have difficulties in sleeping both in getting to sleep through worrying and grieving and in experiencing nightmares or disturbing dreams. The most important thing is to encourage a consistent routine, patience and gentle care. In most cases the problems will gradually ease as children realize that they are safe and the dreams begin to fade.

◆ Practical tips include making South American 'worry dolls': 5 or 6 tiny doll-like figures are held within a tiny cloth bag with a drawstring. South American children are encouraged at bedtime to whisper one big worry to each doll. The dolls are then placed under the pillow and the dolls take over the task of worrying for the night.

◆ Alternatively try 'Dreamcatchers' (these can be made on your own). The Native American legend tells how all the dreams of the world flow over our heads as we sleep. Dreams are caught by the dreamcatcher's web; the bad dreams stick to the strands of the web and the good dreams filter softly down the feathers to the sleeper beneath. Some dreamcatchers have beads woven onto the web – these represent 'heroes' and a child can choose their own heroes to help hold back the bad dreams (for example, one could be Dad, another could be a football star, another could be a friend, etc.).

14.4.6 Anxiety on parting

◆ Partings are also mini-bereavements and so anxiety on parting is very common with pre-bereaved and bereaved children.

◆ The important thing is to make sure that a pre-bereaved or bereaved child has consistent care, and what he or she is told will happen, so that they can gradually rebuild trust and confidence in the world and in people.

◆ When parting, encourage the parent or carer to mention something that will happen after reunion. For example, 'remind me to buy some beans when I collect you'; 'let's stop at aunty's on the way home tonight'; 'let's colour a picture together when you get home'. This glimpse of the future that includes both of them can be comforting.

14.5 Practical help

The following section describes some practical interventions that you can encourage before and after the death in order to help and support the bereaved (or pre-bereaved child). Some of what follows below is adapted from Winston's Wish[8].

14.5.1 Making a memory box

Children who are going to die will often find it helpful to work with their families to put a memory box together before they die. Bereaved children will benefit from collecting items that remind them of the person who has died and times shared with them. These items can be pasted into a book or placed into a box. Examples could be anything, an old piece of clothing with the person's smell, cards received, stones collected together, an old toy with particular memories, drawings done together, a piece of writing describing a fondly remembered event, photographs, flowers from the funeral and so on. Videos or sound tapes are even better, if available (but make sure that the child makes copies if at all possible). It is important that the child chooses, as only he or she will recognize what items generate memories that he or she wants to keep. Encourage the child to turn through the items every now and again, particularly at special moments or anniversaries, or when they are feeling sad, or fearful of forgetting or needing strength. Try and encourage the child to make the box or book 'special' by colouring or wrapping it, and by pasting on it items that make it stand out.

14.5.2 Making a family record

Making a family record can help a child or young person gain a sense of where they and the person who has died fits into the family. This is particularly important when a child is to be removed from their old home, or separated from siblings or cousins, and hence when there is a danger of losing a sense of his or her 'roots'. Try and encourage the child to put together a family tree and include family photographs, documents and certificates and mementoes can be included. Stories about the lives of the people who have died and also about the people from whom the child is about to be separated. The stories are even more powerful if contributed by family members and friends, and this is often a welcome way for them to be involved. What was the funniest thing the person ever did? What was their best subject at school? What was the bravest thing they ever did?

14.5.3 Telling the story

Children love stories, and especially when they themselves are incorporated into the story. Try and help children write or tell (with an adult writing) their story so that they remember clearly what happened. This also gives you and other carers an ideal opportunity to pick up misconceptions and misunderstandings, and put them right. With young children, it is often easier to use dolls, model figures or puppets to tell the story. Older children may prefer to use paper and pens. It is easier if you try and get the child to break the story into five or so pieces:

- What was life like before they died? (some idea of the family before the death)
- What happened just before they died? (earlier in the day, the day before…)
- How did they die? What happened?
- What happened immediately afterwards?
- What is life like now?

14.5.4 Handprints

Hands are powerful symbols of love and care. Encourage a pre-bereaved child to place his or her hand on a piece of paper. Then do the same with the parents and/or other people important to the child so that one or more fingers are touching. Draw around the hands and repeat it so that everyone has a copy. An alternative, even nicer, is to get everyone to paint their palms different colours and then carefully place their palms against the paper, fingers touching, so that actual prints are left. Encourage children to keep it safe (maybe even laminate it if possible) so that they can pull it out whenever they feel the need to be close to their lost one by placing their hand over their handprint and 'feel' the other hand alongside, supporting and encouraging them.

14.5.5 Writing a 'children's will'

Although children may have few material possessions, they will almost certainly have some items that they treasure and might have a clear idea of what they wish to happen to these. They also might have some thoughts about what they want to happen after death and how they wish to be remembered. All of these things can be captured in a will.

14.5.6 Permanency planning

Children need to be clear about what will happen to them (if they are bereaved) and what will happen to their loved ones (if they are to die). Uncertainty can compound the loss felt by the child. Particularly in SSA, where child bereavement is so common, a child may be separated from siblings and may experience frequent shifts from place to place in search of a proper home. Children whose parents do not complete permanency planning are at increased risk of developing emotional and behavioural problems.

14.5.7 The 'bereavement tree'

The Bereavement tree[9] (see Appendix 2 of this chapter) is a practical tool that sensitizes people to the feelings and behaviours of individuals and expectations of society, to create awareness about bereavement in order to encourage community support to all bereaved people. It was developed by Jenny Hunt in Zimbabwe and Nkosazana Ngidi in South Africa. The tool involves looking at how people deal with bereavement issues tracking it over a period of time, firstly immediately after death, then after 6–8 months and then after a year. It looks at how they feel, what they show in terms of their behaviour and how they are expected by society to feel, show and behave. It involves using the analogy of a tree, where the person who was looking after it has died. Children are engaged to talk about what they think the tree feels, what it looks like and what other people are expecting it to do, immediately after the death of the person, 6–8 months after the death and a year after the death. This can later be related to their own experiences of bereavement relating it to the tree. It can be used with individual children or groups.

14.5.8 Other useful activities

If you have internet access, the following activities can be found on the 'Winston's Wish' website (www.winstonswish.org.uk)

- 10 ways to remember someone who has died
  - Some ideas of ways to remember someone
- 10 things to do on Mother's Day
  - Some ideas of ways to remember a mother on Mother's Day
- 10 things to do on Father's Day
  - Some ideas of ways to remember a father on Father's Day
- 15 ways to remember people at important festivals
  - Some ideas of ways to remember people at Christmas and similar festivals
- Calendar of memories
  - Mark important dates connected with the person who has died on a calendar, which you can then share with other people
- Memory shapes
  - Make your own coloured shape of memories

- ◆ Feelings
  - Compare your feelings with our feelings grid
- ◆ Remember
  - Add a star to our skyscape of memories.

14.6 **Questions for you**

1. Which myths about children and bereavement did you hold before you read this chapter? Reflect on how the chapter has affected your beliefs (or not).

2. Reflect on whether you could envisage a situation when it would be acceptable to lie to a child about their prognosis. Think about who you might be trying to protect in such a scenario.

3. Imagine that your own death is approaching. What would you be most frightened of? How would you like to be remembered? What would you put in your own memory box?

Notes

1 Winston's Wish (2003). The Clara Burgess Centre, Bayshill Road, Cheltenham, Gloucestershire, GL50 3AW. Available online at www.winstonswish.org.uk

2 Talking about Death with Children. The Dougy Center, The National Center for Grieving Children and Families, Used by Permission. Available online at http://www.dougy.org/

3 Himmelstein, B.P., Hilden, J. M., Boldt, A. M. & Weissman, D. (2004). Pediatric Palliative Care. *JAMA, 350*(17), 1752–1763.

4 Ministry of Health and Child Welfare. (2006). Palliative Care for Children: A Training Manual for Communities in Zimbabwe.

5 Worden, J.W. (1991). Grief Counseling and Grief Therapy 2nd Edition, Spring Publishing Co., NY.

6 Waechter. E. (1971). Children's Awareness of Fatal Illness. *The American Journal of Nursing, 71*(6), 1168–72.

7 Watson, M., Lucas, C., Hoy, A. & Back, I. (Eds.) (2005). *Oxford Handbook of Palliative Care*. Oxford University Press, Oxford.

8 Winston's Wish. Available online at www.winstonswish.org.uk

9 Nkosazana Ngidi (2006). The Bereavement Tree. Hospice Palliative Care Association of South Africa. Available online at www.hospicepalliativecaresa.co.za

10 'Dream Catcher' by Enchanted Learning. com. Available online at http://www.enchantedlearning.com/Crafts/

Appendix 1: The dream catcher[10]

Dream Catchers are from Native American lore; they trap bad dreams and let the good dreams filter down to the sleeper.

For each dream catcher you will need:

- a bendable twig about 1 foot long
- a few inches of thin wire
- some twine
- beads with large holes
- a few feathers.

Have an adult make a hoop from a twig. To do this, wrap a short length of thin wire around the overlapping ends. Use thin wire to tie the ends of a twig together to make a hoop.

Cut a few feet of twine. Tie one end of the twine to the twig hoop. String a few beads onto the twine and push the beads toward the tied end. Wrap the twine around the other side of the hoop.

String a few more beads on the twine and then wrap the twine around the far side of the hoop. Repeat until you have an interesting webbing design.

Tie a short length of twine on the hoop. String a bead or two on it and then tie a feather onto the end. Repeat this a few times (2 or 3 hanging feather strings look nice). Hang the dream catcher near your bed!

Rainbow Dream Catcher

Appendix 2: The bereavement tree

You can use the analogy of a tree to talk to a child about bereavement. Explain to the child that the person who has taken care of the tree has left or died. Use the pictures below, or draw your own pictures with the child, to help explain and to help the child talk and understand.

Immediate

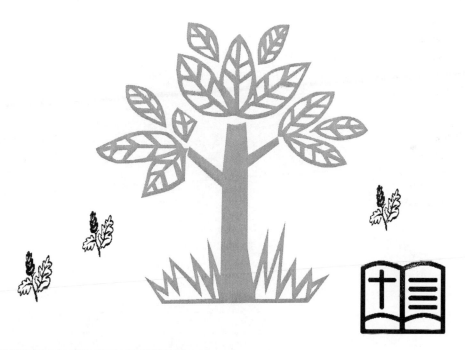

Felt	Shown	Expected
◆ shock	◆ lose colour	◆ expected to; provide
◆ sad	◆ lose leaves	◆ shade
◆ helpless	◆ signs of withering	◆ shelter
◆ alone	◆ no flowers	◆ fruit
◆ scared	◆ unhealthy	◆ look healthy and pretty
◆ angry	◆ no fruit	◆ to protect
◆ worried and confused	◆ not happy	
	◆ no shade	
	◆ no birds	

At 6–8 months

Tree receives a little rain and sunshine (6–8 months).

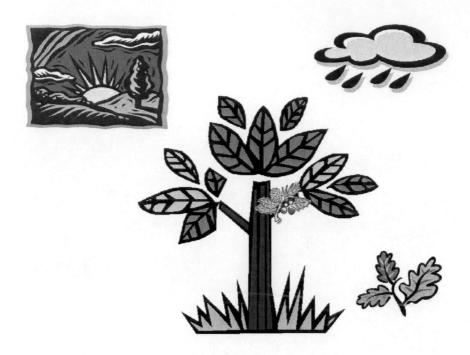

Felt	Shown	Expected
◆ abandoned	◆ leaves are still falling	◆ same as immediate
◆ lonely	◆ still no fruit	
◆ worried	◆ no shade	
◆ angry	◆ no shelter	
◆ deserted	◆ not healthy	
◆ missing a person	◆ starting to grow new roots	
◆ feel some hope	◆ new shoots	
◆ feels I need to look for support	◆ one or two flowers	

A year later

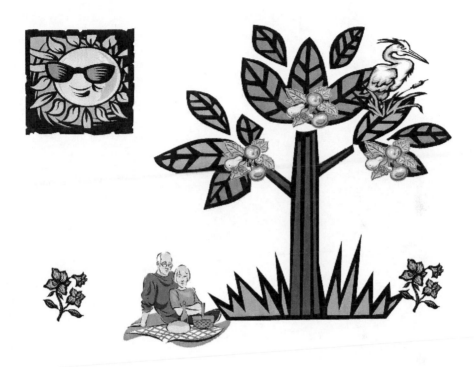

Felt	Shown	Expected
◆ substitute affections	◆ bears fruit	◆ as before but explore rituals, etc.
◆ lonely	◆ birds come to it	
◆ missing the person	◆ provides shade	
◆ angry sometimes	◆ flowers	
◆ sad sometimes	◆ new leaves	
◆ hope	◆ looks healthy	
◆ sometimes happy	◆ new roots	
	◆ more support	

Chapter 15

Spirituality

Justin Amery, Eunice Garanganga
and Carla Horne

Key points

- Spirituality and religion are related but different.
- Children are capable of significant spiritual experiences.
- Children, like adults, need to attribute meaning to illness and death.
- Allow space for mystery and paradox. They may be alien to medicine but they are at the heart of spirituality.
- African traditional and Western beliefs and approaches to health, healing, illness, death and dying weave together in a very complex way around the death of children. You need to have some understanding of how.
- You may feel ill-equipped to answer or deal with some of the awkward spiritual questions that childhood death throws up, but you can learn how to deal with spiritual questions of children and assess their spiritual needs without difficulty.
- Health workers often ignore the spiritual needs of children.
- Assessing a child's spirituality is not difficult if you know what to look for.
- You don't have to pretend you know the answers; you just need to help children express their questions.

15.1 Spirituality and religion: children's palliative care perspective

15.1.1 What is spirituality?

Spirituality is defined broadly as human search for purpose and meaning in life. This search often involves seeking answers to questions such as what matters to us most, what gives us hope, what makes us sad or happy, what we are concerned about and our relationship with others, the earth and the universe. Spirituality is a personal view about making sense of our place in the world. It can often include an idea of something greater than people. There may be many facets to our spirituality[1]: a sense of belonging, of mystery, of connectedness, of meaning, of hope, of the sacred, of morality, of beauty and of acceptance of dying to name but a few. Developing an understanding of how and where we fit into the greater picture appears to be a need common in all cultures and societies and starts when we are young.

Children are very aware and in tune with spiritual issues yet often adults assume that the child is not concerned with these complicated aspects of life. Children are capable of significant spiritual experiences[2] and children, like adults, need to attribute meaning to illness. Because children do not always talk about things the way adults do, we may not 'hear' their spiritual concerns.

15.1.2 Relationship between spirituality and religion

For some people, this self-understanding and sense of meaning is lodged in religious traditions, for others it can be lodged in the sense of freedom and mastery associated with science and problem-solving. For some, it may be related to individual or communal spiritual practises. Whatever a patient's spiritual belief, there is likely to be a search for the meaning of life and a purpose for living.

15.1.3 Relationship between health, well-being and spirituality

Support around spiritual issues is as important to a child's well-being as physical and emotional support. With life-threatening illness common spiritual questions arise for the child and the family. These might include: *'Is there life after death?'*, *'What happens when we die?'*, *'Does God still love me?'*, *'Am I being punished?'*, *'Why me?'* These perplexing questions are not easily answered, yet can cause serious distress. That distress can manifest itself in physical and emotional pain.

15.1.4 Health professionals and spirituality

Health professionals, perhaps unsurprisingly, often do not feel at ease with these types of questions and discussions. But the art of spiritual support is the art of addressing the unknown and the uncertain. Mystery, paradox and connectedness are its core subjects. Answers are not the question. Let yourself be comfortable with that and it will become a lot easier.

Answers are not the question.

15.1.5 Useful concepts in spirituality

You might be disappointed (but not surprised) to know that, just like with medicine and nursing, spirituality has its jargon. Some words and concepts that might be useful to you include the following[3,4]:

◆ **Meaning:** This includes the purpose of life and the reason for an event that happens within life. It may also be sought in a review of life achievements; in a review of relationships; in a moral or spiritual search (especially of life as it was lived); and in an effort to discern the meaning of dying, of human existence, of suffering and of the remaining days of life[5].

◆ **Hope:** When confronted with their own mortality, people often hope initially not to die, and failing that, hope to live and die in a way which is perceived to be good. Spiritual hope may also mean achieving a purpose in life, reconciliation with God, self and others[6].

◆ **Relatedness:** This means being able to relate to and commune with a higher being, God or a system of spiritual faith or belief. It also can include relatedness to a religion or faith community.

◆ **Acceptance:** This concept is also related to forgiveness and reconciliation. It will help in meeting the underlying need to deal with mistakes or misfortunes in life[7] through the eventual acceptance of these.

◆ **Transcendence:** This can be explained as a quality of faith or spirituality that allows the person to move beyond, to transcend, what is happening in their own experience – which in our patient's cases is often suffering as a result of their disease. It can occur as the outcome when spiritual needs are met and can also occur through grace[8].

15.2 **African concepts of 'healing'**

Many people educated in modern schools with inadequate knowledge of African cultural backgrounds, tend to recognize only the Western form of treating the sick, and may see traditional African approaches to healing as 'witchcraft', 'spiritual possession', 'divination', etc. Yet 'healing' is a concept not constrained to any one world view or approach. Traditional African healing is focused on restoring wholeness and peace. God is seen as the ultimate healer and curer and doctor, helped by his divine intermediaries and the good living-dead ancestors, the diviners, who can find the cause, the local doctors who can find the cure and the caring and loving family and community who can make all the above possible. In particular it tries to restore wholeness and peace between the sick person and:

◆ God, the ancestors and the living

◆ the family

◆ the community and its basic beliefs and values.

Ultimately, the African traditional approach to healing aims for sick persons to be completely at peace with themselves, to collect together their fears and overcome them, to be assured that their desires and wishes will be dealt with and that their anxieties and aspirations will be catered for by the one they love. All these modes of healing are necessary for the children who are dying and their families. Together they form part of an integrated healing/holistic approach. It would be naïve for health professionals to think that the above modes of healing can be done in a uniform way, by all societies. Thus, there is a need for a sincere dialogue between health workers, from different cultures and faith backgrounds, who use different definitions of, and approaches to, healing.

Box 15.1 Healing and wholeness

Reflect on the word 'healing'. What does it mean to you?

The word 'healing' comes from the same stem as the word 'whole'. Therefore, 'healing' can also be thought of as 'whole-ing' (or 'making whole'). It is only recently that the word healing has taken on more Western connotations of physical 'pathology' and physical 'cure'. Therefore, Western and African approaches might be more similar than we realize.

Reflect on your own practice. What percentage of your patients do you actually 'cure'? In other words, from what proportion do you completely remove the pathology forever?

The chances are that you actually can 'cure' very few. What do you do with the rest? In what ways do you try and make them 'whole' again? Is there a spiritual element to your care? If not, what might you be missing?

15.3 **Spiritual development**

15.3.1 **Spirituality: where are you?**

Before beginning to discuss and understand spirituality in children, it is important to try and work out our own stage of spiritual development. After all, without some self-understanding, how can we help children and their families understand and interpret their own spirituality? Because children interpret spiritual issues and questions in different ways according to the stage of their development, it is very important for health workers to be able to gauge their own stage of spiritual development. Such spiritual self-awareness will help the health worker to find a level of communication that works for the child. It is not the job of the children's palliative care health worker to evangelize or proselytize to children. Rather the job of the health worker is to help children explore their spiritual concerns in their own way and at their own pace.

While a full discussion of spiritual development is well beyond the scope of this book; it is important to realize that, unlike physical and cognitive development, this is an area that continues from birth through to old age. It is beyond the scope of this book to give anything more than a cursory overview of this area, but it is worth briefly discussing the most influential theory, which is that of Fowler[9].

Fowler describes six stages of spiritual development. Like all 'stage' theories, his theory is open to criticism that not all people go through all stages, that development is not always linear or one-way and that development is multi-factorial and so can rarely be easily categorized into concrete stages. Nevertheless his theory gives an idea of how humans can differ in their approaches to the spirituality. The six stages are as follows. Read through them and try and work out which stage describes your own spiritual stage most accurately.

1. Intuitive-projective faith (usually between 3–7 years): Faith is highly imaginative, influenced by growing self-awareness and an awareness of one's culture's taboos. The strength of the imagination (un-restrained by logic and experiences of older childhood and adulthood) can lead people in this stage to develop powerful senses of terror or (conversely) unrestrained power. Children in this age group are therefore often fascinated by stories of horrible monsters or witches, and also obsessed by (and sometimes imagine themselves to be) super-heroic figures.

2. Mythic-literal faith (usually starting at school age and usually completed by early adulthood, although many people remain in this stage for life): At this stage myths, symbols and rituals begin to be incorporated into belief systems. They may however be taken quite literally rather than as pointers to/descriptors of wider, more abstract concepts. This stage features a strong belief in justice 'an eye for an eye' and reciprocity 'you reap what you sow' or 'karma'. Deities in this age group are strongly anthropomorphic (e.g. God with a beard sitting on a throne).

3. Synthetic-conventional faith: Most people remain in this stage for life. It tends to start in adolescence or young adulthood, when one's search for identity within a frightening and enormous world is a major concern. It is characterized by conformity and/or rebellion against societal norms, but without strong attempts to reflect on this conformity or rebellion critically. Other people are often divided in black and white terms: 'us versus them', and therefore faith at this stage can be quite exclusive (e.g. the saved and the unsaved, the believers and the unbelievers).

4. Individuative-reflective faith: This stage tends to occur in people who begin to be challenged by increasingly obvious contradictions/hypocrisies in authority and authority figures. In this stage one's identity separates from that of the crowd and it therefore often generates strong and unsettling questions about who one is and what one believes. Many people do not reach this stage at all, but those that do usually pass into it during their mid-thirties to early forties. It is a stage where one realizes that one must take personal responsibility for one's own beliefs and feelings, and things that were previously unquestioned are now strongly questioned. Therefore, it is a stage where nothing is certain and everything appears fluid and unfixed. It is a stage of excitement but also of angst, struggle and often despair. People who get stuck in this phase may become bitter and cynical and trust nothing and no one, and give up on spirituality all together.

5. Conjunctive faith: Few people reach this stage, and it tends to occur in later middle age. In this stage one accepts and eventually begins to enjoy paradox. A typical person in this stage may know they believe, but be unable to express this belief clearly in words, preferring to use symbols, myths, rituals and music as routes of expression. Unlike in stage 2, these are not taken literally, but as routes or springboards for expression of deeper meaning. It is a stage where one transcends the limitations and conceptions of one's own specific tradition and culture. It is a stage where symbols talk more loudly than words because symbols point to a deeper, if indefinable, reality behind the symbols. This deeper sense of mystery and unconscious overcomes the cynicism of stage 4 and allows a new vision of a 'bigger picture' beyond the confines of individual cultures and traditions. This stage is often experienced almost as a 'return to infancy', in that it is filled with an almost childish wonder at the world and a radical openness to possibility.

6. Universalizing faith (sometimes called enlightenment): This is a stage that very few people reach. In stage 5, while one sees the possibilities of an ultimate 'one-ness' of the universe, one is torn between the possible interconnectedness and unity of all things and loyalty to the deeply held attachment to the idea of oneself as a concrete, separate entity. In stage 6, this attachment to oneself and one's own ego dissolves and one accepts one's place but a small (though important) as part of a much larger, if mysterious, whole. A typical person in this stage seems very wise, slightly 'other-worldly', accepting of their own mortality but full of a considered optimism and an almost childish delight at people, the world and its workings.

15.3.2 Spiritual development in children

Spirituality in children is related to age, or more specifically, to stages of development (see table 15.1). Whilst for adults spirituality and religion may be closely overlapping concepts, religious beliefs, structures or practises have less effects on children's experience of spirituality than they do on those of adults. For children spirituality is far more likely to be centred around their understanding of life as they experience it day-to-day. Common spiritual concerns for children involve love, forgiveness, safety, hope and legacy (will their life and their accomplishments have made a difference and will they be remembered after they have died). Children are also likely to be concerned by loneliness and separation (from parents, siblings, pets, friends) and from the loss of themselves as a whole (for example no longer being able to go to school or do the things that they enjoy). Children can sometimes talk about 'magical' and non-human beings such as angels, fairies or monsters. Listening to these stories, which may at first seem like childish storytelling, may tell us something about a child's current 'spiritual' thinking and help us to better understand their fears and worries.

Table 15.1 Children's development, stages of spiritual growth and interventions (adapted from Himelstein et al.[10]).

Age range (years)	Characteristics	Spiritual development	Interventions
0–2	Has sensory and motor relationship with environment. Has limited language skills. Achieves object permanence. May sense that something is wrong.	Faith reflects trust and hope in others. Need for sense of self-worth and love.	Provide maximal physical comfort, familiar persons and transitional objects (e.g. favourite toys) and consistency. Use simple physical communication.
>2–6	Uses magical and animistic thinking. Is egocentric. Thinking is irreversible. Developing language skills. Engages in symbolic play.	Faith is magical and imaginative. Participation in ritual becomes important. Need for courage.	Minimize separation from parents. Correct perceptions of illness as punishment. Evaluate for sense of grief and assuage if present. Use precise, non-metaphorical language (e.g. dying, dead).
>6–12	Has concrete thoughts.	Faith concerns right and wrong. May accept external interpretations as the truth. Connects ritual with personal identity.	Evaluate children's fears of abandonment. Be truthful. Provide concrete details if requested. Support child's effort to achieve control and mastery. Maintain access to peers. Allow child to participate in decision-making.
>12–18	Generality of thinking. Reality becomes objective. Capable of self-reflection. Body image and self-esteem paramount.	Begins to accept internal interpretations as truth. Evolution of relationship with God or higher power. Searches for meaning, purpose, hope and value of life.	Reinforce child's self-esteem. Allow child to express strong feelings. Allow child privacy. Promote child's independence. Promote access to peers. Be truthful. Allow child to participate in decision-making.

15.3.3 Children's beliefs

Children will often appear (superficially) to hold the same beliefs as their parents or religious teachers. However, as can be seen from the discussion on spiritual development above, each child's actual personal belief system will be unique. Providing children with spiritual support must be done in a manner that allows for this individualism. Adults often show their spiritual understanding in structured religious beliefs such as traditional beliefs, Christianity and Islam. Young children are more likely to explain how they understand life in their own unique ways, until they learn from their family what to believe. All children have a sense of their belonging within the world around them and find separation and disconnectedness from the family as the start of the journey of spiritual exploration and questioning.

Although understood differently at different developmental stages and expressed diversely in different cultures and religious ways, the spiritual needs of children are universal.

Box 15.2 Early spiritual beliefs

Think back to when you were a child. What terrified you the most? Was it witches, wild animals, the dark or something else?

Then, think back to how you used to comfort yourself. What did you do if no adults were around to comfort you?

Reflect on that fear. What do you think it symbolized?

Reflect on what you used to comfort yourself with. What did that symbolize and how did it work?

15.4 **How to assess the spirituality of a child and family**

Generally speaking, the principles of spiritual assessment are the same as for any other assessment (see Chapter 4). Remember, children speak three languages: verbal, non-verbal and play. Therefore, all three should be used in spiritual assessment. In particular, health workers should observe carefully a child's behaviour, interactions and emotions. The health worker should also involve the child in play and drawings, watching carefully for issues like magic and symbolism, both of which may signal spiritual questioning or distress in the child.

Stoll[11] suggests some guidelines for spiritual assessment which might be useful. The model suggests four broad areas to be explored through questioning. These include:

◆ concept of God or deity

◆ sources of hope and strength

◆ religious practises

◆ relationship between spiritual beliefs and health.

McEvoy[12] suggests a system called 'B-E-L-I-E-F' in evaluating the spiritual and religious needs of child and family. These include the following:

◆ B–Belief system

◆ E–Ethics and values

◆ L–Lifestyle

◆ I–Involvement in a spiritual community

◆ E–Education

◆ F–Future events.

In reality, these models cannot be used simplistically with children. They are more helpful as 'aide-memoires' to help health workers check that they have thought about all the different angles when assessing a child's spirituality.

In practise, assessment of a child's spirituality should include reviewing a child's hopes, dreams, values, life meaning, their view of the role of prayer and ritual beliefs regarding death. What is important to the child should be examined as well as the meaning of the child's life to both the child and their family. It is also important to explore a child's important relationships; these may be with family, friends, God or other spiritual figures.

Here are some ideas that may help you talk with children about spiritual thoughts when illness is affecting them or their family.

15.4.1 Listen to the words

Use the child's words that give a clue about spiritual questions. These may reflect the beliefs of his family. For example: God, heaven, hell, spirit. Explore these thoughts by asking what the word means to him, and what he feels about it. If there is a faith expert (pastor, priest or minister) available, ask the child and family if they wish to see him and if he could be part of the care team. Ask about particular rituals that have meaning for the child and family.

15.4.2 Dreams

The story or fears coming from dreams can give a chance to look at worries that are difficult to look at in 'real' life. Ask the child what the dream means to him. Do not try to explain it yourself.

15.4.3 Feeling words

Words about being lonely, strong or weak, guilty, brave or afraid can be explored further with the child. This may give you a clue how he thinks about the meaning of life and death. For example, you can say, 'tell me more about that' or 'I think I might feel that way too'.

15.4.4 Thinking words

Words that show that the child is thinking deeply can give you a chance to encourage the child to talk about it more. The child may ask 'why me?' or 'I wish ...' or 'I wonder if ...'. You can help the child work this out more by asking 'what else do you wish?' or 'how do you think that may happen?'

15.4.5 Going home or going away

Children who are beginning to sense that they are dying often talk about going home or leaving. Talking about these feelings and exploring the journey with the child is difficult but it needs to be done. You can help by saying 'What is it like for you?' Do not give false reassurance that he is not dying.

15.4.6 Questions for exploration and assessment of children's spirituality

Here are some useful questions which might help get you started[13]:

- What do you believe in?
- Do you belong to a religion?
- How does your religion help you?
- What makes you feel safe?
- Do you have a special place where you go to?
- Who or what do you trust?
- How do you know what is right and wrong?
- Who/what helps you when you need it?
- What will you be like as an adult? What will you be doing?
- Do you have a hero?
- Have you ever had a moment of great joy/wonder?
- Do you ever feel other peoples' thoughts and feelings?

- Who/what is closest to your heart?
- What makes you happy/sad/frightened?
- When you have a good idea what do you do about it?
- What unique/special thing do you offer the world?
- Who are you?
- What is important to you in life?
- What is life about?
- What are you here for?
- What and who do you love deeply?

15.5 Challenges for children's spirituality in children's palliative care

Children may not always speak about things the way adults do, therefore adults may miss the chance to talk to them about spiritual concerns. Adults also often feel ill-equipped to discuss existential and spiritual issues with children. Even if both child and adult are willing to talk, both may feel overwhelmed by the situation and therefore unable to discuss questions fully.

Children who are dying or facing the death of a loved one face a number of different challenges. There are probably as many challenges as there are children, but these are some of the common spiritual challenges that children might face:

- Seeing the world and spirituality differently to adults.
- Finding it harder to communicate spiritual concerns and distress.
- The need to experience unconditional love at a time of imminent separation.
- Fearing separation and worrying about who will look after them once they have died.
- Trying to attribute meaning to their illness.
- Feeling guilty or blameworthy and seeing illness as a punishment.
- Feelings of anger and unfairness of what is happening.
- Feelings of meaninglessness.
- Hoping that they still will have a place in the family even as they realize that their time in the family will soon come to an end.

Children may also have many questions in relation to their illness, death and spirituality. There may be a desire to re-establish links with God or spiritual power, or to develop a relationship with a previously unknown spiritual power. Children may display a sense of guilt, remorse and seek forgiveness as part of an understanding and acceptance of their illness and prognosis.

As a general rule children should be allowed to take part in ceremonies and practises as desired, but of course with the permission of parents or caregivers. They should be given the opportunity to continue to develop meaningful secure relationships. Most importantly the health worker should ensure that the family has time to reflect on life's meaning and purpose and be available for when the family may want to talk, discuss and question and to allow the child's spiritual growth and development.

Working with dying and bereaved children may be a very stressful and difficult work for health workers, as it may make them think about their own beliefs and personal fears. It is important for carers to have their own source of spiritual strength. However, it is not the job of the health worker to evangelize or impose their own spirituality on the child. No matter how strong your faith, you are not the saviour of the family in distress. You can help most by listening as the family tries to make sense of what is happening. Be careful not to impose your beliefs on the family.

Parents naturally have many spiritual questions when they have a child who is facing a life-threatening illness. Guilt and blame are usually felt. Parents are often angry and try to use their beliefs to make sense of their experience. Sometimes they find that this situation forces them to rethink what made sense to them about life and death. What they believed before may not suit them anymore and they may need to find different ways of making sense of what is happening to them. It is not for the caregiver to give answers to spiritual questions but rather to be a support for the family on their journey of understanding.

Families who have an affiliation to a faith community (e.g. church, mosque, synagogue, etc.) may seek spiritual support there. However, even if they do, do not assume that they will receive all they need from their faith community. Be prepared also to give support. This means being able to discuss spiritual questions with the family, not advising them what they should believe in. Faith communities can often bring practical help and this should be encouraged if the family and child are agreeable.

15.6 Helping children address their spirituality and spiritual needs

Overall, the role of the health worker is to act as a facilitator; encouraging the child and family to identify their own questions, issues and needs with support. Just as in other areas, the most important thing is to build trust with the child, and thereby enabling a relationship to develop. This can only come with time, and of course time is one thing you may not have. Nevertheless, it is something that you might be able to do yourself, or (if not) might be able to support volunteers or family carers to do so themselves.

The techniques one can use for helping children are very similar to those used when managing pre-bereavement and bereavement (see Chapter 14 for more detail). These would include the following:

- drawing and art
- poetry (especially with older children)
- using tools such as the bereavement tree to encourage discussion
- praying (allowing the child to lead the prayers)
- memory book keeping
- journal writing
- create learning opportunities
- read, write and tell stories
- circle times
- group worship;
- children's 'thought for the day'
- time/space for confidential support and communication
- celebrations
- display of ideas, pictures, stories, plays, etc.
- reflection times.

Prayers and rituals can be a source of comfort and strength if the child and family are used to praying. Saying familiar prayers or singing familiar hymns can create a bond within the family.

Children often will say things in prayers that they might not say normally. You may do something often that brings you comfort, such as looking at a picture, singing a favourite song or reading something special that helps you feel better. These rituals can help bring meaning and allow children to find comfort in something they can count on regularly.

Children and their families may have many questions in relation to their illness, death and spirituality. There may be a desire to re-establish links with a faith community or spiritual power, or to develop a relationship with a previously unknown spiritual power. Families may display guilt, remorse and seek forgiveness as part of understanding and acceptance of their child's illness and prognosis.

Most importantly the health professional should ensure that the family has time to reflect on life's meaning and purpose and be available when the family may want to talk, discuss and question and to allow the child's spiritual growth and development. It may be that you do not have the time, or feel that you do not have the confidence or competence to address the spiritual needs of the child or family. That is fine, but it is not an excuse for failing to find someone who does have the time and expertise.

If you are in this position, find out which local and culturally appropriate spiritual carer might be available and contact them. Explain the child's illness and prognosis to the child's spiritual carer (with the permission of the family), and then ensure he or she gets involved.

15.7 **Beliefs and practises surrounding death of children in Africa**[14,15]

Africa is probably the 'tree where man was born'[16]. If you believe the mitochondrial DNA evidence for the original site of evolution of man, there is eight times more genetic diversity within African tribes than amongst all of the rest of the tribes of the world put together. There are many different cultures and ethnic groups in Africa (53 in Uganda alone). It is not often realized that there is more diversity between the southern and northern tribes in Uganda than there is between European Caucasians, Australian Aborigines, North American Inuit and South Asian Indians put together.

Furthermore, in modern Africa, there is often a blending of traditional beliefs with 'Western' religion. For example, a family may attend a Christian church or a mosque and hold those beliefs while also consulting with traditional leaders regarding spiritual beliefs such as communication with and veneration of ancestral spirits. Many African funeral rituals stem from traditional rather than Western religious beliefs and practises. This can often cause conflict between members of the family and health professionals. Secrecy around traditional practises can create serious misunderstandings that can hamper delivery of care.

Given this huge diversity, in many ways it is nonsense to talk of 'African practises'. There are, however, some common beliefs that cut across the different cultures in SSA[17], and which seem to have implications for children's palliative care in many diverse African countries and cultures. It is beyond the scope of this book to describe these in great detail, but there are some commonly held beliefs that impact on children's palliative care and therefore are important to mention.

◆ The belief that life is a great gift and therefore its preservation and prolongation is the central duty of every person, family and community:
  • This belief can make it difficult for families to move from a curative to a palliative approach. Children may be subjected to pointless but distressing and/or expensive treatments if health workers do not discover and gently challenge this belief.

◆ The belief that illness and death (especially in childhood) do not come by themselves. Rather some enemy (living or dead) must have caused it.

   • This belief can continue to distract the child and family into searching for external agents and seeking redress rather than using the limited time left to them in a constructive, peaceful and supportive way.

◆ The belief that 'blessings of all sorts come from fulfilling the duty to care for the terminally sick'.

   • This belief sits fairly easily with children's palliative care as it provides a strong spiritual driver for the family to pull together to do as much as they can to care for the child.

◆ The belief that a 'good death' comes in old age, is not sudden and allows the patient to make all the preparations, forgive and reconcile with all, and above all, to be able to see their dear ones and bid them farewell.

   • Death in childhood is rarely seen as a good death. Try and help the family focus on all that has been good in a child's life to show that life has not been wasted. Encourage them to understand that children too have affairs that need to be put in order and farewells that need to be said.

◆ The belief in the importance of death rituals:

   • Traditional African beliefs put great importance on correct rituals after the death of the child. The particular rituals vary, but there are common themes; particularly around burying the dead child close (or within) the family home and around not tempting fate by bringing death of very young infants too close to the mother or surviving siblings (in case further childbirth is prevented or surviving children themselves succumb). In most cases these rituals seem to serve to complete the circle of life, appease ancestral spirits and allow the surviving family to move forward unencumbered by unfulfilled obligations from the past.

   • It is important to enquire about rituals specific to the child and family. Even if you think you know your country well, you might be surprised to find how much rituals and practises can vary.

However, this brief outline cannot do any justice at all to the diversity of practises and beliefs across Africa. It is for the health worker to find out what each family believes and practises. Even in the same tribe and community each family needs to be understood uniquely as distinct entities with distinct belief systems. To try and give a view of ways in which practises of different tribes are similar and different, health workers at Hospice Africa have described below the practises of their own tribes within just one tiny country in Africa, Uganda. These can be found in Appendix 15.1. We hope these will give readers a feeling of the complexities, differences and similarities between different cultures and tribes in Africa, so that they can be more sensitive to and aware of these practises when providing children's palliative care in their own places of work.

15.8 Questions for you

1. Try to explain to yourself what you believe without using any 'jargon'. Don't use terms such as 'God', 'heaven', 'salvation'. Use language that a 5- or 6-year-old might be able to understand.

2. Read through 'Fowler's spiritual stages'. Try and work out which stage you are at. If you are not sure, discuss it with someone who knows you well and whose opinion you trust.

3. Think back to when you were a child. What terrified you the most? Was it witches, wild animals, the dark or something else?

4. Then think back to how you used to comfort yourself. What did you do if no adults were around to comfort you?

5. How would your family deal with the death and funeral of a child? What are the similarities and differences compared to the traditions described from Uganda? What do you think might be the meaning of the similarities and differences?

Notes

1 Galek, K., Flannelly, K., Vane, A. & Galek, R. (2005). Assessing a patient's spiritual needs: A comprehensive instrument in holistic nursing practice. *Holistic Nursing Practice, 19,* 62–9.

2 Brykczynska, G. (Eds.) (1992). Nursing Care. Delmar Learning, Independence, KY.

3 Speck, P. (1998). Spiritual issues in palliative care. In D. Doyle, G. Hanks & N. Macdonald (Eds.) *Oxford Textbook of Palliative Medicine* 2nd Edition. (pp. 805–14). Oxford University Press, Oxford.

4 Kemp, C. (2001). Spiritual Assessment. In B. Rolling Ferell & N. Coyle (Eds.). *Palliative Nursing.* (pp. 407–14). Oxford University Press, Oxford.

5 Speck, P. (1998). Spiritual issues in palliative care. In D.Doyle,G. Hanks & M. MacDonald (Eds.). *Oxford textbook of palliative medicine.* (pp. 805–16). Oxford University Press, Oxford..

6 Kemp, C. (2001). Spiritual care interventions. In B. Ferrell & N. Coyle (Eds.) *Textbook of Palliative Nursing.* (pp. 407–14). Oxford University Press, New York.

7 Kemp, C. (2001). Spiritual care interventions. In B. Ferrell & N. Coyle (Eds.) *Textbook of Palliative Nursing.* (pp. 407–14). Oxford University Press, New York.

8 Kemp, C. (2001). Spiritual care interventions. In B. Ferrell & N. Coyle (Eds.) *Textbook of Palliative Nursing* (pp. 407–14). Oxford University Press, New York.

9 Fowler, James, W. (1981). *Stages of Faith.* Harper & Row ISBN 0-06-062866-9.

10 Himmelstein, B., Hilden, J., Boldt, A. & Weissman, D. (2004). Pediatric palliative care. *New England Journal of Medicine, 350,* 1752–62.

11 Stoll, R. (1979). Guidelines for Spiritual Assessment. *The American Journal of Nursing, 79*(9), 1574–77.

12 McEvoy, M. (2006) An added dimension to the pediatric health maintenance visit: The spiritual history. *Journal of Pediatric Health Care, 14*(5), 216–20.

13 *Palliative Care for Children, A Training Manual for Communities In Zimbabwe,* Hospice Association of Zimbabwe (HOSPAZ) P.O Box, A1822. Avondale, Harare, Zimbabwe 2006

14 Dr. J.M.Waliggo & Fr.Peter Mubiru (2006). *Religious & Cultural Beliefs Surrounding Illness and Death.* Hospice Africa Uganda Health Care Professionals Course Manual.

15 Hospice Afrca Uganda Distance Learning Diploma Course: DPC 213. (2006). Unit 7. Religious and Cultural Beliefs Surrounding Death.

16 Matthiessen, P. (1995). *The Tree where Man Was Born.* Penguin (Non-Classics), New York.

17 Adapted from Hospice Africa Uganda Spiritual Leaders Course handbook.

Appendix 1: Approaches to the death of a child in Uganda

Concepts of childhood death in Busoga District (Northern Uganda)
By Beatrice Juru Bungu

Immediately after the death of a child, mourning starts. The body is bathed, dressed and wrapped in bark-cloth and positioned face up during mourning and then laterally and curled at burial. The body is bathed and dressed and put in a bed or coffin. A newly born child is never carried by the mother, but by an aunt or grandparents. During burial the body is wrapped in a white cloth. The heir of the family hallucinates during the mourning period and the small children of the family are held by their aunts on their laps. During burial a first born is buried in a sitting up position. Other children are buried in a lateral position. The burial is always at the father's home (or paternal relative's home if the father does not have land). A child is never buried at the mother's family home.

The family food is prepared separately from that of other mourners. Matoke (banana) skins are laid over the family's food, which is divided among the family members. This is believed to take away misfortunes and bad spirits. A shade is built for the body. Depending on the age of the child, prayer is said before burial followed by a feast. Cultural rituals are then performed after burial. Twins are believed to be special children with special spirits. Therefore, there is a great fear of the possible impact of those spirits on the remaining family members, especially the surviving twin. A twin is never said to be dead, merely that he/she has flown away. When a twin dies the mother does not mourn, they believe that when she mourns the second twin will also die; the body of a twin child is not passed through the main door to the house. If there is no side door, a piece of wall is broken and the body is brought through that. Surviving siblings are cleaned with herbs to prevent the spirit of the dead from affecting the children as it is believed that they might otherwise become sick and also die.

Concepts of childhood death Buganda People (South Central Uganda)
Florence Nalutaaya and Nabitaka Josephine

In Buganda, any child beyond 4 months gestation is taken to be a child. If a child dies between 4 months gestation and full term, no announcements are made. The body is wrapped in a cloth and the placenta (if any) is separated and wrapped differently. Both are buried together in a hollowed out banana tree in the banana plantation. If a child dies near or at full term, an announcement is made. A coffin can be used (if affordable) and the body buried on the same day as death in an ancestral burial place rather than the banana plantation.

If a younger child dies, the mother is not allowed to mourn or attend the burial as this may curse the other children to die. No announcement is made and the child is buried by the father and other family members at home. If an older child dies, announcements are made either on the radio or by micro-phone around neighbouring villages. The child is buried on the day of death, either at mid-day or 4 pm depending on arrangements. If a child is a twin, the child is not said to have died but to have flown. The relatives are not supposed to mourn or cry because this will make the other twin to die. Twins are buried in the evening around 6 pm.

Before burial a child's body is laid at the side of the room and not the middle. The body is bathed using the scraped out stem of a banana tree. The banana pieces are cut into small sizes and crushed. The close relatives each pick a piece and place it in the face going down to the feet. This is seen as a last farewell by the mother and relatives.

The body is then dressed by the mother. The bodies of all children are wrapped in a new sheet. The sheet used for carrying the baby on the mothers back must not be used as, if it is, the mother will not have any more babies. The mother must make sure that the sheet is always used when lifting the baby. Both parents wrap their own clothes around the child, so it does not become cold in the grave. These clothes must have all buttons, sleeves and hems removed. It is believed that nothing should be tied to the body so that it will be free to enter heaven and to communicate with other spirits, rather than coming back to haunt the living in dreams. The final wrapping of the body is a bark cloth. Sometimes paraffin is injected in the body to prevent the smell. Others may put a coin on the forehead of the child's body.

The body is not supposed to be passed through the main door. Either a side door is used or an opening is made in the wall. The time of burial is between 12 noon and 4 pm. The body of a dead child should never stay overnight, but is buried on the same day unless he/she has died very late. The child is sometimes buried with an egg-plant and a sewing needle in his/her hands. This is to put off cannibals who might otherwise steal the body (because the needle and egg-plant symbolize that the child is still alive – i.e. eating and sewing).

The children are allowed to attend the burial ceremony and some last funeral rites; this helps them to understand and to know the steps followed and done during the burial. This will increase their knowledge and meaning of death.

Concepts of childhood death in the Iteso People (Eastern Uganda)
Mariam Akiror & Josephine Muhairwe

The Iteso traditions vary with the age of the child. Stillbirths and newborn babies who die are buried under the veranda or in the house of the grandparents. No mourning takes place. A baby which lives for few days is mourned briefly only by the mother and in the open. Other people do not mourn but simply pay condolences. If a baby dies after living for more than a few days, he/she is buried at the cemetery. If a child is older than 2, the family and others mourn; but not for long. The surviving siblings of a child who has died of measles are bathed with special herbs including fresh milk from a local cow to stop them from contracting the measles. Lamentions are much greater than in adult death, as the next generation has been lost. Deceased children are buried in cemeteries.

If the child is a first-born and dies at birth, the mother must not cry as the tears prevent the mother from conceiving again. Similarly the grave of the first-born child is not cemented because this is regarded as blocking the chance of further procreation.

Twins are treated differently. Traditionally, the bodies of twins are placed in earthenware pots and placed in a particular place in the swamp. The deceased twin child is said to have flown rather than died. This is because of the belief that since they are twins, the twin sister or brother may die. The surviving twin will later be taken to view the body of the deceased and some rituals are performed. The mother of twins is also respected in the community and people endeavour to avoid annoying her because if she gets annoyed with you, you may get misfortunes.

The bereaved mother is made a necklace of thread with a grass and a needle is put inside the grass. This is worn for 2 weeks and the purpose is to control the breast milk from paining and flowing.

Breaking of news of a death of a parent to a child is done according to the age of the child. If the child is less than 5 years, they are just escorted to see the parent's body in a coffin. If they are older than 5 years, they are taken to a private room and explained in simple terms what has happened. The child is then dressed in something that has black. If they are boys or young girls their hair is shaven. Older girls are given a headscarf to cover their hair. The children are normally seated near the coffin during the funeral services. If they have to travel up county for burial, the children travel in the car that is carrying the coffin. It is believed that there may be some last communication between the deceased and the children.

Two or three days after the burial of the parent, the children are taken to be bathed on the grave of the deceased. This is done by the elder of the clan. They just wash the feet, arms and pour water on the heads. The water is mixed with some herbal plants. This marks the celebration of the first funeral rites.

Concepts of childhood death in the Bakiga people (Central Uganda)
By Charles Byarugaba

When an adult dies, the whole village gathers in the compound and a fireplace is made in the middle of the compound to indicate that this has been the owner of the home. The body is placed in the coffin in the middle of the living room indicating that this has been the owner of the home. The body can stay overnight depending on how the family can afford to look after the people who have come to mourn with them. Those who have some food stuff can bring for people to eat as long as they are there. When time for burial comes he is taken to the ancestral grounds for burial.

However, if a neonate or child dies people are not supposed to mourn and very few people are informed about the death of the child. The burial should take place in the evening of the same day the child has died. The father descends into the grave and receives the body from the mother. The body is not buried in a coffin but wrapped in pieces of clothing.

If an adolescent dies, he or she can be buried in a coffin. People are informed and mourners come. A fire is built, but only at the edge of the compound. A banana tree is planted beside the coffin to assuage the possible anger of the spirit of the adolescent at not having been married.

Chapter 16

Palliative care for adolescents

Justin Amery, Julia Downing and
Collette Cunningham

Key points

- 12 million (30%) of PLWHA worldwide are <25 years old and of these 9 million are between 15–24 and 6 million are young women.
- Adolescence is a time of rapid change: physical, psychological, spiritual and sexual.
- Adolescence is also a time of paradox:
  - it is exciting but also frightening
  - it is a time when one is a child imprisoned in an adults body; but also when one is an adult imprisoned in a world of rules and restrictions
  - it is a time to explore and search, but also a time to set roots and establish an identity.
- In other words: adolescence is not childhood, but it is not adulthood either. Adolescents form a distinct group with their own unique physical, emotional, psychological and social needs that are significantly different from those of adults and children.
- Health workers need to accept and understand these changes and young people's reactions to them, and not allow adolescents to fall into the gap between adults' and children's needs and services.
- In the African context, adolescence is recognized in many communities and cultures and marked with traditional rites of passage when adolescents learn about the expectations of their communities of them as adults.

16.1 Adolescent development

The WHO defines adolescents as individuals aged 10–19 years. In many countries within Africa, adolescents are married at a young age (from 14 upwards) and may themselves have children. In such situations, legally, adolescents may be seen and treated as adults if they have their own children and are therefore able to legally consent to treatment options.

In developmental terms, there are three stages of adolescence – early, mid and late. It is important to note that physical and sexual maturity does not mean there is emotional and cognitive maturity and this needs to be recognized when discussing issues around illness, death and dying.

16.1.1 General developmental stages

In broad terms, adolescent development can be summarized as shown in the table below.

Table 16.1 Adolescent development[1]

Area of development	Early 10–13	Middle 14–16	Late 17 years and older
Physical	Pubertal changes	End of pubertal changes	Sense of responsibility for one's health
Emotional	Wide mood swings Intense feelings Low impulse control Role exploration	Sense of vulnerability Risk taking behaviour peaks	Increasing sense of vulnerability Able to consider others and suppress ones needs Less risk taking
Cognitive	Concrete thinking Little ability to anticipate long-term consequences of their action Literal interpretation of ideas	Able to conceptualize abstract ideas such as love, justice, truth and spirituality	Formal operational thought Able to understand and set limits Understands thoughts and feelings of others
Relation to family	Estranged Need for privacy	Peak of parental conflict Rejection of parental values	Improved communication Accepts parental values
Peers	Increased importance and intensity of same sex relationships	Peak of peer conformity Increase in relationships with the opposite sex	Peers decrease in importance Mutually supportive mature intimate relationships

16.1.2 Factors influencing development of the individual adolescent

Just as in discussions of childhood development, it is very important to be aware that individuals may not fit the mould when it comes to emotional and cognitive development. Perhaps the biggest determinant of these is the individual's own experience.

An adolescent who has had a long-term illness may either have a very well-developed sense of illness, death and dying or, conversely, may suffer with emotional and cognitive delay as a result of their illness. In many cases both things can occur at once. For example, an adolescent may have a very advanced cognitive understanding of her own illness and prognosis, but may revert to a less mature emotional stage as part of an emotional reaction to that knowledge. Adolescents may throw temper tantrums to rival toddlers, but they may do that whilst also knowing and understanding more than their parents or health professionals.

There are of course numerous factors influencing how rapidly or slowly an individual develops. Some of the universal factors are listed below:

Social factors[2]:

◆ The presence (or absence) of close friendships outside the family.

◆ The effect of the peer group and peer pressure.

◆ Concerns about deviation from the perceived 'norms' of the peer group.

◆ The presence or absence of a sexual partner (or potential sexual partner).

Box 16.1 Case scenario – Winnie

Case study: Read the following case story and then try and answer the questions:

Winnie is a 15-year-old girl with HIV/AIDS and Kaposi's sarcoma. She covers the spots with boot polish and has just met a boyfriend. They have started sex. She tried to persuade him to use a condom but he refused; and she was too scared to tell him about her status in case he split up with her. She talks to her counsellor about her fears for him, but gets very angry and tearful when the counsellor suggests disclosing her status to him. It takes the counsellor a long time and several sessions to establish a constructive dialogue and Winnie eventually decides to disclose her status to her boyfriend. It turns out he is HIV positive too. They do not split up.

1. In what ways is Winnie demonstrating an advanced developmental stage?

2. In what ways is Winnie demonstrating a reversion to a younger developmental stage?

3. Even in normal times, adolescents have to deal with many challenges. What are the typical challenges that Winnie is facing, and what additional challenges is she facing as a result of her HIV and KS?

Psychological factors[3]:

♦ The ability of the individual to form a personal identity separate from the family.

♦ Concern about body image (in particular concern about the perceived gap between the way adolescents think they look and the way they would like to look).

♦ Perceived loss of control in the face of uncertainty and demands of the future.

♦ Questioning of and ambivalence towards perceived norms and values of society.

♦ The development of sexual awareness and maturity.

♦ Mood and behaviour changes.

♦ The wish to explore and test boundaries, coupled with a sense of invulnerability (often leading to physical and sexual risk taking).

16.1.3 Adolescents and sexuality

Sexuality includes the interplay of physical, psychological, social and spiritual aspects in the makeup of gender, gender roles, gender identity, sexual orientation, sexual preference and social norms as they affect physical, emotional and spiritual life[4]. Within Africa sexuality is important due to the very clear gender divisions in society.

Adolescence is a time when individuals develop their sexuality and the impact of illness and the prospect of death can impinge greatly on this development. Illness in adolescents may cause a delay in the onset of puberty. Therefore adolescents, in particular girls, may not feel normal or feel that they have failed to achieve societal expectations. Adolescents partake in risk taking behaviour and explore issues with regard to their sexuality and this has particular significance in Africa with the HIV/AIDS epidemic; adolescents who are already sick may run the risk of infecting others or being reinfected.

In many African cultures adolescents are expected to go through various traditional initiation ceremonies as they move from childhood to adulthood[5]. These initiation ceremonies can be difficult for adolescents who are suffering from life-threatening illnesses, and yet they need these to feel normal and included in society. The palliative care team needs to have an appreciation of these culture rituals and norms surrounding sexuality.

Evidence also suggests that adolescents with chronic illnesses are at higher than average risk for STD and pregnancy[6]. Care should therefore include education about family planning, pregnancy-related care and advice on prevention and treatment of STD[7].

16.2 Communicating with adolescents

Effective communication with adolescents is vital in palliative care. However, it can also be challenging. Some of the challenges faced in communicating and counselling adolescents within the palliative care context are as follows :

- It takes time to build trust and communication.
- If adolescents are not aware of their illness and included in decision-making, there is more chance of them defaulting or not adhering to treatment.
- They are less likely to seek health care from other sources so if they are not given the opportunity by health workers to explore the meaning of their illness, then they are unlikely to get this opportunity elsewhere.
- Lack of cognitive development can result in a reduced awareness of the consequences of the illness and decision-making.
- Adolescents have a need for positive responses from health workers even in the face of inappropriate behaviours.
- Adolescents have a need for balance between structure and freedom.

Information about communicating with children and adolescents can be found in Chapters 2 and 16; however, some quick tips for communicating with adolescents are as follows[8]:

- Creating an adolescent-friendly environment.
- Establishing rapport.
- Taking time to build trust and relationships before dealing with issues.
- Using activities, such as art and music therapy to help them explore feelings and difficult issues.
- Being open and honest about illness, death and dying and not making promises that you may not be able to keep.
- Assessing risks and discussing these openly.
- Ensuring that plenty of accurate and relevant information is available and provided to the adolescents.

16.3 The impact of life-limiting illness on adolescents

Adolescents may fully understand their disease, its prognosis and its effects on self and family. However, this understanding can be particularly threatening as they may not have formed fully developed adult defence mechanisms to help cope with the illness and its implications[9]. Defence mechanisms commonly used in adolescents include anger and withdrawal, both of which make communication with family and carers more difficult at a time when communication is crucial.

16.3.1 Illness experience of adolescents

The illness experience of adolescents will vary according to important influences on their life which may include[10–12]:

- An increased need to preserve normality (e.g. school attendance, etc.) even if this seems foolish to adults. Disrupted schooling and education is a particular source of anxiety.

- An increased gap between the perception of their actual body image and their ideal body image due to the physical effects of illness.

- The perception of the loss of personal control is exacerbated by illness and worsened by the tendency of parents to become overprotective at such traumatic times.

- Anxiety and uncertainty about the future are heightened in illness.

- Adolescents' psychological defence mechanisms often include denial, withdrawal and anger. These all mitigate against good and open communication, thus exacerbating the sense of the loss of control and increasing anxiety and uncertainty.

- Partly as a result of these factors, conflict may develop, often between adolescents and parents but sometimes between adolescents and other carers.

- Illnesses lead to changes in social relationships at a time when peer group support and acceptance are particularly important. The maintenance of support from and contact with peers is crucial.

It is worth re-stating that identification with a peer group is important for adolescents. In chronic illness, opportunities for peer group identification are limited due to poor health, changed physical appearance or impaired cognitive function that renders them different from their peers[13]. If adolescents are unable to attend school or join in social activities this can leave them socially isolated and lonely. This isolation can be exacerbated by friends moving on and forming new relationships and peer groups without them. In palliative care when addressing the needs of adolescents, it is important to look at different ways that they can maintain social inclusion with their peers. Whilst it is important for them to interact with other children with life-limiting illnesses, this should not be at the expense of spending time with other 'healthy' peers.

As part of creating their own identity and value systems, adolescence is often the time when young people question the meaning of life and look for reasons for pain, suffering, unfairness and punishment. For those adolescents whose illness may lead to death the prospect of an early death and the loss of future identity often gains increasing significance[14]. Therefore, palliative care for adolescents needs to include spiritual care and allow the adolescent to explore such issues including their lost hope for the future.

16.3.2 Relationships between life-limiting illness and poor care

Unfortunately, while adolescents with life-limiting illnesses need high-quality care, there are certain factors that they may share which actually inhibit good care. Thus, poor care can be made worse by these factors. In the West, studies have shown that adolescents with life-limiting illnesses tend to have particular characteristics which mitigate against good care. In the authors experience there is no reason to believe that these characteristics do not apply in the African setting. They include[15,16]:

- Low expectations for themselves and for their care package.
- Lack of knowledge of existing educational and vocational opportunities.
- Lack of self-advocacy skills.
- Low self-esteem.
- Lower levels of integration with peers.
- Heightened orientation to and dependence upon adults.
- Low educational aspirations.
- Poor knowledge of sexuality.

It is very important that health workers are aware of these characteristics and the negative effect that they can have on palliative care. Tips of how to involve adolescents can be found below; but – for now – take note of the importance of boosting adolescents' knowledge, self-esteem and confidence and also encouraging and supporting them to meet with peers, at every opportunity you get.

16.4 The challenges of palliative care for adolescents in Africa

Adolescents with life-limiting illnesses face grave challenges wherever they live in the world. However, in Africa, adolescents with life-limiting illnesses face huge additional burdens and challenges.

16.4.1 Psychosocial challenges

◆ Child and adolescent headed households: Many adolescents in Africa are heads of their house-holds, often caring for siblings, parents or other relatives. This work inhibits peer group iden-tification and formation, education and development of independence. On the other hand, many adolescents in Africa who are in this position talk of how these experiences can also help them become stronger and wiser (see Simbarashe's Story[17] below).

◆ School dropout: A study of commercial farms in Zimbabwe found that nearly half the orphans of primary school age had dropped out, and none had continued into second-ary school. Children who leave school are less likely to develop the skills necessary to abstain from sex or practise safe sex; they are economically vulnerable and open to sexual exploitation[18].

◆ Financial problems: Adolescents with chronic illnesses place a financial burden on the fami-lies, which may already be very severe due the illness of other breadwinners. These problems may lead to family break-up, with consequent risks to health and safety of all children and adolescents.

◆ Access to health care: In Africa access to health care is very poor, and so many potentially treatable problems go untreated, thereby increasing the burden of the disease.

◆ Stigmatization: HIV/AIDS and cancer carry particular stigmas, and at no time is stigmatiza-tion so painful as in adolescence, when it is essential for young people to make relationships and establish identities outside their families.

◆ In a similar vein: HIV/AIDS and cancer often lead to adverse body changes just at a time when body image is the least settled and the most worrying.

Box 16.2 Case scenario – Simbarashe

Simbarashe's story

Simbarashe Chiparo (18 years) is an orphan who is part of the Dananai supported orphan project, in Murambinda. Both his parents have died, and he lives by himself. He is benefiting from the orphan programme which has 15 members. They are running a gardening project supported by Dananai and he is the team leader being the eldest in the group. 'We as young people know who to help – just equip us and we can get going. I am excited about it and certainly welcome the noble idea.'

Simbarashe Chiparo, Dananai Orphan programme, Murambinda

Permission 1: Reproduced with permission from Jihn Snow International (www.jsiuk.com).

16.4.2 **Sexual challenges**

Adolescents, particularly adolescent girls, are vulnerable to sexual abuse and exploitation. That is not to say that boys are safe. In one study in Uganda, 15% of boys report having been sexually abused, many by teachers[19]. This vulnerability is increased when they are sick, do not have adult carers or have become ostracized or stigmatized in their communities.

It is hard for health workers to have to be alert to these concerns. However, the facts and figures presented below suggest that many of the adolescents we care for are either at risk of being sexually abused or are currently being sexually abused. If we do not recognize this and try and address it, we are not addressing one of the main causes of suffering in their lives. In other words, we cannot claim to be practicing good palliative care.

- In rural Malawi, 55% of adolescent girls surveyed report that they were often forced to have sex[20].

- In Addis-Ababa, Ethiopia, an estimated 30% (about 30,000) of prostitutes are women ranging from 12–26 years of age. The number of adolescent females engaged in informal prostitution may be far greater[21].

- In Zimbabwe, nearly 80% of all young people (age 15–24 years) who are infected with HIV are female[22].

- A study of female adolescents in Kenya revealed that 50% of the girls admit receiving gifts in the form of money, ornaments and clothes from their partners when they engaged in sex for the first time[23].

As if that is not enough, these vulnerabilities are made worse by a variety of societal and cultural factors in Africa. These include:

- lack of social status of young women before childbirth
- tendency for older men to seek younger sexual partners
- poverty and isolation leading to sexual relationship formation[24]
- reliance of young women on male partner for sexual decision-making
- peer pressure on young men to prove masculinity through sex
- limited access to information about sex and STDs
- early sexual relationships
- cultural expectations regarding sex and childbirth
- problems negotiating safe sex
- lack of adolescent-friendly health facilities
- parents with limited knowledge regarding STDs.

Finally, all these factors interplay with the physical and psychological developmental stage of adolescents (particularly adolescent girls) making them even more vulnerable. These include:

- Immaturity of genital tract leading to higher risk of STDs.
- Higher risk of risky sexual behaviour as a result of developmental stage and isolation.
- Exposure to risk behaviours from other infected peers.
- Increased fear and sensitivity to stigma and rejection leading to increased likelihood of seeking close physical relationships.

Box 16.3 A message from Gabelan about stigmatization[25]

I'm a boy of 17 years and I do not like the way people who have AIDS are treated. I have a message for those who have this disease: God will not allow you to have a burden that is too heavy for your shoulders. If you are HIV-positive, it is not the end of your world. AIDS is like any other disease. To those who marginalise these people I say:

"You are not even sure whether you have the disease or not. Do not treat other people like outcasts. Instead be faithful to your partner, use a condom, and be careful with your life. Show support and love to those who are suffering because of the disease."

Gabelan Marcopes Kanakembizi, Mashonaland Central

Permission 2: Reproduced with permission from Jihn Snow International (www.jsiuk.com).

16.4.3 **Challenges with adherence**

Most adolescents seen in the African palliative care setting will have HIV and some will have cancer. It is still too early in the history of ARTs in Africa to know the prognosis for adolescents with HIV, but we can be clear that poor adherence to ARTs will reduce life expectancy considerably. Furthermore, second-line ARTs are rarely available. If an adolescent has cancer (with or without HIV), it may well be that they are prescribed chemotherapy, and where this is available, it is also important to take this regularly and properly; however, in many settings within the region access to both chemotherapy and radiotherapy treatment is limited.

In both HIV/AIDS and cancer care, adherence to medication is crucial. Unfortunately, adherence to medication in adolescence is a problem world over. In the West, it is common for diabetic or epileptic teenagers to go through a phase of poor adherence. Although these lapses can have fatal consequences, this is rare, so the adolescent usually has plenty of time to adapt without serious consequences. In HIV/AIDS and cancer care, this luxury does not exist. With ARTs and chemotherapy, even if the adolescent decides to adhere again after a period of non-adherence; it is often too late. The HIV virus or cancer cells have often become resistant to therapy by the time treatment is restarted.

There are a number of reasons why adolescents are less likely than adults to adhere to treatment. These include the following[26]:

- ◆ Adolescence is a time of rapid development and uncertainty, so it can be difficult to follow strict routines.

- ◆ Drugs are a visible sign of being different at a time when stigmatization and peer pressure are particularly powerful.

- ◆ Adolescents often have a low self-esteem and may well be grieving for the loss of loved ones. These can both lead to the feeling 'what does it matter if I take them? I'm not really worth it anyway'.

- ◆ Use of alcohol and other substances becomes common in this age-group. Alcohol and street drugs make users more chaotic and may adversely interact with medications.

- ◆ Fear of the disease and of the treatment may cause adolescents to go into denial, and stop taking the drugs.

- ◆ Lack of understanding: health education and access to health information tend to be very limited in Africa. This can lead to a lack of awareness of consequences of defaulting.

16.4.3.1 Tips for improving adherence

Research in Uganda[27] with regard to adherence found that complete disclosure and strong parental relationships were related to good adherence in both children and adolescents at the Mildmay Centre in Uganda. Complete disclosure for adolescents was a key in their motivation for adhering to treatment and an understanding of reasons behind this. Thus, issues around disclosure of disease status for adolescents are important with regard to overall adherence to treatment.

The strategies for maximizing adherence are fundamentally aimed at giving as much control, information and autonomy to the adolescent as possible, thereby enabling him or her to make informed choices and also demonstrating that you trust him/her, which can boost self-esteem and confidence. Tips would include:

- Make it clear that you are giving responsibility for medication to the adolescent.
- Give plenty of age-appropriate education and information.
- Get them to document their medication, perhaps asking them to design and develop their own diary for the purpose.
- Set up support structures such as school teachers, parents, carers, friends.
- Ensure disclosure to key supporters so that they can keep a distant and supportive eye out.
- Connect to PLWHA adolescent support groups if they are available.
- Give plenty of positive feedback and encouragement.

16.4.4 Adolescents as carers

With the advent of the AIDS epidemic coming on top of the huge challenges posed by poverty, disease and poor nutrition, adolescents in Africa arguably have to face up to greater challenges than their age-mates anywhere else in the world. Challenges within the provision of palliative care for adolescents are not only found in providing the care for the adolescents themselves, but also in supporting the adolescents who are caring for their parents or who are heading households and caring for sick siblings. Maxwell's story is a common one.

Box 16.4 Written by Maxwell Chambari, Advocacy Officer for Hospice Association of Zimbabwe (HOSPAZ)[28]

Maxwell's story:

After the death of my mother I realized that I could have done things differently; I could have taken care of her and been of greater assistance to her before her death. Unfortunately, there was no one to prepare a teenager to care for a sick parent at home. Her illness came as a surprise and to me, death was a distant shadow. When my mother fell ill, our roles reversed, and I became the caregiver. This meant doing all the household chores, deciding what to eat, even taking her to the hospital. I found work and had to support us both. I was confused, life came to a standstill, and I felt trapped. As the days went by she got worse, and finally she died. . . . Of course I pray that AIDS will disappear from Zimbabwe, but I know that it is here for a while. I only hope that other children won't have to go through what I did – the pain of caring for a loved one on their own – but that they will be given the support they need.

16.5 **General principles of palliative care for adolescents**

The general principles of palliative care for adolescents are similar to those for adolescents with chronic illnesses.

Palliative care should aim to help adolescents to[29]:

- ◆ have the best possible quality of life despite their illness
- ◆ be in control as much as possible
- ◆ be clear about their personal identity
- ◆ accept their new body image
- ◆ gain and maintain some freedom from their parents without losing their support and open communication
- ◆ develop a personal value system.

These aims are difficult to achieve in health-care environments because of a number of factors, including[30]:

- ◆ the restriction of physical activities due to ill-health and health-care environments
- ◆ the threat of change in body image posed by illness and treatment
- ◆ the lack of privacy
- ◆ the threat to life of illness and treatment
- ◆ the use of anger, withdrawal and denial as defence mechanisms
- ◆ the change of environment and the effects of illness and treatment cause loss of independence
- ◆ professionals being caught between parents (who want to protect) and adolescents (who want independence and respect)
- ◆ separation from peer groups which can generate fear of rejection and undue dependence upon family and care professionals.

Palliative care should address the needs of the adolescent in a holistic manner. Health care workers should try to find out what is important for the adolescent and to focus on improving the quality of life. It is important that the adolescent is involved in decision-making for their care as much as possible and their assent should be sought for any treatment-related issues.

In the same way, you can maximize privacy and autonomy by getting the adolescent to undertake as much of his/her own care as possible (e.g. self-medication, etc.). At times tensions may arise between the adolescent and their parents and family so a balance needs to be sought to involve the parents but maintain the independence of the adolescent.

It is important to provide honest and realistic information about the effects of illness and treatment on body image and support given to help the adolescent adapt to any changes that might occur. Support may also be needed for peers to help them to accept their friend's illness and possible changed image and to involve them in caring for and supporting their friend. The palliative care team needs to be sensitive to the needs of adolescents to explore their fears, anger and other emotions as they come to terms with their illness in order to help boost their sense of control and independence. Adolescents may express the need for privacy and this should be respected where and when possible. As previously mentioned, adolescents present unique palliative care needs and these should be carefully assessed and care planned in accordance to these needs in such as way so as to facilitate normality as much as possible.

Education remains an important aspect of the adolescents care as school plays a unique role in our society and their development. Even when an adolescent is not expected to live long enough to complete their schooling, it is important that they be given the opportunity to continue learning and to maintain normalcy so that they can continue to 'fit in' with their peers.

Body image is always important, but never more so than in adolescence. Where a disease or treatment may have an adverse effect on body image, this should be disclosed and discussed honestly and realistically, emphasizing ways in which the body remains unchanged.

Finally, remember that adolescence is a frightening time even without having to cope with a life-limiting illness. Adolescents seek comfort from both their family and their peer group; so it is important that peer groups are involved wherever possible. One great fear that always needs to be addressed is fear of rejection. Therefore friends should be included in activities, events organized and a 'buddy system' utilized (using role models with similar conditions).

16.6 **Care of dying adolescents**

The aims of palliative care remain the same for dying adolescents as for that of children and adults. In other words, to provide the best possible care to adolescents is to enable them to die in peace, comfort and dignity.

The basic practise of providing palliative care to adolescents is also the same as in children and adults. In other words:

◆ establish good communication and rapport

◆ perform a thorough and holistic assessment

◆ draw up a problem list of physical, psychological, social, spiritual and financial concerns

◆ draw up and agree a management plan to address each of these problems.

However, given that adolescents have unique needs, there are some specifics pertaining to caring for the dying adolescent. Carr[31] noted the following specific issues that need to be taken into account. The study was on a Western population, but the authors' experience in Africa would suggest the same principles apply. These works seem to suggest that the needs of young adults with terminal illnesses are similar to those of young adults with chronic illnesses. However, there are some differences that need to be highlighted:

◆ Clinical depression is prevalent amongst dying adolescents (17%).

◆ Most dying adolescents are aware of their prognosis, yet often this is not discussed.

◆ Adolescents are capable of discussing their prognosis, but need to be able to set the pace of such discussions.

◆ Hospitalization and illness reinforce social isolation. This can lead to prolonged dependence of adolescents upon their parents.

◆ In order to counter the tendency of parental overprotection, the dying adolescent should be given opportunities to spend time and develop relationships outside the immediate family group.

◆ Adolescents have a great need to explore their emotions and fears, so a 'permission giving' atmosphere and staff who can facilitate this are vital.

◆ Practical issues such as will-making, funeral planning and writing good-bye messages seem to be very useful.

◆ Sibling relationships in this age group are often very strong, so good sibling care is important.

◆ There are frequently many professionals and carers involved in the care of a dying adolescent. Adolescents will however often select only one person with whom they will communicate, therefore adequate communication between carers can be a problem.

When setting about care-planning for adolescents with life-limiting illnesses, we recommend that you try and follow the following principles:

- Adolescents tend to need to seek and find reasons and are happier when they have them. Therefore try and help adolescents to find reasons and meaning.

- Adolescents need to feel some degree of control over what is happening, so involving them as far as possible in decision-making during life and helping them to plan for their death and funeral are important parts of the care package.

- Try to allow adolescents to ventilate and explore their concerns and fears. This should give them a degree of control[32].

- In early stages of illness, try to facilitate and encourage social contact. However, adolescents often have contradictory social needs as death approaches; they need to maintain a sense of belonging but they also seem to prefer to withdraw to a closer set of family and friends in order to focus upon their most significant relationships[33]. You might need to give 'permission' for adolescents to withdraw as death approaches and facilitate communication and sharing amongst their chosen intimate family and professional contacts at that time.

- Make sure that you give plenty of opportunities for discussing prognosis. Most dying adolescents are aware of their prognosis, yet often this is not discussed.

- Sibling relationships in this age group are often very strong, so good sibling care is important[34].

- Adolescents often use symbolic rather than direct ways to communicate their feelings and concerns: so 'play' or occupational therapy is important as in younger children. Drama, poetry, music and art are particularly appropriate for these age groups.

16.7 **Practical tips**

In many ways, the practical things you can do with adolescents are not that different from those you can do with children. However, perhaps the key differences are as follows:

- Adolescents usually want to involve peers.

- The fact that adolescents are able to think abstractly and symbolically means that music, drama, poetry and art are particularly helpful.

- The fact that adolescents like to seek meaning, reasons and patterns mean that opportunities to learn and discussions (especially in peer groups) are crucial.

16.7.1 **Making a memory box**

Adolescents may well find it helpful to work with their families to put a memory box together before they die. Meaningful items can be pasted into a book or placed into a box. Examples could be anything. See Chapter 14 for more details.

16.7.2 **Making a family record**

Making a family record can help a young person gain a sense of where they fit into the family and therefore their 'legacy' within the family after they have gone. Try to put together a family tree and include family photographs, documents, certificates and mementoes. Stories about the life of the dying adolescent and also about the people from whom the adolescent is about to be separated should be included. The stories are even more powerful if contributed by family members and friends, and this is often a welcome way for them to be involved. What was the funniest thing the person ever did? What was their best subject at school? What was the bravest thing they ever did?

16.7.3 Writing an 'adolescent's will'

On one hand, adolescents may have few possessions. On the other, adolescents may lead whole households. In both cases, but particularly the latter, it is important to discuss thoughts about what they want to happen after death and how they wish to be remembered. All of these things can be captured in a will. Where siblings or other people under the care of the dying adolescent will be left behind, it is vital to talk and plan what will happen to them, involving statutory agencies if needed.

16.7.4 Peer groups

Young people usually like to be together, particularly with others with similar concerns and problems. Try and arrange such a group and agree a programme of activities. These should include opportunities to:

◆ Learn and discuss important factual topics, e.g. about the diseases, transmission and treatments. You can use pictures or captions of common everyday situations to stimulate discussion (see the 'discussion starter' picture of the embracing couple below).

◆ Learn and discuss about broader issues, e.g. sexuality and safe sex, adherence and domestic violence.

◆ Discuss and share experiences of illness and health in order to enable mutual support.

◆ Fun activities within the abilities of the group.

◆ Symbolic play, art, poetry, music and drama: encourage poetry writing and reading, singing, praying, drama groups – all perhaps using the individual experiences of group members as spring-boards.

◆ Games: you can make up a number of games relevant to the group: two examples are shown below.

Box 16.5 Couples and sexuality: discussion starter[35]

Pretend you can hear what these young people are saying to each other. Discuss in groups what they might say to agree to not have sex yet but still cope with their sexual feelings, negotiate using a condom, agree to get tested and what would happen when they get their results. Be realistic. Explore what people really say and what can be said in reply.

Permission 3: Reproduced with permission from Jihn Snow International (www.jsiuk.com)

Box 16.6 The Wow Game[36]

Materials

Collect a wide range of materials and put at least five unrelated items into individual bags. You will need one bag for each small group. Suggestions: condom or other contraceptive, bottle cap, hat, diaper, kitchen item, food item, school item, tool, bus ticket, video or cassette tape, toy car, nature item (leaf, flower, stick, rock), etc.

Box 16.6 The Wow Game[36] *(continued)*

Play

Small groups must make up a health or sexuality related story using their items. They can act out their stories using their items. They can act out their stories to the larger group, with a prize to different categories, e.g. most creative, most educational, most realistic, and most dramatic. In order to encourage players to make up more compelling stories, present them with a simple story invention tool developed by author Mary Amato, called WOW, which stands for Want, Obstacle, Win (or Lose). That is, most stories begin with Want: something, goal or desire of the main character(s). An Obstacle creates excitement and interest in the story. At the end, the character(s) either Wins (or Loses) in their quest.

Discussion

What themes are common in the stories? Are they realistic stories? What do they say about our society? Have any of you ever experienced a situation like one of these stories? Do you think people in other countries would make up the same stories? How might they be different, and why?

Permission 11: Reproduced with permission of Program for Appropriate Technology in Health (PATH) 2002 - Copyrighted

16.8 Questions for you

- ◆ Think of the last time you cared for an adolescent with a serious or life-limiting illness. What do you think you did well and what do you think you did not do so well?

- ◆ Having read this chapter, what would you do differently if the same situation were to recur?

- ◆ Try playing the WOW game by yourself and then reflect on the story you have created. What does your story say about you, your beliefs and your values. Have these changed since you were an adolescent? How?

Notes

1 Tindyebwa, D., Kayita, J., Musoke, P., et al. (Eds.) *African Network for Care of Children Affected by HIV/ AIDS (ANECCA) Handbook on Paediatric AIDS in Africa.* (Revised Edition 2006). Available online at www.anecca.org

2 AIDS Relief and Catholic Relief Services: *Psychosocial Care & Counselling for HIV Infected Children and Adolescents: A Training Curriculum.* Catholic Relief Services 228 W. Lexington St. Baltimore, Maryland 21201-3413 | 888-277-7575 | info@crs.org. January 2008 (in press).

3 Coleman, J. (1984). The Nature of Adolescence (3rd Edition). Methuen, London.

4 Module 7: Working with Adolescents in AIDS Relief and Catholic Relief Services: *Psychosocial Care & Counselling for HIV Infected Children and Adolescents: A Training Curriculum.* Catholic Relief Services 228 W. Lexington St. Baltimore, Maryland 21201-3413 | 888-277-7575 | info@crs.org. January 2008 (in press)

5 Tindyebwa, D., Kayita, J., Musoke, P., et al. (Eds). *African Network for Care of Children Affected by HIV/ AIDS (ANECCA) Handbook on Paediatric AIDS in Africa.* (Revised Edition 2006). Available online at www.anecca.org

6 Choquet, M., Du Pasquier, F.L. & Manfredi, R. (1997). Sexual Behaviour among Adolescents Reporting Chronic Conditions: A French National Survey. *Journal of Adolescent Health, 20*(1), 62–7.

7 Viner, R. & Keane, M. (1998). Youth Matters. Evidence-based Best Practice for the Care of Young People in Hospital. Caring for Children in The Health Services. London.

8 Module 7: Working with Adolescents in AIDS Relief and Catholic Relief Services: *Psychosocial Care &*
   Counselling for HIV Infected Children and Adolescents: A Training Curriculum. Catholic Relief Services 228
   W. Lexington St. Baltimore, Maryland 21201-3413 | 888-277-7575 | info@crs.org. January 2008 (in press)

9 Evans, M. (1993). Teenagers and Cancer. *Paediatric Nursing, 5*(1), 14–5.

10 Evans, M. (1993). Teenagers and Cancer', In *Paediatric Nursing, 5*(1), 14–5.

11 Denholm, C. (1987). The adolescent patient at discharge and the post-hospitalisation environment.
   Maternal Child Nursing Journal, 16, 95–101

12 Viner, R. & Keane, M. (1998). Youth matters. Evidence-based best practice for the care of young people
   in hospital. Caring for children in the health services, London.

13 Stevens, M. (2005). Care of the dying child and adolescent – Family adjustment and support. In Doyle,
   Hanks, Cherney & Calman (Eds.). Oxford Textbook of Palliative Medicine. (3rd Edition). Oxford
   University Press, Oxford.

14 Stevens, M. (2005). Care of the dying child and adolescent – Family adjustment and support. In Doyle,
   Hanks Cherney & Calman (Eds.). Oxford Textbook of Palliative Medicine. (3rd Edition). Oxford
   University Press, Oxford.

15 Blomquist, K.B., Brown, G., Peersen, A. & Presler, E.P. (1998). Transitioning to independence:
   Challenges for young people with disabilities and their caregivers. *Orthopaedic Nursing, 17*(3), 27–35.

16 Stevens, S.E. et al. (1997). Adolescents with physical disabilities: Some psychosocial aspects of health.
   Journal of Adolescent Health, 19(2), 157–64.

17 Young People We Care Programme Zimbabwe HIV and AIDS Programme Available online at www.
   jsieurope.org/docs/young_people_we_care_v2.pdf

18 UNICEF, UNAIDS & WHO. (2002). *Young People and HIV/AIDS: Opportunities in Crisis.* UNICEF,
   New York.

19 Sebunya, C. (1999). Child abusers face mob justice. Aids Analysis Africa, 6(3), 15.

20 Njovana, E., Watts, C. (1996). Gender violence in Zimbabwe: A need for collaborative action.
   Reproductive Health Matters, 7, 46–52.

21 Bohmer, L. (1995). 'Adolescent Reproductive Health in Ethiopia: An Investigation of Needs, Current
   Policies and Programs. Pacific Institute of Women's Health, Los Angeles, CA.

22 WHO World Health Report (2003). Shaping The Future. WHO, Geneva. Available online at www.
   Who.Int/Whr/2003/Chapter1/En/Index2.Html Department For International Development (DFID).

23 Wjau, W. & Radeny, S. (1995). Sexuality among Adolescents in Kenya. Association for the Promotion
   of Adolescent Health, Nairobi, Kenya.

24 Mulemi, et al. (2008). Relief and Catholic Relief Services: Psychosocial Care & Counselling for HIV
   Infected Children and Adolescents: A Training Curriculum. Catholic Relief Services 228 W. Lexington
   St. Baltimore, Maryland 21201-3413 | 888-277-7575 | info@crs.org. (in press)

25 Young People We Care Programme Zimbabwe HIV and AIDS Programme. Available online at www.
   jsieurope.org/docs/young_people_we_care_v2.pdf

26 Relief & Catholic Relief Services. (2008). Psychosocial Care & Counselling for HIV Infected Children
   and Adolescents: A Training Curriculum. Catholic Relief Services 228 W. Lexington St. Baltimore,
   Maryland 21201-3413 | 888-277-7575 | info@crs.org. (in press)

27 Bikaako-Kajura, W., Luyirika, E., Purcell, D.W., et al. (2006). Disclosure Of HIV status and adherence
   to daily drug regimens among HIV-infected children in Uganda. *AIDS Behaviour, 10* **Suppl1** (7),
   85–93.

28 Young People We Care Programme Zimbabwe HIV and AIDS Programme Available online at www.
   jsieurope.org/docs/young_people_we_care_v2.pdf

29 Weller, B. (1985). Paediatric Nursing and Techniques. Harper Row. London.

30 Mackenzie, H. (1988). Teenagers in hospital. Nursing Times, *84*(32), 58–61.

31 Carr-Gregg, M., Sawyer, S., Clarke, C. & Bowes, G. (1997). Caring for The Terminally Ill Adolescent.
   MJA, 166, 255–8.

32 Corr, C. & Balk, D. (April 1996). Handbook of Adolescent Death and Bereavement. Springer, New York.

33 Papadatou, D. (1989). Caring for dying adolescents. *Nursing Times, 85*(18), 28–31.

34 Papadatou, D. (1989). Caring for dying adolescents. *Nursing Times, 85*(18), 28–31.

35 Young People We Care Programme Zimbabwe HIV and AIDS Programme Available online at www.jsieurope.org/docs/young_people_we_care_v2.pdf

36 Story Taken From Games For Adolescent Reproductive Health – An International Handbook. Available online at Path.com. www.path.org/files/gamesbook.pdf

Chapter 17

Ethics and law

Justin Amery, Joan Marston
and Nkosazana Ngidi

Key points

- Ethics in children and adults can be different in very important ways.
- There are three key questions in children's palliative care. These are
  - What needs to be decided?
  - Who decides?
  - How do they decide?
- The most important principles in medical ethics are those of autonomy and informed consent. But children are (often) neither fully autonomous nor fully able to give consent.
- Health professionals may be as influenced (subconsciously) by prejudice and emotion as they (consciously) are by logic and rationality when it comes to decision-making in children's palliative care.
- Many of our decisions are based on ultimate beliefs of what is 'right'. However, ultimate beliefs are irrational in that – by definition – one cannot rationally support them.
- Therefore, in practise, most medical ethical dilemmas are resolved using a consequence-based approach.
- The problems with consequence-based ethics is that we cannot foresee all the consequences of our actions, and those we can foresee have arguable moral values.
- Children have rights, and the duty of health professionals is to uphold and protect those rights as far as possible.
- Many of the ethical dilemmas we face in children's palliative care in Africa are decided for us because we don't have the resources to carry out the ethical therapeutic options that are theoretically possible.
- By far and away, the most important skill in ethics in children's palliative care is the ability to communicate under pressure.

17.1 Introduction

In principle, ethics should apply equally to adults as to children. But in practise, ethics in children and adults can be different in very important ways. In comparison with adults, children may not fully understand their illnesses and treatments, and even if they can, they may not be able to communicate fully their thoughts and wishes. Children tend to have more developmental potential as well as quantity of expected life than adults, so the lives of children are sometimes argued to be of more value than those of adults. On the other hand, children's rights are rarely as well respected as those of adults, and so in some ways they are less valued. Children tend to arouse stronger feelings of protectiveness and empathy than adults. On the other hand, children are also more vulnerable to abuse and neglect. All of these factors can affect how decisions regarding children are made and communicated. In the children's palliative care setting, these decisions are absolutely crucial to the child's wellbeing, and often even life and death.

It might seem like a question with an obvious answer, but why should health workers understand the principles and practise of ethics? Well, firstly, all health workers have a duty to respect the life and health of their patients. In children's palliative care, where children's lives are coming to an end, this duty can often become very hard to carry out rationally and fairly. Health workers also have a duty to perform to an acceptable standard. This applies just as much to the ability to make and communicate difficult decisions as it does to the ability to diagnose and to treat our patients. We have a duty to maximize benefits for our patients and to minimize harms. Yet what is beneficial and what is harmful is not always clear or agreed in the children's palliative care setting. We have a duty to respect 'autonomy' (i.e. the ability to decide for oneself) of our patients. But in children's palliative care, we are dealing with children, who have varying degrees of autonomy. Finally, we have a duty to act rationally, honestly, fairly and professionally, all of which can be particularly difficult when in the midst of the emotional upheavals that often surround the death of a child.

17.2 Ethics in children's palliative care: the key questions

This handbook is intended to be a practical guide for health workers in Africa. In ethics it is sometimes difficult to hold the line between what can be quite an esoteric theory and philosophy and the need to have clear and simple guiding principles on which to act. However, in the author's experience, ethics in children's palliative care becomes a little bit clearer if you make sure that you can answer three key questions:

- What needs to be decided?
- Who decides?
- How do they decide?

Box 17.1 Case scenario – ethics

In this chapter, to illustrate the issues, we will follow the real-life case of a 6-year-old little girl we will call Esther (not her real name). Esther was referred to Hospice Africa by a community volunteer who was worried about her. Charles (our Children's Services Coordinator) and I visited her in a small brick house with no running water or power on the outskirts of Kampala. We were told that she lived with her mother, who was separated from the father, and that she had no siblings. We were also told that she had advanced HIV/AIDS.

When we arrived we found the house shut up and locked. We assumed the family were out until we heard a faint crying from within. On asking the neighbours we eventually found that one held a key and so we let ourselves in. The neighbour informed us that the mother had gone out to the shop and would be back soon. We found Esther in bed in the dark, in a dry nappy. She was small for her age, with fixed contractures in her arms and legs, lying on her side and crying and moaning faintly. She had frequent myoclonic jerks and regular shakes that probably signified some low-level seizure activity. She did not obviously register our presence but her moaning did settle when she was picked up and cuddled. When we examined her we found that her chest, cardiovascular system and

Box 17.1 Case scenario – ethics *(continued)*

abdomen were clear. Her neurological system was grossly abnormal. She had fixed flexion of the arms and extension of the legs, with marked clonus in the ankles. She had occasional spinal spasm with arching as well as localised and generalised seizure activity. We could not assess her vision but she did startle to loud sounds, suggesting her hearing was at least partially intact. We found packs of ARTs and some anti-epileptics in the house which had been prescribed by a local clinic, although most were out of date.

After examining her I made a provisional diagnosis of advanced HIV encephalopathy with global neurological regression. After discussions with the neighbour we satisfied ourselves that there were no acute symptoms to manage. We debated whether or not to prescribe something for her dystonia, but, in view of the relative ineffectiveness and frequent side effects associated with treatment for dystonia, decided it would be in Esther's best interests to wait until we had a chance to assess her with her mother and get a fuller history. We told the neighbour to ask Esther's mother to bring her to hospice the next day.

When they visited as planned, we were able to get a better history from Esther's mother, who we shall call Mary (not her real name). Mary was HIV positive and very poor, surviving on less than $20/month from a cleaning job. She told us that Esther was diagnosed HIV positive after she began to develop seizures and recurrent chest infections at around two years old. Since then she had begun to lose all her skills. She could no longer walk, talk, bathe or feed herself. She had difficulty swallowing and tended to choke on food, also suffering with recurrent chest infections. Mary had no local family, having been excluded from her family back in the village. She could just make ends meet with her small wage, but could neither afford to give up work nor to afford a carer. Therefore she was forced to leave her at home under the care of the neighbour, even though she knew the neighbour did not take good care of Esther. She told us that a benevolent expatriate had originally funded her to visit a local clinic, where the doctor had started Esther on ARTs and anti-epileptic. Unfortunately, the benefactor had recently stopped funding and Mary could no longer afford to see the doctor or to buy medications.

17.3 **What needs to be decided?**

This is probably the most important step in trying to manage ethical dilemmas. If we are not clear about the dilemma, it becomes very difficult to manage the case properly. Therefore, when faced by an ethical dilemma, always try and define the ethical questions (there are usually more than one).

Box 17.2 Case scenario – ethical and legal questions

The Ethical and legal questions in the case of Esther

In Esther's case, there were a number of different ethical and legal questions that we had to answer. These included:

- *Should we break into a locked house?*
- *Should we report this as child neglect to the relevant authorities?*
- *Should we divulge who we are to the neighbour?*
- *Should we discuss Esther with the neighbour?*
- *Should we immediately take Esther into care or leave her in the care of the neighbour?*

> **Box 17.2 Case scenario – ethics and legal questions** *(continued)*
>
> ♦ *Should we examine Esther in the absence of her mother?*
>
> ♦ *Should we go through the house to try and find medications or medical notes in the absence of Esther's mother?*
>
> ♦ *After diagnosing Esther with advanced HIV encephalopathy, how should we break the news to the mother?*
>
> ♦ *Should we start new medications for Esther, either immediately or on review?*
>
> ♦ *Should Esther's ARTs be withdrawn?*
>
> ♦ *Should Esther continue to be fed, either by mouth or artificially?*
>
> ♦ *Should we give Mary some money from the Hospice's small and limited 'comfort fund' (intended for destitute patients) to help her with living expenses?*
>
> ♦ *Is what we are doing in the best interest of Esther?*

17.4 **Who decides?**

In medical ethics, perhaps the most important principle is that of informed consent[i]. That is that health workers must give patients sufficient information that they can make an informed choice about what they want to do.

17.4.1 **Can children decide?**

To be autonomous you need to have several attributes. Exactly what these are can be argued. However, for the purposes of this chapter, in the medical setting (and in the UK law)[1] an autonomous person needs to be able to:

♦ understand relevant information

♦ believe this information applies to him or herself

♦ remember this information

♦ use the information to make decisions

♦ communicate the decision to other relevant people.

A person that has all these attributes is said to be *competent*. It will be immediately clear to readers that, when it comes to children, some or all of these attributes may be lacking. Children's ability to understand, believe, remember, use and communicate information is influenced

---

[i] For those that are interested, the principle of informed consent comes from the principle of the primacy of human autonomy (Greek: auto = self, nomos = law, therefore autonomy is the ability to govern/decide for oneself). Health workers have a primary duty to respect the wishes of their patients, even if the patients wish to take an option that the health worker thinks is not in the patient's best interests (for example, a patient who refuses to take ARTs for advanced HIV/AIDS because he prefers traditional herbal remedies). These principles were first described by Kant (see endnote), who argued that we should treat persons as an end not means (a powerful argument against slavery, servitude, forced conscription and other issues very relevant in his day) and also by Mill (see reference in endnote) who argued that if people are to be free to act, their actions should be unconstrained by others (a powerful argument for the rule of law and equality).

by many factors including their age, development, illness, awareness, understanding and their communication skills. In other words, very often, children are not fully competent to give informed consent to medical investigations or treatments.

However, that is not to say that children lack all competence; merely that their level of competence may not reach a level sufficient for the law. Health professionals still have to do what they can to inform and consult children whenever they can. A useful guide to the duties of health professionals is that of the Royal College of Paediatrics and Child Health (UK)[2]. It describes four aspects of child involvement in decision-making that health professionals should ensure are addressed wherever possible. These include the child:

- being informed
- being consulted
- having views taken into account in decision-making
- being respected as the main decision-maker.

Box 17.3 Case scenario – who decides?

Esther and competence

Esther was only 6 years old and, even if she had been aware and intelligent, it would have been difficult to argue that she was fully competent to decide for herself. Given that she had severe global neurological regression, and could not communicate except by moaning or crying, we had to conclude that Esther was not competent to decide for herself and had to look for other ways of making decisions about her care.

17.4.2 Essential 'ethical competencies' in CPC

Reading through the attributes of a competent person in the section above should also make you realize that competence also depends partly on the health worker, and in particular on the health worker's ability and willingness to *communicate* with children. As can be remembered from Chapter 2 – Communicating with children and their families, this is not an art health workers often excel at. When judging a child's competence, we should also turn the microscope on ourselves and check that we have fully carried out the duties that are vital if a child is to be given every chance of understanding and communicating their wishes. These would include the following (often neglected) duties that all health workers should be competent in:

- Understand how a child's understanding and awareness of health issues varies with age and experience.
- Know how to communicate with children of different ages and abilities.
- Be conversant in the child's language or have access to a competent interpreter.
- Know how to help the child retain and interpret health information.
- Know how to facilitate children's decision-making processes.
- Be prepared and willing to have difficult and painful conversations regarding life and death issues with children and parents.
- Help children communicate their wishes to others, especially family members.
- Be aware of their country's relevant laws relating to children.

Generally speaking, the evidence is that health workers tend to underestimate desire for information but overestimate desire to participate in decision-making[3]. The Institute of Public Policy Research[4] has recently argued that even children as young as 5 years old can have some limited self-awareness and understanding of the dilemmas surrounding their health care. On the basis of this claim, they argue that children above the age of 5 years should at least have their views taken into account when decisions concerning them are taken.

17.4.3 Proxy decision-makers

In the event that children are unable to decide, or (more commonly) that they can take part in the decision-making process but are not fully competent, other people have to make the decision for them. These people are sometimes known as 'Proxy decision-makers'.

Proxy decision-makers sometimes have a clear legal authority to make decisions and can over-ride the advice of health workers. In many countries though, proxy decision-makers do not have ultimate authority in decisions concerning a child. In these cases, it is the senior health worker that has ultimate responsibility for making the decision, even in life or death matters. Law varies from country to country but, in the UK, since Lord Donaldson's ruling on 'Baby J' in 1990[5] it is legal in the UK for health workers to decide to withhold or withdraw treatment from severely ill children, if it is considered that there is no hope of recovery. You should check the law in your own country. However, in most circumstances, even if the law gives you authroity to decide, health workers would be unwise to go against the wishes of the family, especially in life and death matters. There may also be gender issues related to proxy decision-making. Women may not be allowed to make decisions in some cultures. If there is a chance of a significant dispute, it is wise to seek advice from your government legal office.

One of the practical problems with proxy decision-making is that it is not always obvious who the proxy decision-maker(s) should be. If it is clear, there are sometimes more than one, each with different views. However, in most cases, it soon becomes obvious who the proxy decision-makers are once the health worker gets to know the family. Usually, it is the parents who act as main proxy decision-makers. Sadly, in Africa it is not at all uncommon for both parents to have died, leaving the question of who exactly has parental responsibility unclear. Even if both parents are alive and together, they might not agree with each other. Or, there may be other proxy decision-makers. In some cultures, extended family members, particularly paternal grandparents or uncles, may be very influential or even have a veto over important decisions regarding the health and treatment of a child. It has been our experience in hospice that, even once a chosen plan is agreed with the parents, a grandmother or uncle appears late in the day and either changes the plan or, in extreme cases, even takes the child away up country and out of reach of health services. It is therefore very important to work out who the main decision-makers and opinion formers are in each child's family early on, and to make sure that these people are included in the discussions as much as possible. Remember that there may be conflict between who the legal guardian is and who are seen as decision-makers within certain cultures.

It is also important to understand the limitations of Western ethics. The beliefs, values and conceptual frameworks used by other cultures must be considered when making decisions with families. The most appropriate source of information is the family itself as there will be considerable variability within cultural groups. There is some benefit however in understanding how ethical principles are applied in different cultural settings[6,7].

Box 17.4 Case scenario – consent

Case study on consent – Samantha

Eleven-year-old Samantha is a bright, loving child who was treated for osteosarcoma in her left arm. The arm had to be amputated, and Samantha was given a course of chemotherapy. She has been cancer-free for 18 months and is doing well in school. She is self-conscious about her prosthesis and sad because she had to give away her cat, Snowy, to decrease her risk of infection. Recent tests indicated that the cancer has recurred and metastasized to her lungs. Her family is devastated by this news but do not want to give up hope. However, even with aggressive treatment Samantha's chance for recovery are less than 20%. Samantha adamantly refuses further treatment. On earlier occasions she had acquiesced to treatment only to struggle violently when it was administered. She distrusts her health care providers and is angry with them and her parents. She protests, 'You already made me give up Snowy and my arm. What more do you want?' Her parents insist that treatment must continue. At the request of her physician, a psychologist and psychiatrist conduct a capacity assessment. They agree that Samantha is probably incapable of making treatment decisions; her understanding of death is immature and her anxiety level very high. Nursing staff are reluctant to impose treatments; in the past Samantha's struggling and need to restrain her upset them a great deal. Nevertheless, Samantha is included in discussions about her treatment options, and her reasons for refusing treatment are explored. Members of the team work hard to re-establish trust. They and Samantha's parents come to agree that refusing treatment is not necessarily unreasonable; a decision by an adult patient would certainly be honoured. Discussions address Samantha's and her parents' hopes and fears, their understanding of the possibility of cure, the meaning for them of the statistics provided by the physicians, Samantha's role in decision-making and her access to information. They are assisted by nurses, a child psychologist, a psychiatrist, a member of the clergy, a bioethicist, a social worker and a palliative care specialist. Discussions focus on reaching a common understanding about the goals of treatment for Samantha. Her physician helps her to express her feelings and concerns about the likely effects of continued treatment. Consideration is given to the effects on her physical well-being, quality of life, self-esteem and dignity of imposing treatment against her wishes. Spiritual and psychological support for Samantha and her family is acknowledged to be an essential component of the treatment plan. Opportunities are provided for Samantha and her family to speak to others who have had similar experiences, and staff are given the opportunity to voice their concerns. Ultimately, a decision is reached to discontinue chemotherapy and the goal of treatment shifts from 'cure' to 'care'. Samantha's caregivers assure her and her family that they are not 'giving up' but are directing their efforts toward Samantha's physical comfort and her spiritual and psychological needs. Samantha returns home, supported by a community palliative care programme and is allowed to have a new kitten. She dies peacefully.

◆ What are the likely consequences of continuing and resuming aggressive treatment on both her quantity and quality of life?

◆ What do you think about the decision that Samantha does not have sufficient capacity to give fully informed consent?

◆ What do you think was the most important competency of the health workers caring for Samantha and why?

17.4.4 **Facts, rationality and emotion**

Another practical problem with decision-making in the children's palliative care setting is that of dealing with the heightened emotion and the psychological defences of all involved in the care of the child. The theory of ethics might seem clear enough in the pages of a book, which can be read at leisure and in peace. However, in children's palliative care decisions are rarely made in such a conducive atmosphere.

For a start, for a good decision to be made, all decision-makers need to be in possession of all the facts. Without facts, decisions can become speculative and subjective. But, as any health worker will know, it is rare, particularly in an African setting, for all the facts to be available. Diagnosis and hence prognosis are not always clear, patients often have no medical records of previous consultations, investigations are either unavailable or unaffordable, language and cultural barriers are common, deference to doctors is widespread and may interfere with open disclosure and discussion. All of these, and many other factors, serve to cloud the picture and make decision-making very difficult indeed.

Box 17.5 Case scenario – proxy decision-makers

Esther and proxy decision-makers

It was clear almost immediately that Esther was incompetent to understand the dilemmas or to make her own decisions. However, when we met her for the first time, we were alone except for the neighbour, who clearly was not that interested in Esther, and so could hardly be a useful proxy decision maker. Therefore, we had to make our own decisions about whether to take her into care and whether to start new drugs. Later on, when her mother came to see us with Esther, it was clear she had Esther's best interests at heart and so she became Esther's main proxy decision maker. She certainly knew much more than us about Esther, her health and her happiness. However, even her mother could not act as a sole decision maker at that point, because she was not clearly informed of all the facts regarding possible treatment options. She had no record of previous consultations or tests, and she could not recall them clearly. Even later, when both Mary and we had a much better understanding of Esther, the problems and the management options, could any of us really have understood what life was like for Esther? In practise, proxy decision-making can be a very inexact art.

Even if everyone involved does have all the facts, making rational choices in emotionally painful and taxing situations is not easy, as empathy and psychological defence mechanisms invariably come into play. In any culture, the death of a child is a very difficult and painful thing, not just for family members but also for health workers. Do we really have the ability to make considered, rational, unprejudiced decisions in the heat and rush of the real world of providing children's palliative care in Africa?[8] Parents who have just been told of the possible outlook for their child may deny the problem altogether, or become wildly optimistic, or, conversely, sink into such desolation and despair that they are simply not capable of the careful and exacting logical analysis required to make a rational decision. Even health workers may not be as rational or fair as they would like to think either. In a study to determine on what basis paediatricians either withhold or withdraw care from sick infants in special care baby units, only 65% placed the best interests of the child at the head of their deliberations, 2% cited cost to society and 0.5% cited cost to the departmental paediatric budget[9]!

This brief discussion has shown up both the strengths and weaknesses of drawing on the principle of autonomy in ethical consideration of a particular case. What is clear is that we need a framework around which to decisions about what is in the best interests of a child. It is important to question to what degree children are competent to decide, and to question who should be the proxy decision-maker if they are not competent. It is important to question on what basis decisions by proxy decision-makers are made. In the heat of such painful human dramas, there is a danger that little consideration is given to the broader ethical picture and that decisions are made 'on the hoof', without adequate reflection and discussion. This is an issue that we must remain very vigilant for, and do our utmost to remain as objective, rational and fair as we can be.

17.5 **How do we decide?**

Once the dilemma has been clarified and the question of who should be involved in the decision has been settled, the final step in the ethical decision-making process is to decide how to decide. This may seem simple, but in reality the basis of how we make decisions for other people in the children's palliative care setting is far from clear.

In ethical theory, decisions can be of five sorts. These are as follows:

- decisions based upon beliefs, e.g. the belief that all life is sacred
- decisions based upon duties, e.g. the duty to act in your patient's best interests
- decisions based upon consequences, e.g. the premise that it is best to act in a way that will be likely to do more good than harm
- decisions based upon values, e.g. that health workers should act out of compassion, honesty and fairness
- decisions based upon rights, e.g. that the child has a right to the best possible treatment.

At first glance, there does not appear to be any problem. Most health workers believe in the sanctity, or at least uniqueness, of each life. Most health workers would agree that their prime duty is to act in the best interests of the child. In deciding what is in the child's best interests, most health workers try to calculate the consequences of the various treatment options available, and to choose the one that is likely to do the least harm (known as *non-maleficence*) and most good (known as *beneficence*) to the child. The health worker tries to be motivated by values such as compassion, honesty and fairness, and to repress such values as carelessness, laziness and greed. Finally, at all times the health worker tries to uphold the rights of the child to the best possible care available.

However, in practise (even ignoring the fact that many decisions we take are far more rushed, subjective and speculative than we care to admit), things are rarely that simple. In practise, we find that many of these factors can conflict with each other in children's palliative care.

17.5.1 **Making ethical decisions using a beliefs approach**

Regarding beliefs, one health worker might believe that all life is sacred[10], while another might believe that the value of life is based upon its quality[11,12], and therefore there are times when a person is better served by being dead than alive. This can leave health workers with a difficult dilemma and an ambivalent attitude which may go on to undermine their attempts to be rational and fair. So for example, in one study, 72% of senior paediatricians felt that 'there could never be circumstances in which it is morally permissible to actively take the life of an infant with severe defects'. On the other hand, 95% of the same sample had actually withheld or withdrawn treatment in cases of severe and multiple defects.

Question for you:

What are your beliefs regarding the sanctity of life? Do you believe the taking of life is wrong and that you should always do everything in your power to preserve it? Or do you believe there are circumstances where it might be legitimate to take life (for example late abortion for severe congenital abnormality or euthanasia for a child with incurable, unbearable suffering) or perhaps that it can be legitimate not to act to keep people alive in all circumstances (e.g. withholding or withdrawing tube feeding in a child who is dying and suffering)?

Box 17.6 Case scenario – ultimate beliefs

Esther and moral beliefs

In Esther's case, my own beliefs on the sanctity of life did not prove helpful; possibly because they are a bit confused. In general, I believe in the overall sanctity of life, and in general I have difficulties with abortion. I do not believe that it is ever right to actively kill a child, and therefore do not believe that euthanasia is morally right. On the other hand, there are circumstances in which I believe that a child's quality of life is so bad, and the outlook for improvement so remote, that it might be morally right to allow the child to die a natural death rather than intervening to keep the child alive. Esther was a case in point. She had a disease which had severely damaged her brain and all her faculties. She had distressing symptoms and no reasonable hope of recovery. On the other hand she could potentially have been kept alive with long-term intensive supportive care. However, my personal belief system led me to the conclusion that Esther's interests would be best served by being allowed to die. Other people might not agree with this. Some people who believe that life is sacred do not accept it is ever right to allow a child to die. They would argue that the fine moral distinction between possible acts (i.e. actively killing) and omissions (i.e. omitting to do everything possible to keep the child alive) is so fine as not to exist at all. They would argue that pushing someone into a river so that they drown is no worse than refusing to throw a drowning person a life belt[13]. In other words, they believe failing to keep someone alive is morally as bad as actively killing someone[14]. What do you think?

*** Rachels. (1975) Active and Passive Euthanasia. *New England Journal of Medicine* (1975, January 9th), 78–80.

17.5.2 Making ethical decisions using a duties approach

Regarding duties, it is clear from our training and from the Hippocratic Oath[15] that all health workers have a duty to protect life. But similarly, we all have a duty to act in the best interests of our patients. In a children's palliative care setting, these duties may conflict. For example, the best interests of a child might be that the child is better off being allowed to die peacefully than to be kept alive by painful and pointless treatments.

Box 17.7 Case scenario – duties

Esther and duties

Our duty towards Esther was clear, but the outworking of that duty was not. As health workers, we had a duty to act in her best interests. But what were her best interests? Obviously, there was no question that we had to do all we could to relieve her suffering and to ease her symptoms. But should we strive to keep her alive, or should we allow her to die naturally? Which was in her best interests?

17.5.3 Making ethical decisions using a consequences approach

Another way of trying to decide what is the right decision is to try and look at all of the management options available and then trying to predict the consequences of each. Using this approach, the 'right' thing to do is the course of action which involves the least harm (*non-maleficience*) and the most benefit (*beneficience*) to the patient.

This is the approach that health workers use so often; we are probably often unaware that we are doing it. Every time we prescribe a drug (all drugs are poisons, albeit useful poisons) we do two things. Firstly, we try and *predict* the future for our patient with and without the drug. Secondly, we make a *calculation of value*. In other words, we calculate as to which option carries the least risk and the most benefit. Sometimes, we even give extremely dangerous drugs which we know will make our patients very ill and may even kill them (e.g. chemotherapy) because we predict that the future with chemotherapy is less harmful and more beneficial than the future without it.

As can be seen, this approach, while very useful and pragmatic, is an inexact science. Firstly, none of us can clearly see the future, and so we may make mistakes (for example unintentionally kill our patients with our prescriptions when in fact they would have survived without them). This is known as the *problem of unforeseen consequences*.

Secondly, calculating the value of life is a subjective art. One person might think that a life without mobility, speech or eyesight is a life of such limited value as to not be worth living at all. Another person might calculate the opposite. In children's palliative care we are always trying to make this calculation of value of life on behalf of the child, yet we can never be sure that their calculation of value would be the same as ours.

Thirdly, there is an important ethical debate about whether foreseen but unintended consequences have the same moral value as foreseen but intended consequences/effects. For example, one might decide to give high-dose morphine and sedatives to a child who is in pain, breathless and nearing the end-of-life. The intent here is to relieve pain and breathlessness. The foreseen consequences/effects would include relief of symptoms but also respiratory suppression to the point the child stops breathing and dies. The former is a foreseen and intended consequence/effect; the latter is a foreseen but unintended consequence/effect. In other words, you wanted to relieve pain; you did not want to cause death, but death was the consequence/effect of your desire to relieve pain.

This dilemma is called 'double effect' (because there are two sets of effects from the same action: intended and unintended). The solution to the dilemma is called the Doctrine of Double Effect (DDE). The DDE asserts that a bad effect, such as the patient's death, may be permissible, if it is not intended and occurs as a side effect of a beneficial action.

The DDE has been recognized by commonwealth law since 1957 which states that DDE may only be used:

- if the patient is terminally ill
- if the treatment is right and proper
- if the treatment is recognized by a responsible body of medical opinion
- if the motivation was to relieve suffering
- if the hastening of death may or may not be foreseen, but it is never intended.

Provided that appropriate drugs are given for appropriate medical reasons and in appropriate doses, this is not euthanasia. In practise, this dilemma is less of a problem than lay-people believe. It is actually very rare in children's palliative care to see respiratory arrest from sensible use of analgesia or sedatives, and in fact good palliative care does not generally have a life-shortening effect. Effective symptom control is just as likely to extend as shorten life.

Box 17.8 Case scenario – consequences

Esther and consequences

With Esther, we first had to try and predict how the future would look. After discussing her case with experts in the field of HIV/AIDS neurology we established that it was extremely unlikely (to the point of certainty) that she would recover any significant neurological function. If she continued her ARTs, she might remain alive for a long time whereas, if she stopped them, it was likely that the HIV/AIDS would progress and she would die sooner than if she continued. If her HIV progressed, it was likely that she would suffer with Opportunistic Infections and other AIDS complications, including pain and other distressing symptoms. On the other hand, she might well have suffered with pain and distressing symptoms even if she continued ARTs. Either way we had a reasonable hope of controlling them using palliative approaches. Furthermore, continuing ARTs would involve increased costs for Mary, her mother. Even if she could access free ARTs, she would still have to pay for transport to clinics, and other incidental costs. Either way, Mary would have a very difficult time ahead of her, caring for a very disabled child with no support and minimal financial resources.

Overall then, we predicted two possible futures, as follows:

Future with ARTs	Future without ARTs
Likely to live longer	Likely to die sooner
Likely to have distressing symptoms	Likely to have distressing symptoms
ARTs and anticonvulsants interact	Esther needs anticonvulsants
ARTs have adverse effects	Stopping ARTs stops the risk of side effects
Costs of treatment higher	Costs of treatment lower
Mary to carry heavy burden of care alone	Mary to carry heavy burden of care alone

If the first step in this consequentialist approach is difficult (predicting the future) the next step is even harder. That is – trying to place a net value on possible futures on someone else's behalf. Remember Esther herself could not tell us which future she would prefer. So we had to do the next best thing and

Box 17.8 Case scenario – consequences *(continued)*

ask her mother, giving her all of the (distressing) information outlined above so that she could make an informed choice. She ultimately decided that the future without ARTs was preferable. Her reasoning was that both choices involved suffering and costs, but that the suffering would be likely to be longer and the costs higher if Esther continued ARTs. She therefore decided to stop them. She did not have ultimate say as, at least in Ugandan law, the ultimate decision must rest with the clinician (or the courts if the decision is disputed). However, we had no reason to argue with Mary, or not to believe that she was the person best placed to make a decision on Esther's behalf.

17.5.4 Making ethical decisions using a rights approach

Regarding the rights of the child, in children's palliative care we are all trained (and hopefully believe) that we must try to uphold the rights of the children we care for, as have been enshrined in the UN Convention of the Rights of the Child[16] and the World Medical Association codification of those rights which are relevant to health care settings[17]. At the level of principle, these rights cannot be disputed. Children must have the right to be consulted about their care and treatment and also the right to have their views considered. They have the right to be protected from harm and abuse and they have the right to achieve their full potential. They have the right to expression, rehabilitation, privacy, freedom from discrimination, family life and to hold religious beliefs. Ultimately they have the right to the highest attainable standards of care.

However, in practise, rights-based ethics are not so easy to apply. In children's palliative care, most health workers have many more than one child to care for, and so it is far from easy to make sure that each has the highest attainable treatment. Even if resources allow, health workers are not supermen or superwomen, and achieving the highest attainable care might occur at the expense of burnout and consequent failure to care well for future patients.

Box 17.9 Case scenario – rights

Esther and rights

On paper, Esther had many rights: the right to have her best interests guarded by her health workers, the right to be consulted, the right to be protected from harm and the right to the best attainable care. But, in the African setting, the sad fact is that we were unable to uphold any of these rights in any meaningful sense. So, for example:

How could we calculate the best interests of Esther, who could not communicate and whose experience of life was so markedly different from those who are deciding for her?

How could we consult Esther when we could not communicate with her?

How could we protect Esther from neglect, even though she was being left home alone so her mother, alone and coping without support, could earn some crucial money, in the absence of any meaningful children's social and welfare systems or financial & social safety net?

How could we honestly say that Esther was receiving the best attainable care when she had missed out on potentially life-saving ARV treatments because her mother could not afford them in time, and who also was missing out on even basic support care, again because her mother was so poor?

17.5.5 Making ethical decisions using a values approach

In some ways, values are easier to apply in practise than duties, consequences and right-based ethics, largely because value-based ethics focus on motivation rather than outcome. In value-based ethics, 'it ain't what you do it's the way that you do it'[18]. Health workers are expected to act out of compassion, competence, honesty and justice. According to value-based ethics, if we act with these motivations and within those parameters, we should find that our actions are moral, whatever the outcome. Indeed, value-based ethics is a very reassuring and grounding approach to ethics, but in practise, it cannot provide easy answers to specific dilemmas. For example, we may be genuinely motivated to act out of compassion, but, in caring compassionately for one child, we might find it hard to ensure that we care fairly and equally for all of them. We might want to be honest about situations and scenarios that are unpleasant, but we also want to be compassionate in protecting our patients from receiving and coping with distressing information.

Box 17.10 Case scenario – values

Esther and values

Hopefully, both Charles and I are motivated out of values that are appropriate to children's palliative care health workers. We are, we hope, compassionate people and had genuine empathy for Esther and Mary. We wanted to be honest with them, and did not shirk from sharing all the relevant information, even though some of it was distressing for Mary. We tried to be fair, ensuring Esther had all the resources she was entitled to, and also checking to make sure Mary and Esther genuinely qualified for financial support payments from our very limited 'hospice comfort fund'. But, overall, it didn't make the decisions any easier. On the other hand, it probably did help Mary and both of us feel that we had gone about things the right way and had done what we could. This feeling should not be underestimated, for patients, families or health workers. The feeling that 'we did everything we could' is a very powerful comforter for both families and health workers in the years following the death of a child.

17.5.6 Justice in African children's palliative care

One particular value is particularly hard to apply in the children's palliative care setting of Africa, that is, *justice*. Aristotle wrote that we have a duty to treat equals equally[19]. Health workers should seek to maximize benefit for patients within the limits of the resources available. But while few people would argue that medical treatment should be justly provided, there is far less agreement about what this actually means in practise. For example, how should finite resources be allocated? On which 'property' should judgement be based? Should it be 'an equal share to all', or 'to each according to need'? Who is to be treated equally and what does equally mean? Take for example a child born with multiple disabilities. Should he be treated in the same way as a fit and healthy child? If they both fall ill, who has more claim on resources?

One argument states that the greatest net increase in the quality of life will ensue by treating the healthy child because the quality of life available to the handicapped one is necessarily limited. This is a kind of 'don't throw good money after bad' argument. The opposite point of view states that the handicapped child has a greater claim because he has a greater need. If he does not receive the resources ahead of the healthy child, he is caught in a position of 'double jeopardy'. On the one hand, he needs more resources because he is sick, on the other hand, his very sickness renders his claim to greater resources less valid. So, while justice is difficult to argue with in theory, in practise justice is often in the eye of the beholder. What is just to one group of people (e.g. health ministries) may not be at all just from the perspective of another (e.g. parents of children with multiple disabilities).

Box 17.11 Case scenario – justice

Esther and justice

As Esther's case shows, without adequate resources, the health worker has very limited room for manoeuvre in most ethical dilemmas. He might have a duty to act in the best interests of the child. But with limited drugs, health workers and health facilities, children may go without even simple preventative, curative and palliative treatments. Children on one side of the globe are dying from diseases related to malnourishment and poverty, while children on the other side are dying from diseases related to obesity and affluence. The health worker might be able to calculate all of the possible consequences of starting particular treatments, but if the patient cannot afford the treatments, lives too far away to access them or has never been told about them, such calculations are only intellectual exercises with no benefit for the child. A health worker might want to act compassionately and fairly but, if her day-to-day work involves watching endless children die needlessly for want of resources sooner, or later her compassion will run dry and she will become burnt out and worn out. Perhaps the greatest lesson that Esther teaches us is that justice of resource allocations is probably the greatest challenge to ethical practice in children's palliative care in Africa.

17.6 Ethics and communication

The authors have many years of experience of dealing with children's palliative care cases and have had to deal with many difficult dilemmas, often involving life and death decisions and often in the most painful circumstances. Thankfully, in most of these cases there have been very few times where serious problems or disagreements have arisen.

Where problems have arisen, in our experience the most common cause has been where there is a pre-existing family conflict or split, with key decision-makers on either side of the divide. Another common theme is when difficult decisions have had to be made quickly, without proper time to inform, reflect and discuss the issues with patients and their families. Finally, problems within the care team have sometimes arisen where there has been a decision to withdraw life-sustaining treatment (particularly feeding treatments) and the child has then taken a long time to die.

In reflecting on 'what went wrong' with these cases, there is one theme that emerges each time. In each case there was a problem with communication. So many people are involved in dilemmas in children's palliative care: the child, the parents, the siblings, grandparents, uncles, carers, nurses, doctors, managers, volunteers, community workers, even sometimes lawyers and local leaders. Even though it is the child's own view that carries most weight, and then the parents', each of these people has a valid point of view, and each person needs to hear and to be heard.

What is more, some of the decisions that need to be made are complicated. Many require some technical understanding of the various medical options and treatments available. Almost always, people need time for the problems to sink in, and yet more time to reflect. Different people will be at different stages of understanding and acceptance. Peoples' emotional responses will be different.

> *This is perhaps the most important lesson of ethics in children's palliative care: communicate, communicate, communicate.*

We therefore suggest that there are some additional guidelines that, arguably, are even more important than an understanding of the ethical theory. These are as follows:

Tips for maximizing communication in children's palliative care:

◆ Involve everyone whose view counts in the dilemma.

◆ Be completely honest and open with all, within the confines of each person's intellectual and emotional ability to understand.

◆ Be absolutely rigorous: go through all possibilities and scenarios with all the relevant people.

◆ Don't shirk from difficult conversations, however difficult or distressing that might appear to be.

◆ Look for hidden agendas: people make decisions with their heads and their hearts, so look for the hidden agenda as well as the expressed agenda.

◆ Be absolutely fair: give each person a say, do not discriminate against anyone (especially the child) because of age, sex or background.

◆ Be compassionate but be fair: empathize, try and put yourself in everyone's shoes; but try to avoid siding with those people whose emotional approach most closely mirrors your own.

◆ And, most importantly, take *time*: all of this takes time. Take as much time as you can without being unfair on other patients or yourself.

17.7 Particular dilemmas in children's palliative care

17.7.1 Withholding and withdrawing life-sustaining treatments

Esther's case provides an example of a dilemma about whether or not to withdraw a life-sustaining treatment (LST). This is a very common and difficult dilemma in children's palliative care. In Esther's case, the potentially life-sustaining treatments were anti-retroviral drugs. Although there was little hope that they would improve her neurological problems or the quality of life, there was good reason to expect that they would help her fight off opportunistic infections and other HIV-related complications, and thus increase her life-expectancy. LST's don't just have to be drugs however. They might include chemotherapy for children with cancers, tube-feeding for children that cannot swallow, operations for children with tumours or congenital abnormalities, radiotherapy for cancers or intravenous fluids or drugs for children who cannot maintain their hydration or cannot take oral medication.

In these cases, it is the consequences approach which is usually the most useful. The health worker has to help the child and family understand all the different possible future scenarios and guide them in coming to a decision as to which future scenario is in the child's best interests, even if this scenario involves allowing the child to die. In the UK, the Royal College of Paediatrics and Child Health[20] issued simple guidelines as to the kind of cases where it might be appropriate to withdraw LST. These might be helpful here:

◆ Brain stem death

◆ PVS: where the child has a persistent vegetative state

◆ No chance: where the child has no chance of self-directed activity (most often severe neurological pathologies)

◆ No purpose: where the treatment has no purpose (e.g. in children with cancer where chemotherapy has little or no chance of curing the child)

◆ Intolerable life: where the burden of staying alive is arguably greater than that of death itself (for example where a child can survive only by being connected to ventilators and feeding tubes and with significant and distressing symptoms).

Box 17.12 Case scenario – witholding and withdrawing life-sustaining treatment

Case Study: Withholding and withdrawing life sustaining treatments – Themba

Themba was severely asphyxiated at birth. He took more than 30 minutes to breathe. He developed seizures immediately after birth, which were difficult to control. The initial cranial ultrasound revealed severe cerebral oedema. Subsequent cranial ultrasound showed severe leukomalacia (holes in the brain). Clinically, he had signs of severe neurological damage. He had to be fed with a nasogastric tube for a long time. At the age of 3 months, the parents were requested to give consent for a gastrostomy feeding tube (larger tube that goes directly into the stomach through the abdominal wall). This would also help in giving the child better nutrition and make feeding easier and safer for the family when the child was discharged. At the age of 4 months, Themba developed severe stridor for which he was taken to high care. This subsided without needing ventilation. During this period it was decided that he would not be ventilated even if the need arose. He became oxygen dependent. He then developed several infections, including pneumonia. Septic work up was done and each time infection was suspected and antibiotics started. The first gastrostomy started leaking and was taken out. The parents were requested to give consent again for a second gastrostomy, for which they refused. They said the first one did not work and they are therefore not willing to go through that again. The infant was now 10 months old, blind and probably deaf. The parents lived in an informal settlement and they therefore could not take him home, especially because he required home oxygen. The health care providers looked for a hospice where Themba could be referred but all the places contacted were full or could not cope with a child with a nasogastric tube. His parents kept on visiting him in hospital throughout his hospital stay. At the age of one year Themba died in hospital still weighing less than 5 kg.

Questions

◆ If you were part of the health care team, how would you have managed this child? You are in a busy, overcrowded public hospital with limited resources.

◆ Would you have intubated him when he had severe stridor, assuming that he needed ventilation?

◆ Would you continue doing invasive procedures and giving him antibiotics? For how long?

◆ Are the parents justified in refusing to give consent for the second gastrostomy? Support your answer. Would you consider a legal route?

◆ When would you start discussing palliative care with this family?

17.7.2 Euthanasia

Most discussion in paediatric palliative care centres around passive non-voluntary euthanasia or 'selective non-treatment' in which 'death is produced as a secondary effect by withholding or withdrawing the ordinary means of nutrition or treatment for the subject's condition'. It is important to draw a distinction here between good medical care and euthanasia. Good medical care involves making a judgement based on whether a given intervention is in the best interests of the patient. If it is not (based on benefits/burdens proportionality) then it should be withdrawn or withheld. The medical practitioner may predict that death will result but this is not the intention. Euthanasia (be it passive or active) centres on the intention to bring about the death of the patient.

Health professionals do not wish to actively end patients' lives. On the other hand, they do not wish to contribute to suffering by continuing therapies which are unlikely to benefit the patient.

'When a dying patient is receiving palliative care, the underlying cause of death is the disease process. In euthanasia, the cause of death is the intended lethal action'[21].

17.7.3 Child protection

Child abuse is an area that most of us feel very uncomfortable dealing with. The idea of children being abused is horrible, the difficulties in obtaining evidence considerable and the issue of having to accuse potential abusers in a family is something that few health workers have the training or experience to do.

Nevertheless, child abuse is frighteningly common (see Chapter 13 – Psychosocial and family care). According to some estimates, over one-third of children in Uganda are subject to physical, emotional or sexual abuse. Most of this abuse takes place within the family and by a family member.

It follows that a considerable proportion of children who use children's palliative care services are victims of abuse of one sort or the other or of a combination. Yet in the authors' experience, this is an area that almost never comes up in hospice care. The worrying conclusion that we are forced to is that health workers in children's palliative care tend to avoid the problem, or at least collude with avoidance of the problem.

Yet, ethically speaking, it is impossible to justify inaction. We have a duty to protect children from harm, being abused is not in the child's best interests, children have a right not to be abused and to be protected from abuse, and a compassionate, just and courageous health worker would not avoid or collude with avoidance.

For all these reasons, most particularly because of the issue of health workers' subconscious or conscious avoidance and denial (which led to the terrible case of the torture and death of a little girl called Victoria Kilimbie in the UK), all institutions in the West now are legally obliged to have child protection policies, to provide child protection training to all staff and finally to screen all staff for criminal records pertaining to child abuse.

One of the main problems facing child protection initiatives in SSA is the relative weakness of social and child welfare services in many countries. Even if one does identify a child who is being abused, often there is no infrastructure which can protect the child, prosecute offenders and rebuild a caring and safe environment for the child. However, just because the solution might be difficult, it is not an ethical or moral reason for not to act. All hospice and palliative care institutions in SSA should have child protection policies and provide child protection training for their staff.

Note that the most important directive in these policies is that health workers are expressly forbidden from using their 'discretion' in cases where abuse is alleged or suspected. In all cases, all staff members have to inform their line-manager who, in turn, has to inform the child protection officer, who, in turn has to inform the police, social and child welfare services. This compulsory chain, while possibly appearing dictatorial and heavy-handed, has been found to be the only safe way of getting round the problem of collusion, avoidance, denial and poor communication which undermine child protection efforts.

17.8 Conclusion

In one notable case, the author cared for two separate children with near identical terminal conditions at near identical stages and with near identical treatment options. To add to the tension, the children were in adjoining rooms in a hospice. In one case, we opted to continue life-sustaining treatment, and in the other we opted to withdraw it. In both cases, to both families, and to the care team involved, it felt that we had made the right decisions. How can this be?

It is sometimes thought that the study of ethics enables health workers to resolve ethical dilemmas more easily. Hopefully, as this chapter shows, the study of ethics actually throws up more questions than it answers. Each ethical approach has its strengths and weaknesses. None is a panacea.

However, the study of ethics is important because it gives health workers tools with which to begin to approach dilemmas. They may not make decision-making easier or even (as the example above demonstrates) more consistent. But they should make decision-making more objective, thoughtful, rigorous and thorough. In other words, they should help us to make better decisions.

Remember, dilemmas are only dilemmas because there is no easy answer. In trying to resolve ethical dilemmas, your view is important, but other people's views are important too. You may be a technical expert in the field of medicine, but when it comes to morality and ethics, every person's view is equally valid, so you should try to avoid using your status to influence the outcome (even though you may well be pressured into that by both family and colleagues). Most of all, while it is important to understand the theory, it is even more important to remember that good communication is at the heart of good ethics, and that good communication takes trust, time, openness, empathy and courage.

17.9 **Questions for you**

◆ Do you always seek the views of children over the age of 5 before starting treatments? If so, how competent do you feel in the list of essential competencies for health workers in children's palliative care?

◆ Do you know the law regarding the status of proxy-decision-makers in your country? If not, you should find it out.

◆ Are you just, or do you discriminate? We are sure that you would never knowingly discriminate against anyone on the basis of background, colour or sex. But what about age? Do you give children the same chance to express their views as adults? Do you spend as long making sure that they understand? Do you sometimes assume that you know what is best for them, or jump to conclusions? Do you sometimes hide information from them, even only to protect them? How would you feel if a health worker acted in those ways to you?

◆ Would you consider withdrawing or withholding treatment as euthanasia?

◆ Have you ever been involved in a case where child abuse was alleged, suspected or confirmed? What happened? Was the child successfully protected? Do you have a child protection policy in your institution? Have you been trained in child protection? Would you know which authorities to turn to if you came across a case of suspected or actual child abuse?

Notes

1 Legal case R, C. (1994). 1 All ER 819, in Ethics. *Oxford Textbook of Children's Palliative Care 2006.* (p. 56). Oxford.

2 Children's Palliative Care Guidelines. Royal College of Paediatrics and Child Health, London.

3 Barnes, J. et al. (2000). A qualitative interview study of communication between parents and children about maternal breast cancer. *British Medical Association Journal, 321,* 479–61.

4 Anderson, P. & Montgomery, J. (1996). Health Care Choices: Making Decisions With Children. Institute of Public Policy Research, London.

5 Dunn & Peter. (1993). Appropriate care of the newborn. *Journal of Medical Ethics, 19,* 82–4.

6 Gatrad, A.R. & Sheikh, A. (2001). Medical ethics and Islam: Principles and practice. *Archive of Disease in Childhood*, *84*, 72–5.

7 Da Costa, D.E., Ghazal, H. & Al Khusaiby, S. (2000). Do not resuscitate orders and ethical decisions in a neonatal intensive care unit in a Muslim community. *Archive of Disease in Childhood*. *86*, F 115–9. (Fetal and Neonatal Edition) .

8 Savlescu, J. (1994). Rational desires and the limitation of life-sustaining treatment. *Bioethics*, *8*, 191–222.

9 Outterson, C. (1993). Newborn infants with severe defects: A survey of paediatric attitudes and practices in the UK. *Bioethics*, *7*, 420–34.

10 Meilander, G.C. (1995). Body, Soul and Bioethics. (p. 50). University of Notre Dame Press, Notre Dame.

11 Glover & Jonathan. (1977). Causing Death and Saving Lives. Penguin, London.

12 Engelhardt, H. & Tristram. Jr. (1986). The Foundations of Bioethics. Oxford University Press, Oxford.

13 Beauchamp and Childress (pp. 115–126).

14 Sumasy, D. and Sugarman, J. (1994) Are Withholding and Withdrawing Therapy Always Morally Equivalent. *Journal of Medical Ethics* 1994, *20*, 218–222.

15 Hippocratic Oath. (1967). Ancient Medicine. In O. Temkin & C.L Temkin (Eds.). John Hopkins University Press, Baltimore.

16 UN Convention of The Rights of The Child. (1989). General Assembly Of The UN Convention on The Rights of The Child. The Stationery Office London.

17 World Medical Association Declaration of Ottawa on The Rights of The Child to Health Care. (1998). 50th World Medical Assembly Ottawa.

18 The Bangles: Audio CD. (1999). The Best of The Bangles

19 Aristotle (1959). Aristotle's Principle of Justice Shellens, Aristotle on Natural Law. Natural Law Forum, *4*, 72–100.

20 RCPCH (2004). Witholding or Withdrawing Life-Sustaining Medical Treatment in Children: A Framework for Practice. RCPCH; London.

21 HPCA Introduction to Paediatric Palliative Care Manual: Hospice Palliative Care Association of South Africa. Available online at http://www.hospicepalliativecaresa.co.za/index.htm

Section 4

Bringing it all together – caring at the end of life

By now, you will hopefully have a good and broad understanding of the physical, psychological, familial, social, cultural, spiritual and ethical issues that need to be addressed in helping a child and family achieve a 'good death'.

The next section deals with the final step in that process: the child's death itself. You may find that some of the content of previous chapters is repeated, but that is necessary for the sake of clarity. And clarity at this stage is vital. At the end of life, things have a habit of speeding up, just at the time the child and family are feeling most alarmed and vulnerable and just at the time when the health worker is feeling most anxious and lacking in confidence.

However, if you remember the four rules, you should be fine:

1. *Don't panic!*

2. *Immaculate assessment*

3. *Hope for the best, prepare for the worst*

4. *Treat what you can treat*

Chapter 18

Caring for children at the end of life

Michelle Meiring and Justin Amery

Key points

- It is often difficult in children to accurately determine the 'end-of-life' stage. Don't worry if you get it wrong, it happens to the best of us.
- Good palliative care neither hastens nor postpones death.
- The best way to manage end-of-life symptoms is to anticipate them and to prepare both family and staff for them.
- At all times maintain open and honest communication with the child and his/her family.
- Don't be scared to increase the morphine dose for pain as required.
- Don't be scared to increase other drug doses as necessary either. Remember the child is dying. Your priority is to try and ensure that he or she dies in comfort and dignity.

18.1 Introduction

In many ways, using the term 'end of life' is misleading. There is no clear cut off between 'middle of life' and 'end of life'. Sometimes people move from one to another seamlessly, sometimes suddenly, sometimes rapidly and sometimes slowly. The principles and practise of management of the child at the end of life is no different to that described in previous chapters.

However, as a child moves towards the last few days and hours of life, there is a different 'feel' to the experience for child, family and health workers. Everyone becomes aware that death is imminent, emotions become heightened, symptoms can develop quickly and the levels of fear and anxiety can rapidly mount unless things are handled well. Ultimately, this is the time everyone will look back on when deciding whether the child had a 'good death' or a 'bad death'.

For all these reasons, palliative care health workers tend to focus particularly on this stage, and it is sensible to write a special chapter for it.

18.2 What makes a good death?

The aim of care at the end of life is to ensure that the child has a 'good death'. As far as we are aware, we do not have any research identifying what children consider to be a 'good death'. Neither do we have any research in the African context (although see Chapter 15 – Spirituality for African interpretations of a 'good death'). However, research in adult palliative care suggests that patients think there are five components to a good death[1]:

1. Adequate pain and symptom management
2. Avoiding inappropriate prolongation of dying

3. Achieving a sense of control

4. Celieving burden

5. Strengthening relationships with loved ones.

The experience of managing death is of course different for health professionals than for patients and families. It is therefore not surprising that Western health workers focus more on how to avoid a 'bad death'. These are the factors that they think contribute towards 'bad deaths'[2]:

- Health worker time constraints
- Staffing patterns
- Communication challenges
- Treatment decisions that were based on physicians' rather than patients' needs.

Anecdotally, the results of both of these studies accord well with African children's palliative care. Children and their families here also look for a peaceful, quick, pain-free death, in which they feel in control and without fear, with their families around them and with having said everything that needs to be said. Similarly, we have seen bad deaths occur particularly because of lack of health worker time to spend with children and families; because of poor communication between health workers and both patients and colleagues; and because management plans are made without consulting adequately with the child or family.

18.3 How do I know when the child's life is ending?

It may seem obvious, but the first step in good end-of-life care is recognizing that the child has reached the end of his or her life. If you don't recognize a child is dying, you won't have time to make the necessary assessments and draw up the necessary plans. Without such assessment, anticipation and planning, it is far more likely that the death will not be a good one.

Such 'prognostication' may sound much easier in theory than it is in practise. Determining the end-of-life stage for a child with a non-curable condition can be extremely difficult. Unlike elderly people (whose vital organs have often degenerated with age) children can be remarkably resilient and will often surprise caregivers and health professionals alike by surviving what we may have deemed to be 'the last event'. On the other hand, children can also decline very rapidly and unexpectedly.

With advances in modern medicine, the 'end-of-life' can also be postponed through various interventions, especially in resource rich countries. Sometimes the end of life is preceded by a period of aggressive efforts to save the child's life which may make it difficult for the family to accept that the child has reached the end stage.

18.3.1 Patterns of dying

As far back as 1968, different patterns of dying were described. Glaser and Strauss described three patterns of dying[3]:

- Abrupt and sudden death.
- Expected death of varying duration (both short-term and lingering).
- 'Entry–reentry' deaths involving frequent acute deteriorations, often with hospital admissions, with an underlying steady decline.

Knowing the usual trajectory for both treated and untreated disease may help somewhat to determine the 'end-stage'. The disease trajectory for most malignant diseases no longer responding to treatment is fairly well defined. Once anti-cancer treatment stops working or is withdrawn the patient moves from following a pathway of slow overall decline in function to a pathway of fairly rapid decline just before death. These expected deaths are likely to have a fairly predictable terminal phase. In many non-malignant diseases, a trajectory consisting of periods of acute deterioration followed by improvement (usually due to treatment) but with a general underlying downward trend may make it more difficult to determine the terminal phase.

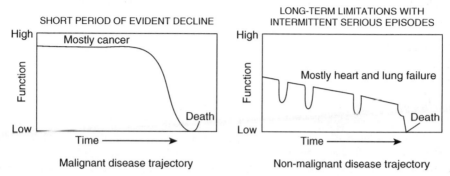

Fig. 18.1 Different disease trajectories.

18.3.2 **Prognostication in cancer conditions**

Prognostication in childhood malignancies is particularly well described, with certain malignancies having worse prognoses than others. Poor prognostic factors (age, sex, stage, genetic markers, etc.) have also been identified for most paediatric malignancies.

The survival rate for childhood cancers has improved dramatically in developed countries over the past 30 years due largely to advances in treatment. Sadly in sub-Saharan Africa and other resource constrained countries almost 60% of children with malignancies die[4]. Many are never diagnosed or are diagnosed too late. Even if timely diagnosis is made, treatment options are often limited. It is estimated that only 20% of the worlds' children with cancer have access to treatment.

18.3.3 **Prognostication in non-cancer conditions**

In contrast to children with non-curable malignancies, the end-stage of several non-malignant non-curable conditions is often less well defined. HIV/AIDS is an example of a non-malignant non-curable disease in sub-Saharan Africa where the disease trajectory can be significantly modified by the use of anti-retroviral treatment. There is also a subset of children (particularly in countries with diagnostic limitations) where the exact cause of a clinical syndrome (e.g. liver failure) is unknown, which makes prognostication very difficult.

18.3.4 **Indicators of poor prognosis**

Apart from statistical indicators of prognosis, there are other physical, behavioural and psychological indicators of impending death. These include:

◆ deteriorating vital signs
◆ loss of interest in surroundings
◆ decreased interaction with others
◆ loss of appetite
◆ decreasing urine and stool output

- increasing periods of sleep and/or withdrawal
- worsening laboratory tests (if being monitored).

Many professionals who have worked in hospice environments develop their own ways of knowing when patients are going to die. There have even been reports of hospice pets (e.g. Oscar the Rhode Island Cat) being able to correctly indicate which patient was going to die by curling up in the bed next to them a mere two hours before they died (animal behaviouralists believe that cats are able to smell some type of odour that is released by dying persons). Sometimes however, especially with children (who have remarkable resilience), we may get it wrong. Don't worry if this happens, it happens to the best of us. In addition sometimes children who we do not expect to die do so suddenly and without warning.

18.3.5 **Attitudinal barriers to accurate prognostication**

Apart from the abovementioned indicators of the 'end-of-life', there are several 'attitudinal barriers' that make identification of the 'end-stage' difficult. Deaths of children are still regarded as unfair[5] and there is still widespread belief that death is a failure rather than a natural event. Paediatricians in particular see the death of a child as a personal failure[6]. Since death in childhood is not regarded as normal, there is often denial on the part of the family and health care providers alike that the child is actually dying. Where the underlying diagnosis or prognosis is uncertain the reluctance to 'let go' and to still try numerous (both proven and unproven) therapies is still a strong driving force. When death does occur in such cases, it comes as an unnecessary and painful shock to the family.

18.3.6 **Importance of accurate prognostication**

Probably the biggest barrier to providing good end-of-life care is failure to recognize that the child is at the end of his/her life. Without a recognition that the child has reached the end of his or her life, there can be no discussion with child and family, no planning for management and follow up and reluctance on the part of both parents and health care providers to use certain drugs (which often become necessary at the end of life) for fear of 'causing death'. These myths need to be dispelled, and open lines of communication between the treating professionals and the family need to be maintained at all times. The dictum 'good palliative care neither hastens nor postpones death' should help guide most palliative care decisions at the end of life.

18.4 **What on earth do I say?**

At the end-of-life your communication skills need to be at their most attuned and sensitive. You will need to read the different verbal and non-verbal cues that the child and family are giving you; and then take the time to communicate carefully in order to assess their needs, anticipate problems and prepare for their management.

The aims of communication with the child and family at the end of life are to:

- ensure that the family (and usually the child as well) understands and accepts that the child is at the end of life
- ensure that the child and family have an opportunity to say and do what needs to be said and done before death

♦ ensure that the child, family and health professionals have planned for all (especially worst-case) scenarios and are aware of what to do (and when to do it) as and when these scenarios occur.

18.4.1 Breaking the news

> # Box 18.1 Case scenario – Joseph
>
> You are working in a medical centre. You have been looking after Joseph, who comes from up-country and who has osteosarcoma, with widespread metastases. Last week he started fitting and you suspect intra-cranial tumour, although you have no access to imaging. The fits are becoming more frequent and more prolonged. Over the last week he has gone off his food, become increasingly sleepy and his pulse has quickened and become more thready. From time to time he becomes confused and he often moans in pain. You are fairly sure that he has reached the end stage of his life. You know that his parents want him to die at home. You sit down to try to work out what you need to discuss with his parents. You decide that there are three big issues to discuss:
>
> ♦ To make sure that they understand that Joseph has only a short time to live.
>
> ♦ To make sure that they have a chance to say any final words to Joesph and make any final preparations.
>
> ♦ To discuss with them how they should manage some of the possible serious physical symptoms that might develop as he dies.
>
> How would you go about discussing these issues?

As can be seen from the case scenario of Joseph, all of these issues are effectively 'chunks' of bad news. The principles for dealing with these discussions are the same as for any other form of breaking bad news. Similarly, the principles of dealing with difficult discussions with children are the same as at other times. We will not return to the principles here, but you can remind yourself in Chapter 2 (Communication).

18.4.2 Discontinuing treatment

Very often, a child entering the end-of-life will be on drugs or other treatments which no longer serve any useful purpose. They will not stop the child dying and they are not relieving symptoms. In such a case, the sensible thing is to stop them. However, in practise, it is not always so easy. Both child and family may be reluctant to let go of what are powerful symbols of the fight for life, be fearful that harm will come to the child or be worried that stopping treatment amounts to a form of euthanasia.

The issue of withholding and withdrawing treatment is dealt with in Chapter 17 (Ethics and law), so we will not go into detail here. Your role is to help the child and family understand all the different possible future scenarios and guide them in coming to a decision as to which future scenario is in the child's best interests, even if this scenario involves allowing the child to die. In practise, you may decide to stop certain drugs which, strictly speaking, serve no purpose, as long as they are not actually contributing to the symptom burden the child is suffering. If they are, then you may have to explain your concerns more vigorously. In the end though, it is very rarely worth damaging your relationship with the child or the family at such a crucial time by forcing an argument about withdrawing treatments. If you need to beat a graceful retreat, now is the time to do so.

18.5 **How can I relieve the burdens of the child and family?**

What happens at the time of death has profound implications for surviving loved ones. A painful, traumatic death may leave survivors feeling guilty, angry and traumatized. A 'good death' can help survivors to look back on the positives of a child's life rather than being not tortured about the painful moments of death. Therefore, management at the time of death is crucial. Yet it is precisely the time when health workers often feel least confident and most out of their depth. This section aims to help you minimize the trauma of witnessing a loved one die.

18.5.1 **Remember the rules**

At no time are the four rules of good children's palliative care more useful than at the time of death. In case you have forgotten them they are as follows:

1. Don't panic

2. Immaculate assessment

3. Hope for the best, prepare for the worst

4. Treat what you can treat

Relieving the burden for children and families at the end of life is all about rules 1, 2 and 3: don't panic, keep assessing and planning and hope for the best and prepare for the worst. We will see no. 4 surface in the section on symptom control below.

18.5.1.1 **Don't panic**

- You might feel very nervous, even out of your depth.
- But however you feel, the child and family will feel much better if you look calm and in control (even if you don't feel that way inside).
- Calm is catching, as is panic. Panic helps nobody, so try and ooze calmness. It really works.
- If you feel like panicking, make an excuse to go outside for a bit (a mock phone call is always useful) until you calm down.
- Above all, remind yourself that:
  - the child is dying and there is nothing you can do to stop it;
  - it is a very sad experience for all, and you are not going to stop that either;
  - it is extremely unlikely you will make things any worse;
  - there are almost certainly symptoms you can control and comforting words you can say;
  - even if you feel there is nothing you can do, and however useless you feel, just by being around you are helping and making the experience easier for the family. So stick to it.

18.5.1.2 **Immaculate assessment**

Just as at any other time, the key to good symptom control is good assessment (please see Chapter 4 for a fuller discussion). At the end of life, things usually speed up and events can change rapidly. Therefore, whereas you might have been ok assessing weekly, you may need to start assessing daily or even hourly. Robert Twycross used to describe the 'rule of threes', based upon how quickly you think that the patient is deteriorating:

- If a patient is deteriorating every day: assess every 3 days.
- If a patient is deteriorating every hour: assess every 3 hours.
- If a patient is deteriorating every minute: assess every 3 minutes.

We realize that this might be impossible for you, particularly if the child is not dying where you are working; but you should at least pass the same advice on to whoever will be caring for the child at death.

18.5.1.3 Hope for the best, prepare for the worst

◆ The best thing you can do is go through all the worst case scenarios in your head in advance and practise exactly what you will do for each.

◆ We repeat … the best thing you can do is go through all the worst case scenarios in your head in advance and practise exactly what you will do for each.

◆ Have you done it yet?

◆ If not, do it now!

18.5.2 Offer choices and control to the child

◆ The child may or may not be conscious and aware at the time of death.

◆ If they are aware, try to do everything you can to give them choices and control.

◆ Talk through in detail what might happen (best and worst case). For each scenario, explain and agree exactly what the plan is.

  • e.g. *'You might start to get breathless over the next few days. That is to be expected and we can easily deal with it by giving you some medicines. Do you want to ask anything about that?'*

◆ Try to involve them in any plans so that they will keep active.

  • e.g. *'If you start to feel breathless I need you to help me. Can you do that? Good. What I need you to do is to concentrate on those special breathing exercises I taught you. Shall we practise them again now?'*

18.5.3 Offer choices and control to the family

◆ In exactly the same way, you need to do everything you can to give the family choice and control (don't forget the siblings).

◆ Talk through in detail what might happen (best and worst case). For each scenario, explain and agree exactly what the plan is.

  • e.g. *'Moses might start to get breathless over the next few days. That is to be expected and we can easily deal with it by giving him some medicines. Do you want to ask anything about that?'*

◆ Try to involve them in any plans so that they will keep active.

  • e.g. *'If Moses starts to feel breathless I need you all to help me. Mum, I need you to cuddle him so that he feels reassured, but not too tight. Try and make sure he can always see you. Dad, I want you to make a fan and gently fan Moses' face so he feels that there is plenty of air around. Esther, I want you to help Moses think about something else by doing his breathing exercises with him, and maybe singing him some songs when he gets tired. Can you do that? Good!'*

18.5.4 Remember

◆ Fear of the unknown is always greater than fear of the known.

◆ The whole experience will be completely new to the child, and probably to the family too.

◆ They will watch you like a hawk, constantly checking to make sure that you are able to guide them through the process with as little trauma as possible.

- The more they know and understand what is happening, the calmer they will be.
- So commentate on everything you do and think.
  - *e.g. 'Ok, I am noticing that Moses is starting to get a bit breathless, but I am not concerned as we can easily manage that. Mum, Dad and Esther, remember what we agreed for you all to do? Ok, go ahead. I am just giving Moses some medicine called diazepam. It will help him feel less breathless when it starts working in about 15–20 minutes. He will probably fall asleep too. If it does not completely work, I will give him some more. While we are waiting for it to work I will stay around, so don't worry. Do you have any questions?'*

18.6 How can I make sure the child dies without suffering?

As described in Chapter 4, at the end of the assessment process you should have a comprehensive problem list for the child who is coming to the end-of-life. As things can change rapidly, the list will probably need regular updating. However, you need to list the problems to ensure that you, your colleagues and the family keep track.

18.6.1 Checklist of things you might need to cover in the end-of-life management plan

In Chapter 4 (Assessment and management Planning) we gave an example of the 'PEPSI-COLA' management plan used in the UK as part of the Gold Standard Framework. This is an excellent tool for end-of-life care. We won't repeat it in detail here, but the main areas it suggests that you need to cover in a holistic management plan are as follows:

- Physical issues: e.g. functional, symptoms, drugs.
- Emotional issues: e.g. understanding, expectation, fears, relationships.
- Personal issues: e.g. family relationships, play, isolation, spiritual/religious needs.
- Social issues: e.g. nutrition, financial, housing, caring for carers, practical support.
- Information: Does everyone know what they need to know for the plan to work?
- Control: place of death, dignity, involvement in treatment options, will-making.
- Out of hours/emergency: Who will the family call in an emergency? What will happen? Do the family know what to do? Have they got enough drugs and information?
- Late: What is the end-of-life management plan? Has non-palliative treatment stopped?
- Afterwards: bereavement support for family, audit of your performance, opportunities for debrief and support for the team.

18.7 Symptom control at the end of life

Some symptoms that are seen at the end-of-life are intensifications of pre-existing symptoms. Management of these symptoms is covered in other chapters and will not be repeated here.

There is however a range of symptoms that occurs particularly towards the end-of-life. These include distressing and acute terminal events, pain, respiratory rattle, respiratory panic, seizures and terminal restlessness. We will also cover bleeding at the end-of-life, and the issue of artificial feeding.

18.7.1 Distressing acute terminal events

There is a generic approach which fits pretty much all these conditions[7] and it is described below.

The main aims of treatment of distressing terminal events are to:

♦ reduce pain

♦ reduce fear

♦ reduce the level of awareness of the patient.

Make sure that you (or the family) have the following available to be given immediately if such an event occurs:

♦ Diazepam PR (or midazolam IM/IV if available);

♦ Parenteral opiate (if available) or high concentration morphine for buccal or oral use (if not);

♦ If the child is already on these, simply give a larger additional dose.

Give strict instructions that these should be given if such an event occurs and make it clear to the person likely to give the drugs that *they will not be killing the child*. The child is dying from the underlying condition. The drugs are helping that death be less distressing. If you think they have doubts, either get someone else to take over or keep talking to them until they are persuaded. In the authors' experience, initial reluctance can lead to 'freezing' at the critical moment – and the worst of all worlds: the child dying a painful, distressing death.

18.7.2 **Controlling pain at the end-of-life**

Pain control at the end of life follows the same general principles as presented in Chapter 5.

In opioid naïve patients who present with pain for the first time at or near the end of life or who have not been appropriately treated for pain earlier on in their disease, it may be necessary to get rapid control over acute or chronic pain. This is best done using short acting morphine starting at the usual starting dose but titrating rapidly against pain (increasing by 1/3 of previous dose) with every dose if necessary. Remember also to prescribe additional breakthrough doses and to increase the amount of morphine in the breakthrough dose as the regular 4 hourly morphine dose is increased. Occasionally sedation with a benzodiazepine such as diazepam or midazolam may be necessary to assist with rapid pain control especially in very anxious patients.

Don't be scared to increase the morphine dose rapidly as required. Remember there is no maximum dose for morphine for pain, and events can change rapidly in the end-of-life stage. Also be prepared to anticipate and manage any side effects of morphine (nausea, vomiting, constipation, etc.) that may occur. In addition arm yourself with the necessary facts as discussed in Chapter 5 to dispel the myths that families and professionals alike may hold regarding morphine use at the end-of-life.

In many Sub-Saharan settings the only opiate preparation available (if any) will be oral morphine. If the child can swallow, this is usually all that you need. If the child is not able to swallow, you can have it made up to the highest concentration possible (100 mg/ml) and give it buccally or rectally. Another alternative is to give morphine via a nasogastric tube.

Some countries have modified-release morphine available, and this can be helpful. Remember though to still prescribe breakthrough doses of short acting morphine. Sustained release tablets should not be crushed to give them via a nasogastric tube, or the release will no longer be sustained!

18.7.2.1 **The syringe-driver**

In many instances dying children become less able to take medication orally and alternative routes of administering analgesics need to be found. Where available, the most common and convenient route used in children's palliative care settings is the subcutaneous route. The syringe driver is commonly used to ensure steady drug levels over 24 hours. A further advantage of this device is that the child does not need to be disturbed every 4 hours to administer analgesics by mouth and the parent (if he/she decides, for instance, to care for the child at home) does not need to worry about giving analgesics 4 hourly especially through the night.

For children previously on oral morphine, the total daily dose of oral morphine is calculated and divided by two to give the total amount of morphine to be added to the syringe driver. In addition to morphine, other drugs (e.g. diazepam, haloperidol and hyoscine) can also be added to the syringe driver to control other distressing symptoms at the end of life. Additional doses of morphine for breakthrough pain can still be given either by giving a pulse dose of morphine through the syringe driver or an additional oral dose. Please see the appendices of this chapter for further information.

18.7.2.2 Trans-dermal opioid patches

In addition to the syringe driver fentanyl or buprenorphine patches may sometimes be used in opioid experienced patients with chronic pain at the end of life. Unfortunately, the cost and lack of availability of these patches precludes their use in most resource constrained settings. The advantage of patches is that they only need to be changed infrequently and may be easier for some families to use above the syringe driver. Unfortunately, the smallest patches available are sometimes too strong for small children, and fentanyl patches cannot be cut. They are also rarely useful for controlling acute pain in the opioid naïve patient.

Please see the formulary for further information on using buprenorphine patches.

Converting from oral morphine to fentanyl patches is done using the table below. As the level of fentanyl takes 12 hours to reach therapeutic plasma levels, if you are converting from 4 hourly oral morphine continue to use morphine for 12 hours. If you are converting from slow release morphine (MST), then apply the patch at the same time as the last oral dose.

Table 18.1 Morphine to fentanyl conversion

Dose conversion of fentanyl patches							
4 hourly oral morphine (mg)	<20	25–35	40–50	55–65	70–80	85–95	100–110
Fentanyl patch Strength	25	50	75	100	125	150	175
24 hour oral morphine dose (mg)	<135	135–224	225–314	315–404	405–494	495–584	585–674

Breakthrough pain needs still to be managed in patients on opioid patches. The simplest and cheapest is to use oral morphine, if that is still an option. Otherwise other routes must be used – such as buccal, intranasal, subcutaneous or rectal (see Chapter 5 – Pain). Once the total amount of oral morphine (or equivalent) given for breakthrough pain over a 24 hour period equals or exceeds 135 mg an additional 25 µg Fentanyl patch can be added.

18.7.2.3 IV Morphine

In the hospital setting the intravenous route is more commonly used for patients unable to take orally as many hospitals do not have subcutaneous syringe drivers. To convert from oral to intravenous morphine, the total daily dose of oral morphine for 24 hours is divided by three. Intravenous morphine should only be given through an accurate intravenous pump by staff experienced in its use and able to monitor for side effects.

18.7.3 Noisy secretions: 'the death rattle'

Noisy secretions are caused because the child is no longer able to cough or swallow secretions in the large airways, usually because the child's level of consciousness is dropping prior to death. It can be very distressing to the family, who can think that their child is choking or drowning in his/her own secretions. In fact, it is almost certainly not a cause of distress for the child, and this needs to be explained.

18.7.3.1 Management

Table 18.2 Practical management of the 'death rattle'

Condition	Management
All patients	◆ Position the child with his or her head low, so that secretions can drain from the mouth.
	◆ Ensure that pulmonary oedema is excluded or treated with furosemide.
	◆ If you suspect that the child is distressed or breathless, treat with opioids and/or benzodiazepines as per the instructions in the section on breathlessness.
Where secretions remain a problem	◆ Consider using hyoscine butyl bromide (Buscopan) subcutaneously to reduce the production of secretions.
	◆ Review after 30 minutes and repeat.
	◆ You can repeat the doses every 4 hours.
	◆ Only use suction in unconscious children and only very gently.

18.7.4 Respiratory panic

Although less common in children than adults, respiratory panic often occurs at the end of a long illness. It is an episode of acute respiratory distress usually caused by a pre-terminal event such as airway obstruction, SVC obstruction, pulmonary embolism, left ventricular failure or aspiration. It is not a hysterical episode as some may believe.

18.7.4.1 Management

The quickest relief from this symptom is to use parenteral benzodiazepines. Oral or rectal benzodiazepines are appropriate where these are not available. Another option is to use nebulized morphine.

18.7.5 Seizures at the end of life

There are several causes of seizures at the end of life:

◆ underlying disease, e.g. primary or secondary brain tumours;
◆ metabolic derangements;
◆ hypoxaemia;
◆ acidosis;
◆ hypoglycaemia;
◆ liver and renal failure;
◆ precipitated by drugs (occasionally by morphine).

18.7.5.1 **Management**

Management of seizures is covered in Chapter 9 Neurological symptoms. However, a brief reminder is appropriate here. As with many other terminal symptoms, seizures at the end of life are often more distressing to the child's family than to the child him/herself. The child's family or caregivers need to be warned about the possibility of seizures at the end of life, particularly in high-risk cases.

Rectal diazepam usually helps to gain rapid control over seizures and may be administered regularly by the family themselves if the child is being cared for at home. Occasionally subcutaneous infusions of phenobarbitone or midazolam may need to be used.

18.7.6 **Terminal restlessness and agitation**

Sometimes, in the last stages of life, a previously calm and symptom-free child becomes 'agitated'. Conscious patients may not be able to keep still or get comfortable and may cry out or become emotional, hallucinate and delirious. An unconscious patient may become restless, start moaning or talking incoherently and appear generally uncomfortable

Terminal agitation and restlessness may have many causes. Often they may be due to the underlying condition itself, or metabolic changes due to the underlying condition about which you can do little. However, try and rule out the following:

◆ uncontrolled hidden pain (especially bed sores)

◆ urinary retention

◆ severe constipation

◆ hidden infection

◆ medication.

The only drug that has strong evidence to support its use for agitation in the palliative care setting is haloperidol. Many clinicians still use benzodiazepines but there is some doubt about their efficacy, in particular they may mask the symptoms from the observer, but 'lock in' the child with his or her ongoing delirium or frightening hallucinations[8]. However, there is a place for benzodiazepines (such as rectal diazepam or sci midazolam) as an add-on therapy for haloperidol.

18.7.7 **Massive bleeding/haemorrhage**

Although rare, massive exsanguination may be the terminal event in some diseases or their complications (e.g. Fanconi's Anaemia, bleeding varices in end-stage liver disease, bone marrow failure, etc). Decisions should be made in advance as to when hospital admission and emergency haematological support are going to be withdrawn.

A massive bleed can be extremely frightening to the child and the family alike. Where massive haemorrhage is a possible mode of death, families should be counselled and adequately prepared for it. Many will worry that the child is dying an agonizing death but fortunately in most cases of rapid bleeding, the child loses consciousness quickly and does not suffer. With less rapid bleeding, consciousness may not be lost and the use of sedatives (e.g. midazolam, diazepam or lorazepam) may be indicated to relieve the child's anxiety. It is important to explain to families that the sedative is not being used to hasten or cause the child's death but to relieve anxiety from what could be a very distressing symptom.

It is a common practise in palliative care settings to use dark sheets and pyjamas which makes the blood loss less apparent than if white linen is used. Other conservative treatments used for less severe bleeding at the end-of-life include tranexamic acid, Vitamin K and topical adrenalin for cutaneous or mucosal bleeds. Nasal plugs or ribbon gauze should be available in palliative care settings as part of emergency stock to manage epistaxis.

Given the high incidence of HIV in sub-Saharan Africa, all staff and caregivers in palliative care settings should know how to apply 'universal precautions' in the event of a massive bleed. Gloves should be readily available as should post-exposure prophylaxis in the event of accidental high-risk exposure.

18.7.8 Artificial feeding at the end-of-life

Withholding or withdrawing feeds at the end of life is a difficult and controversial topic. Further discussion on the subject can be found in Chapter 17 – Ethics and law. Feeding children arouses particularly strong nurturing feelings in parents and doctors alike, and withdrawing artificial feeding is probably the hardest of all treatments to withdraw. As an illustration, in a survey of paediatricians,

- 98% could deal with decisions not to resuscitate;
- 86% could deal with decisions to withdraw ventilation;
- only 42% could face a decision to withdraw feeds/fluids.

When artificial feeding is not available, the natural dying process sees a child's oral intake naturally decrease, and the reduced blood sugar contributing towards a reduced conscious level, which most people would see as a beneficial effect at the end-of-life. Most dying people are *not* hungry. Terminal anorexia is part of the normal patho-physiology of dying.

Artificially administered fluids can actually be detrimental in the dying patient, they can prolong dying and increase the likelihood of excessive secretions/pulmonary oedema. There are potential benefits in not artificially feeding a dying patient. These include:

- decreased metabolic rate
- decreased urea load
- decreased respiratory secretions, less cough and noisy breathing
- less nausea and vomiting
- less diarrhoea
- fasting releases endogenous endorphins which have an analgesic effect and actually increase pain threshold
- ketosis decreases hunger
- acidosis and ketosis depress the level of consciousness, decreasing pain and other distressing symptoms
- most patients 'slip away' quietly.

If you feel that artificial feeding is no longer indicated and might even be causing distress (e.g. vomiting, reflux, abdominal pain, diarrhoea and so on), the following questions might be discussed with family and colleagues:

- If a child who is able to swallow refuses food, should we force-feed against their will?
- Is artificial feeding going to hasten or prolong death and suffering?

The key to deciding when to withdraw fluids and feeds is to correctly predict the 'dying stage'. A more natural way of withdrawing feeds is to initially 'feed for comfort' if one feels that the child is hungry. As the child's level of consciousness decreases, the amount of feeds and fluids given will naturally decrease until feeding is completely stopped. Parents need to be sensitively counselled through this process and need to be assured that the child is not hungry and is not being starved to death.

18.8 **Checklist of things to cover**

However experienced you are, you will almost certainly find this all quite challenging. To try and help, we have suggested a checklist of things you might want to cover below. These would include:

- Assess the child and family: Carefully assess the physical, psychological, family, social, spiritual and practical issues that might prevent a good death.

- Identify the relevant decision-makers: Remember that, if you don't get everyone on board, someone might derail even the best-laid plans at a crucial moment; perhaps when you are not around to set things straight.

- Set the agenda for a meeting: Make sure that you 'name' all the issues early on, even if you don't cover them all in one go. It is important that all the decision-makers understand what needs to be discussed, and make time to do it. The meeting doesn't have to be formal, but it does need to happen, sooner rather than later.

- Meet and impart all the necessary information: In order to plan effectively, all decision-makers need to be in possession of all relevant facts. This is also an ethical obligation for you (see Chapter 17). Everyone needs to know what you know, what you don't know and what you suspect about the main issues on the agenda. If the information you have might be painful, use the WPC Chunk method in Chapter 2 to help. Don't be frightened about owning up to uncertainty. Children and their families know by now that you are not God, and they might have good ideas to share, even when you don't. Now it is not the time to get marooned on a pedestal.

- Agree which decisions need to be made by the child, by the family decision-makers and by the health professional decision-makers.

- Get the decisions made: If you think, for example, that one of your clinical colleagues might not want treatment withdrawn, or might not want the child to be discharged, you don't have much time left to get that sorted out. Busy as you might be, now is the time to grasp the bull by the horns. The worst thing you can do is allow a death to go badly simply through indecision.

- Talk about the quality of life: Explain how the child's quality of life might be adversely affected as death approaches and agree how you are going to manage these possibilities.

- Draw up a management plan: Where would the child and family like it to be? What processes of care will be needed to support the plan? What social and spiritual support would they like? What private conversations need to be had? Do any 'children's wills' need to be drawn up?

- Think about withdrawal of life-sustaining and other unnecessary treatment: There may be drugs, artificial feeds or other treatments that are no longer necessary. Do the child and family want to continue these? If so, does it matter? If it does matter, you need to explain why and reach a conclusion.

- Implement the plan: Get everything you need in place. Make sure that everyone has access to the relevant drugs and equipment. Check that everyone is in place and prepared, that the location is sorted out and that everyone knows who is doing what.

- Communicate, communicate, communicate: The chances are that the plan you come up with will involve many people: the child, close and extended family, friends and carers, professionals and others. Does everyone know what they have to do and when? *This is the area that most frequently goes wrong, so don't leave it to chance.*

- Plan for the worst: Safety-net. Give yourself a moment of peace to think about what could go wrong? Have you left any gaps? Is everyone clear? Do they have the necessary drugs and equipment? Who calls who if things go wrong?

- Give yourself a reward: When all is done and dusted, whether things went well and according to plan or not, give yourself a reward. What you have just done was emotionally and physically exhausting, frightening and often lonely. Even if it went badly, it probably would have been much worse had you not done what you did. Whatever it is you do to unwind (see Chapter 19 'Caring for Yourself') – do it and enjoy it!

18.8.1 The Liverpool Care Pathway

A useful checklist for end-of-life care has been developed in the UK, called the Liverpool Care Pathway. A version adapted for children's palliative care in Africa is laid out in the table below. It is recommended that each child and family has one of these checklists kept with them (either at home or in hospital) with a written care plan attached. The care plan should clearly and plainly identify which symptoms the child either is or is likely to suffer from, and a guide for how to manage those symptoms. We recognize that not all families will be able to read these plans, but often families can find others that can help. Ultimately, the benefits of doing this will be as follows:

- You will remember everything that you need to.
- You will remember to plan and discuss all eventualities with the child and family.
- The child and family will be clear about what the potential problems might be and what the plan is for managing these.
- Any other carers (family, voluntary or professional) who become involved while you are not around will have a clear idea of what the plan is and will (hopefully) stick to it.

Table 18.3 End of life care plan (adapted from Liverpool Care Pathway)[9]

Diagnosis and basic demographics	
Name	
Main family/carers	
Diagnosis	
Mother tongue	
Physical assessments	
Swallowing?	Y/N
Nausea/vomiting?	Y/N
Constipation?	Y/N
Confusion?	Y/N

(continued)

Physical assessments	
Agitation?	Y/N
Restlessness?	Y/N
Distress?	Y/N
Consciousness?	Y/N
UTI?	Y/N
Catheter?	Y/N
Resp tract secretion?	Y/N
Breathlessness?	Y/N
Pain?	Y/N
Other? (specify)	Y/N
Comfort measures	
Medication assessed and non-essential drugs stopped?	Y/N
Oral drugs converted to non-oral route?	Y/N
Has required medication started and are the family aware how to use it?	Y/N
Analgesia?	Y/N
Sedative?	Y/N
Anticholinergic?	Y/N
Anti-emetic?	Y/N
Anxiolytic/muscle relaxant?	Y/N
Stop inappropriate interventions? (tests, IV fluids etc.)	Y/N
Resuscitation status agreed and recorded?	Y/N
Syringe driver considered/set-up?	Y/N
Insight	
Child aware that he/she is dying?	Y/N
Family aware that child is dying?	Y/N
Spiritual	
Child's spiritual needs assessed?	Y/N

Family's spiritual needs assessed?	Y/N
Communication with family	
Who are the key family members needed for decision-making?	
How can these key people be contacted?	
Communication with other professionals	
Who are the key professionals involved and how can they be contacted?	
Care plan	
Has the care plan been discussed and agreed with child & family?	Y/N
Has the care plan been written down and left with the child & family?	Y/N
Do the child & family understand the care plan?	Y/N

CARE PLAN: Write each existing problem or likely potential problem below and describe the plan for managing each
PROBLEM 1(EXAMPLE): PAIN: Isaac may develop pain in his leg or chest. If he does, increase his morphine dose by XX ml every 4 hours, and review. If the pain is still present, increase it again by XX every four hours. Keep reviewing and increasing until the pain is relieved.
PROBLEM 1:
PROBLEM 2:
PROBLEM 3:
PROBLEM 4:
PROBLEM 5:

Notes

1 Singer P.A., Martin D.K., Kelner M. (1999). Quality end-of-life care: Patient's perspectives. *JAMA 281*(2) 163–8.

2 Beckstrand, R., Clark Callister, L., Kirchhoff, K. (2006) Providing a "good death": Critical care nurses' suggestions for improving end-of-life care.' *American Journal of Critical Care. 15*, 38–45.

3 Glaser, B.G. & Strauss, A.L (1968). *Time for Dying*. Aldine, Chicago

4 Dose, D. (2007). A day in the life of Oscar the Ct. *New England Journal of Medicine. 357*, 328–9.

5 Sheldon, F. & Speck, P. (2002). Children's hospices: Organizational and staff issues. *Palliative Medicine, 16*, 79–80.

6 Khaneja & Milrod, B. (1998). Educational needs among pediatricians regarding caring for terminally ill children. *Archives of Pediatrics and Adolescent Medicine, 152*, 909–914.

7 West Midlands Palliative Care Physicians. (2003). Palliative Care – Guidelines for the Use of Drugs in Symptom Control. Compton Hospice, Wolverhampton, UK.

8 BMJ Clinical Evidence Online – Delerium At The End Of Life. Available online at http://Clinicalevidence.Bmj.Com/Ceweb/Conditions/Spc/2405/2405.Jsp

9 Ellershaw, J. & Wilkinson, S. (Eds). (2003). Care of the dying: A pathway to excellence Oxford. Oxford University Press, Oxford.

10 Satbir Singh Jassal. (2006). '*Basic Symptom Control in Paediatric Palliative Care – The Rainbows Children's Hospice Guidelines*'. (6th Edition) (free for download at http://www.act.org.uk/content/view/100/1/)

11 North Cumbria Palliative Care. Syringe Driver Drug Compatibility Chart. Last Updated June 2006.

Appendix 1: Protocol for subcutaneous drug administration in palliative care

Adapted from the protocol written by Anita Phipps, RSCN Rainbows Children's Hospice[10]

Aim

+ Safe, effective administration of drugs for palliative care via subcutaneous route.

General points

+ Ensure that the child and parents/carers have been prepared. The aims of the syringe driver, the drugs to be administered, the siting of the butterfly, appearance and 'sounds' from the driver should all be explained to the child and carers by the doctor, with the nurse present if possible. The child and carers should be given the opportunity to ask any questions; anxieties should be acknowledged and reassurance given where appropriate.
+ The drugs to be administered, including the diluent, should be checked by two nurses who are trained in the use of the relevant pump.
+ Check that the following details on the drug chart are correct prior to setting up equipment and check against child's records: date, time, child's name, child's date of birth, weight in kg.
+ Check that the prescription is rewritten and signed by the authorizing health professional.

Drugs

+ Check that the dosage is appropriate by comparison with previous levels of oral medication or by comparison with the preceding 24 hours dosage administered via the syringe driver. Refer to pharmacy literature and check with prescribing doctor if in doubt.
+ As a general rule, on commencement of the syringe driver, the dosage of diamorphine over the first 24 hours equates to one third of the previously required total daily dosage of oral morphine, e.g. 20 mg diamorphine is equivalent to 60 mg oral morphine in the preceding 24 hour period.
+ The maximum recommended dose of diamorphine when used as the sole agent in a syringe driver should not exceed 400 mg/ml although such levels are unlikely to be used in a paediatric setting.
+ If more than one drug is to be used check compatibility by reference to Table 6.2. Where possible, the number of drugs used should be kept to a minimum, usually no more than two or three.
+ Check diluent suitability. Water for injection is the preferred diluent for most drugs except non-steroidal anti-inflammatory drugs, which mix better with 0.9% saline.
+ Dilute diamorphine prior to mixing with other drugs.
+ Do not use 0.9% saline to dilute cyclizine because of the high risk of precipitation.

Instructions for use of Graseby syringe drivers

This is the most common type of syringe driver, so instructions are included here as a general guide. You should however always refer to the manual provided with your own syringe driver before giving any drugs.

1. Assemble equipment:
   a. Syringe driver
   b. Battery

    c. Locking syringe (i.e. one in which the giving-set line can be screwed and locked into place 0 – usually 10 or 20 ml)

    d. Giving set

    e. Fine-gauge butterfly

    f. Clean dressing

    g. Diluent

    h. Drugs prescribed

2. Insert correct sized battery – alarm will sound for a few seconds.

3. Press start/boost button. Motor will run for a short while as safety circuits are checked.

4. Release start button.

5. Set the rate of delivery (see box below).

6. Draw up prescribed amount of medication in a 10 ml locking syringe and dilute with sterile water for injection. If using diamorphine, draw this up first by dissolving the contents of the vial in a known amount of sterile water for injection and discarding any excess amount of drug if necessary, i.e. calculate the correct volume of dissolved diamorphine required to obtain the dose required.

7. Once all of the required drugs have been drawn up, make the volume up to the correct amount with sterile water for injection. The total volume in the syringe is usually 8–9 ml which gives a volume infusion length of 48 mm. In calculating the total volume, sufficient water needs to be drawn up to allow for priming of the giving set, i.e. filling the whole line including Luer connectors. For most sets, this 'dead space' accounts for 0.5–1 ml.

8. Site butterfly – the reader should refer to the protocol for insertion of subcutaneous butterfly needle.

9. Start driver by pressing start/boost button. The light will flash every 20–25 seconds. Note that the driver can only be switched off by removing the battery.

10. Protect mixture from light and apparatus from accidental damage by using a holster or carry case.

Calculation of delivery rate
This depends on the make of pump. For the Graseby pump the calculations is based upon the length of the contents in the syringe (in *millimeters*) per *one hour*. Some pumps use *milliliters* and others use volume per *twenty four hours*, so take great care that you use the correct calculation. You risk overdosing the child, if you get it wrong.

Care of the infusion

♦ Check at intervals that the device is functioning correctly, i.e. the light flashes at regular intervals and those connections have not come loose.

♦ Check that the child remains comfortable and has an adequate degree of symptom control and an acceptable level of side effects.

Managing breakthrough symptoms

1. For breakthrough pain the start dose of diamorphine is the equivalent 4 hourly dose, i.e. 1/6th the total diamorphine dose over 24 hours.

2. Do not alter the rate of the syringe driver once set up. This makes it difficult to calculate the dose of drug that has been administered and can potentially lead to excessive doses of one or more of the syringe driver constituents being given. Either administer additional drugs orally or via bolus subcutaneous, intramuscular or other appropriate route or set up a new syringe driver containing an adjusted dose of drugs. Similarly, use of the boost button is not recommended on more than an 'occasional' basis.

3. Check the butterfly site for signs of infection or inflammation. Change the position of the butterfly each time the butterfly is replaced.

4. Check for cloudiness or discolouration of the infusion at regular intervals (indication of degradation of the drug or precipitation). If this occurs, discard and replace the infusion immediately.

Drug compatibility[11]

Generally there are few compatibility problems with common two and three drug combinations containing:

- Diamorphine
- Cyclizine
- Haloperidol
- Metoclopramide
- Levomepromazine
- Hyoscine hydrobromide
- Midazolam.

However there can be problems with:

- Cyclizine with diamorphine: Once diamorphine dose exceeds 200 mg/24 hours, cyclizine can cause precipitation with saline. This can be solved by using water as diluent. At higher diamorphine doses, either put cyclizine in a second syringe driver or use levomepromazine as a single daily SC injection instead.

- Hyoscine butyl bromide (Buscopan) is occasionally incompatible with cyclizine: Levomepromazine could be given as a single daily injection in place of cyclizine.

- Ketorolac has many incompatibilities: The main ones are with haloperidol, midazolam and cyclizine. Using a separate syringe driver is recommended.

- Dexamethasone has common/unpredictable precipitation: It also inactivates glycopyrrollate. This problem may be solved by using hyoscine hydrobromide instead of glycopyrrollate. Alternatively, dexamethasone could be given as a separate once daily injection.

Caring for yourself

No matter what drugs or techniques you use in children's palliative care, by far and away the most important tool you will use is yourself. It is you who communicates, you who assesses, you who analyses and plans and you who implements the plan. As a professional, you know that you would only use drugs that are fresh and effective. But how fresh and effective are you?

On the ancient Temple of Apollo were inscribed two sayings, believed to sum up the wisdom of all of the ancient philosophers. These were

'Know thyself'
and
'All things in moderation'

Do you?

Read on and find out ….

Chapter 19

Caring for yourself

Justin Amery, Mary Bunn, Susie Lapwood and
Gillian Chowns

Key points

- Children's palliative care is rewarding but puts a heavy burden on health workers.
- Being a professional is more than being technically competent. It is about being able to understand yourself, your strengths and your weaknesses.
- Burnout is damaging to yourself, your team and your patients.
- Each of us has built-in resilience, and we can strengthen our resilience just like we can strengthen our muscles or stamina.
- Building resilience is mostly common sense: but it's amazing how often health workers don't apply their common sense to their own health and well-being.
- There are easy-to-use tools for assessing how strong your resilience is and techniques for developing it further. This chapter describes some.

19.1 Introduction

Practising children's palliative care in Africa is a wonderfully rewarding and privileged job. Like all rewarding jobs it is also challenging and, at times, difficult and stressful. Dealing with dying children and their families means sharing a painful and heavy burden, and occasionally that burden can begin to affect us, our work and ultimately our happiness itself.

Being a professional is more than just being technically competent. It is about being able to understand yourself, knowing your strengths and your points of weakness, being able to pace yourself and mastering the tools you need to keep yourself sharp, enthusiastic and happy in your work. This chapter is intended to describe some of the pitfalls that can trap us as we carry out our work, and then make suggestions as to how we can avoid the pitfalls, survive and ultimately thrive.

19.2 What makes us happy?

Before we can start discussing how to prevent our becoming unhappy in our work, it makes sense to discuss what makes us happy. The BBC recently commissioned a major international survey analyzing exactly this[1]: what is happiness, and what makes us happy?

The survey suggests that, assuming people have their basic needs met, there are three key components necessary to have a happy life. These are:

- loving relationships
- challenge (but not more than our ability to cope)
- a sense of meaning and purpose.

People who score highly on life satisfaction tend to have close and supportive family and friends, whereas those who do not have close friends and family are more likely to be dissatisfied. This is probably why the loss of a loved one can have such a negative effect on one's happiness.

People who feel that they are challenged by an important role and/or chasing important goals (whether at home, at work or at school,) also feel the most happy with their life. When people feel that they are involved in dull, meaningless activity or when jobs start going poorly, this can adversely affect happiness.

Finally, a third factor that influences the happiness of most people is a sense of meaning and purpose. It seems to be important that we should feel a connection to something larger than ourselves. People who feel that they are part of some bigger picture, in a spiritual or philosophical sense, and who thereby feel there is some ultimate meaning or purpose, tend to be happier.

Money is an interesting one. It is difficult to be happy if you don't have enough but, once you have enough (and for happiness, enough is probably not that much – just enough to give secure food, shelter, health care and schooling); more money doesn't make us any happier.

The practice of children's palliative care is undoubtedly challenging, and most of us would feel that it is an important and meaningful work. Many health workers in palliative care have strong religious beliefs, and many have close working and home relationships.

If you are like us, you have probably had many encounters with people who think that the work we do must be depressing, and like us, you may sometimes feel a bit guilty that you actually quite enjoy it. However, realizing that practising children's palliative care gives us opportunities to be challenged, work within a good team and feel like we are doing something that has some meaning and purpose, perhaps we shouldn't be surprised that we enjoy it. In fact, practising children's palliative care might actually make us likely to be happier, rather than less happy, despite the burden of pain and suffering that we witness and partially share.

19.3 Job satisfaction in palliative care

There is no research looking specifically at how satisfied children's palliative care workers are in Africa, but we might learn something from looking at the studies that are out there.

The research is remarkably consistent. Despite the general assumption that working with death and dying should lead to higher levels of burnout in children's palliative care workers, in fact that appears not to be the case[2,3]. Palliative physicians have significantly higher levels of job satisfaction compared with consultants working in other specialties. Helping patients through controlling symptoms and having good relationships with patients, relatives and staff are the most highly rated sources of job satisfaction for palliative physicians.

Levels of job satisfaction are generally high among British nurses, but significantly higher among clinical nurse specialists and hospice nurses than district nurses, midwives, ward nurses and health visitors. Clinical nurse specialists describe personal relationships with patients and their relatives, and having the time to develop these, as the greatest source of satisfaction in their work. Other patient-related sources of satisfaction for clinical nurse specialists are controlling pain and symptoms and improving the quality of life and death for patients. Nursing dying patients and supporting their families are an important source of satisfaction as long as nurses feel that they have the time, staff and knowledge to do it well. And most social workers, psychologists and other health and social care workers in the field of palliative care would endorse this too.

The research also suggests that part of the reason for this counter-intuitive infrequency of burnout is the rewarding nature of the work; the high-quality staff support programmes usually available in PC settings and the centrality of team working. PC workers seem to find relationships with colleagues and other health professionals and teamwork very valuable (and conversely find team conflicts particularly stressful)[4].

19.4 Prevalence of mental health problems in children's palliative care in Africa

Where problems do occur, evidence from general palliative care settings tends to confirm that, again, working in palliative care is not particularly worse than working in any other medical specialty. The prevalence of mental health problems in palliative physicians is 25%, similar to that reported by consultants working in specialties in acute hospitals, junior house officers and medical students. Palliative physicians report lower levels of specific work-related distress or 'burnout' than other consultants. Similarly, hospice nurses in the United States have significantly lower levels of burnout than intensive care nurses. Hospice nurses in Britain have a lower prevalence of psychiatric morbidity than Macmillan (community palliative care) nurses and ward nurses, who in turn have a lower prevalence than general community nurses[5]. Therefore, it appears that the stress associated with caring for dying people may be counterbalanced by the satisfaction of dealing well with patients and relatives. Certainly there is no evidence that we need fear mental health problems any more than our colleagues working in other health disciplines.

19.5 Burnout and stress

That is not to say that we should be complacent. There are many reasons why we could become unwell as a result of what we do, and a rate of 25% is still quite high. When we become unwell as a result of work-related issues, we tend to go through a spectrum of reactions, usually starting with so-called stress, then progressing to so-called burnout and finally ending with serious mental health problems such as depression, neuroses and alcohol and drug abuse (a report from the BMA in the UK[6] stated that over 7% of doctors were addicted to alcohol and/ or other chemical substances, and that 23% of GPs had increased their drinking in response to stress).

19.5.1 Stress

Most of us are familiar with the sensation of feeling stressed. Work-related stress is characterized by *overengagement* with our work. We tend to become urgent and over-reactive (even hyperactive). We may lack concentration, have poor timekeeping, poor productivity and difficulty in comprehending new procedures. We might become uncooperative, irritable or aggressive. Importantly for our work, we may start to make mistakes.

19.5.2 Burnout

Ultimately, if stress continues beyond our ability to cope, we begin to burnout. Unlike stress, which is a syndrome of mental and physical overengagement, burnout is more characterized by *underengagement*: mental and physical withdrawal and shut-down. According to Maslach and Leiter[7], burnout is the degree of 'dislocation between what people are and what they have to do'. It is a syndrome of emotional exhaustion, depersonalization, low productivity and feelings of low achievement. Although it can occur in a range of occupations, burnout has been found to occur most amongst professional people in the caring professions of medicine, nursing, social work, counselling and teaching[8]. It manifests itself in the form of chronic exhaustion, cynical detachment and feelings of ineffectiveness. Burnout reduces our productivity and saps our energy, leaving us feeling increasingly hopeless, powerless, cynical and resentful. The unhappiness burnout causes can eventually threaten our job, our relationships and our health.

19.5.3 Impact of stress and burnout on the team

Usually, the first people to notice when someone is burning out are family and friends. Later, the worker tends to give up trying to hide it at work, and the problems become apparent to colleagues. Usually, the worker avoids showing signs to patients until the effects are advanced. Stress and burnout can damage the dynamics of the team as they can cause:

- irritability
- paranoia
- argumentativeness
- slow working
- poor working and mistakes
- resentment
- poor communication.

19.5.4 Impact of stress and burnout on patient care

Health workers who are stressed or burnt out usually are able to hide this from patients until quite late on[9] (and well after they start affecting interpersonal and team relationships at work). Nevertheless, ultimately patient-care will begin to suffer and effects can include:

- making mistakes: even in high-risk areas such as prescribing and dispensing;
- poor time-keeping and sickness
- loss of patience and loss of empathy
- inability to listen fully to patient concerns
- poor communication with other health workers.

19.6 Resilience and coping

19.6.1 Resilience, coping and personality

Two themes that are emerging from research into stress and burnout are resilience and coping. Each of us have an inbuilt buffer which helps us cope with stresses that are an inevitable part of daily life. This buffer is known as our resilience. When we are being put under pressure, we use a variety of coping strategies to help us defend our resilience. It is when our coping strategies become overwhelmed or weakened that we become vulnerable to stress and burnout.

However, one person's ability to cope, and ways of coping, can vary significantly from those of another. These variations seem to be at least partly to do with aspects of our personalities[10]. Read through some of the coping strategies listed below and try and decide which ones you prefer:

- **People who are 'open with their emotions'** often prefer emotional methods of relieving stress, e.g. crying, losing their temper, 'talking it out'.
- **People who are 'extroverted'** often prefer to cope by joking, talking, seeking reassurance from others and looking for peer support.
- **People who are more 'open' to new things and change** tend to cope by doing something creative, looking at the problem in an artistic or philosophical perspective or giving up and doing something totally new.

- **People who are 'agreeable'** tend to cope by putting their faith in their God (or equivalent), or by putting faith in others, often refusing to allow themselves to get emotional or lose their perspective.

- **People who are 'practical and conscientious'** tend to cope by identifying and trying to solve problems, seeking to learn and become better and stronger and by concentrating on the next steps.

If these theories are right, it is clear that there cannot be 'one size fits all' technique for helping people cope with stress. People who prefer practical solutions might not find talking about how they feel useful. People who tend to emotional coping might not find writing poetry or painting helpful. People who prefer to look to God and the bigger picture might not find practical tips or problem-solving helpful. Also, of course most of us will use more than one strategy, often at the same time.

It is useful to try and work out what kind of coping strategies you use and how you can put those strategies into practice, if and when work begins to become stressful. It is also important in a team for each person to recognize and respect differences, and not look down on the coping strategies of others simply because they do not seem to be useful to us.

19.6.2 **Factors that can affect our resilience and coping: traumatic childhood events**

There is evidence to suggest that health workers have significantly increased incidence of past psychosocial trauma compared to the general population[11–14]. Many health workers (perhaps most) have a history of personal loss (such as close family bereavements) or traumas (such as abuse, neglect or alcoholism) or parents/carers suffering from severe mental health problems. At first sight, one might think that these factors might undermine and weaken our resilience. However, it seems to be a bit more complicated than that.

Papadatou[15] postulates that most people who go into the caring professions do so partly because of events or relationships in their pasts that have hurt them in some way, and for which they are grieving. She does not see this as a weakness, but as strength, using the story of the 'wounded healer' to argue that it is these wounds that make health workers empathic and able to understand and communicate with people who are sick or dying. However, this history is a double-edged sword. Unless health workers are aware of this underlying hurt or loss and can come to terms with it to draw on it as a strength rather than a weakness, we can end up repressing this 'shadow side'. Our shadow side can negatively (and subconsciously) influence us – usually in one of two directions, both of which have negative impacts on ourselves, our colleagues and our patients. These are:

- **The overwhelmed care worker**: Overwhelmed care workers begin by identifying too strongly with the suffering of patients, and feeling their pain and suffering as if it is their own. They find it difficult to set personal boundaries – often staying later and coming earlier, working extra shifts and being unable to switch off at home. Gradually, they lose their boundaries and sense of perspective, eventually becoming unable to cope and unable to deal with their own loss and grief. They become ever more exhausted and fearful of their work and end up burnt out or suffering with mental health problems.

- **The perfect care worker**: These are the 'supermen' and 'wonderwomen' of health care. They are obsessive, compulsive perfection-seekers, who believe strongly in themselves and their own abilities[16,17]. They perceive unpleasant or adverse events in the lives of their patients as personal failure. They can be very tough on colleagues and gradually lose the ability to see the world through anyone else's eyes, even their patients'. Ultimately such health workers burnout, suffering with what is commonly known as 'compassion fatigue', looking at their patients and their own work negatively, becoming cynical and ever more distant from patients and colleagues.

However, where a care worker can recognize and come to terms with his or her past trauma and use this as a foundation for *building self-awareness*, he or she can use it to develop into a much more resilient and effective health worker than one who does not have a similar experience of trauma. This is known as:

- **The good-enough health worker:** These are health workers who are aware enough of their own vulnerability and losses to empathise with patients and colleagues, but who are able to distance themselves enough to allow the patients to die without a sense of personal failure. They set boundaries that are strong enough for personal protection, but leaky enough to allow flexibility as patient needs and work circumstances change. They are able to accept their own strengths and weaknesses, without becoming obsessed by the former or overwhelmed by the latter. They recognize that, whatever they do, they will never make more than a tiny difference in the face of the magnitude of suffering in the world, but are also content that they are making a difference for that small number of children; they do have the resources to care for, as long as they can pace themselves. They recognize that children's palliative care is a marathon, not a sprint, and are set for a long and rewarding career in palliative care.

19.6.3 Factors that can affect our resilience and coping: personal factors[18,19]

These are factors which seem to have an impact on our resilience and ability to cope with stress. Most of them are common sense. They include:

- **Age:** The word 'burnout' suggests that a time factor is important – that the longer we work the more likely we are to burn out. In fact (counter-intuitively), the highest risk of burnout tends to occur in the first 2–3 years of a new job. Probably, as we get older, we learn more about ourselves and learn stronger and better ways of coping or simply move on to another job where we feel more comfortable.
- **Health and energy:** If we eat well, sleep well and exercise well, we keep ourselves fit and energetic. If we are fit and energetic, we are much better able to resist the pressures of our work.
- **Positive belief (e.g. optimism):** Those who see the glass as half-full rather than half-empty seem to be more resilient. It is not easy to change the way we look at the world, but we can try to see the best rather than the worst in things.
- **Problem solving skills:** People who are able to break problems down into chunks small enough to tackle, and then plan how to face these problems, tend to be more resilient. If you are not like this, try and speak to people who are, share your issue and learn from them as they assist you in solving problems.
- **Social skills:** People who have better social skills are better at winning people round to their way of thinking, recruiting people to their cause and motivating others to stay with them. You may not have ideal social skills, but they can be improved through getting feedback, advice and coaching from colleagues.
- **Assertiveness:** We all need to be able to say no to the demands placed on us. There is more suffering and there are more patients in the world than any of us can possibly help with. Demands are endless and at times overwhelming. Those who can remember their own needs among the crush of those of their patients are better able to cope.

19.6.4 **Factors that can affect our resilience and coping: environmental factors**

Our personal circumstances change with time, and these have a significant impact on our resilience and coping. Important factors include the following:

♦ **Resources:** If you don't have enough money, time or help from others, it goes without saying that you will struggle more than people who do. You might not be able to do much about your personal circumstances, but you can choose which problems you can realistically take on with the resources that you do have.

♦ **Degree of personal control:** If you feel out of control, it is natural to be fearful, and fear weakens our resolve. You might be stuck in your situation, but often there are ways out, either by trying to tackle the problem or to walk away from it altogether. A job is just that: a job. It's not worth losing your health over.

♦ **Being unmarried and/or not having children:** Being married and having children seem to be protective (again counter-intuitively to those of us who feel at wits end coping with our families!).

♦ **Caring for others at home:** The evidence suggests that people who work in PC tend also to be carers at home. This is probably even more so in the African setting, where the AIDS epidemic has meant that many people require care, and there are a huge number of orphans. People who care for others at home (not surprisingly) tend to have higher rates of burnout than those who don't[20].

♦ **Social support:** Being lonely is a major cause of unhappiness, and people who are lonely have fewer sources of support and also fewer people to distract them and share their problems[21].

19.6.5 **Factors that can affect our resilience and coping: organizational factors**

Organizations that provide children's palliative care have a particular responsibility to provide support and supervision for their staff and to ensure that the team is well managed. While we have not been able to find specific evidence for the PC setting, there is evidence from general organization theory, and strong anecdotal evidence from the author's experience in children's palliative care, that there are several organizational factors which, when managed poorly, can significantly increase job stress and reduce team and individual resilience. These are:

♦ **Work overload:** Every individual and every team has a limit to what they can do in the time allocated. Even the most efficient and effective team will get exhausted eventually. Good managers need to limit overtime and on-call, ensure adequate meal breaks and discourage 'stay-late' syndrome (which is very common in the 'superman/wonderwoman' care type). PC work is not regular, there are peaks and troughs of activity. Management needs to plan not just for the average workload, but also for the extremes, and build in sufficient tolerance.

♦ **Role clarity:** When team members' individual roles are not clear, not understood or blurred, conflicts and burnout are more likely to arise. We need to know the limits of our job, if we are to set boundaries. Without clear boundaries, we cannot plan our time or energies properly.

♦ **Loss of control:** This is partly related to role-clarity. When your work demands are outside your control, or where our managers are not good at listening to problems that arise in the team, we can feel out of control and fearful. Fear is a potent inhibitor of performance, and also a potent drain on energy and personal resources.

- **Home-work boundaries:** Like role clarity, we need to know how long we are to be at work, when we can go off and when we have to be on-call, so that we can plan our resources. Often hospices and palliative care teams slip into using 'family' metaphors for the team. *But palliative care teams are not family groups* (thank goodness!). They have different tasks, different roles and different rules. We should not blur the boundaries between the two.

- **Resource constraints:** These are inevitable in any health care setting, particularly in Africa. However, knowing that we could offer more to a dying child if only we had more money, equipment or time is very demoralizing.

- **Fear of job loss, discipline, bullying or other abuse at work:** As mentioned above, fear is a very destructive element in children's palliative care teams. Managers need to take care to create a supportive, non-abusive and encouraging environment. High-blame environments do not support good children's palliative care.

- **Change:** High rates of staff turnover, frequent policy changes and other changes are unsettling. We should also remember that resistance to change is a feature of early burnout. The combination of the two means that managers have to take great care introducing and implanting change, ensuring that change is agreed with the team and that it is introduced within the abilities of the team to absorb it.

- **Unrealistic goals:** Teams, like individuals, can set themselves unrealistic goals. Mangers also can expect too much. Good managers recognize the capacity of their team, build in some tolerance and only allow their teams to fight battles which they have a realistic chance of winning. Teams and individuals need some challenge, but not too much either.

19.6.6 Factors that can affect our resilience and coping: team factors

One factor that seems particularly important in children's palliative care is the functionality of the care team. Teams provide a very important *holding environment*[22]. Papadatou[23] describes the function of the children's palliative care team as one which is built to contain grief and hold within itself the suffering of its members. When the team becomes unable to contain and hold the members, either because the degree of suffering is too great (for example when the team has been overstretched or dealing with particularly difficult or many cases) or because there are problems with team cohesion (e.g. due to organizational or personal factors) the team can begin to split. Classically, these team splits can show themselves in a number of different ways:

- **Scape-goating:** Where team-members demonise an individual and project all their negative emotions onto him or her.

- **Sub-group (or clique) formation:** Where the team splits into different sub-groups, each with different agendas and values.

- **Psychological 'splitting' of the team:** A bit like scape-goating, but involving projection of negative emotions onto sub-groups rather than individuals (i.e. where one subgroup demonises another subgroup).

- **Change-avoidance:** Where team members stick rigidly to the familiar, even where improvements are needed.

- **Team burnout:** Which shows itself as poor morale, poor quality of care, chronic in-fighting and team divisions.

When teams begin to split, and conflicts develop, this has a serious negative impact on our sense of job satisfaction and job stress of individual team-members. In Amery and Lapwood's study[24], it emerged as one of the top sources of concern amongst children's palliative care workers.

19.6.7 **Factors that can affect our resilience and coping: patient factors**

Perhaps counter-intuitively, coping with death and dying does not emerge as a major source of job stress among health workers[25]. However, there are certain patient factors which are more likely to overwhelm our defences. These are the following:

+ when the patient is young
+ when the patient reminds us of someone close to us, or something/someone from our past
+ when the death is traumatic
+ when the health worker has formed a close relationship with the patient
+ when several deaths occur in a short space of time.

19.7 **Strengthening your resilience: how to care for yourself and the team**

In the preceding sections, we have had to focus on the things that can go wrong and those factors that make things more likely to go wrong. Almost certainly, you will have spotted several risk factors for burnout that apply to you. Most of us are not 'good enough' carers. Most of us have some history of trauma. Most of us do not work in ideal supportive teams. Most of us do not have perfect managers. And most of us are wrestling with numerous challenges and problems, both inside and outside work. Looking at things like this, it seems to be a small miracle that any of us is sane at all! So, the chances are that by now you might be feeling pretty pessimistic about your chances of hanging in there!

But *remember the power of positive thinking*. The glass is half-full not half-empty. If all of the above applies to you, and you are still turning up for work for more than simply to pick up the pay-cheque, you must have tremendous powers of resilience. If you have got to where you are in reasonable shape, the chances are you will go on from strength to strength, as resilience increases with age and experience.

But, it is important not to get complacent either. A carpenter keeps his tools sharp. A soldier keeps his gun oiled. A cook keeps her fire hot. In children's palliative care, you are your own tool. Therefore, you have a duty to yourself, your family and your patient to stay healthy, enthusiastic and whole.

The rest of this chapter will focus on things you can do to boost your resilience and develop a broader and deeper range of coping strategies. Remember that different personality types will prefer different strategies, so it is unlikely that you will find all of them attractive. So, look at them as a restaurant menu. Choose 2 or 3 that appeal to you. But, whatever you do, don't fall into the superman/wonderwoman trap. None of us is perfect. We will all wobble from time to time. In the words of the song, 'We all need somebody to lean on!'

19.7.1 **Strengthening your lifestyle**

Lifestyle factors are so obvious that they should not really need saying, especially to health workers. But we health workers have never been good at practising what we preach. So a reminder: the old adage 'eat well, sleep well, drink well, live well' is not only true, but it is being increasingly backed up by scientific research.

19.7.1.1 **Have fun**

When we get burnt out, we tend to withdraw and become inactive which is the opposite of what we should be doing. Having fun is a great antidote to stress at work. Remember 'all work and no play makes Jack a dull boy'. So, what do you enjoy doing? Are you doing it? If not, why not? Remember – a little bit of what you fancy does you good!

19.7.1.2 Laugh

Laughter triggers the body's release of endorphins, which kill pain and boost mood. Are you laughing much these days? If not, why not? Who makes you laugh? Meet up with them. What makes you laugh? Do it.

19.7.1.3 Know your limits

If you are working too hard, stop it. If you don't absolutely have to for financial reasons, ease up. If you consistently push yourself over the limits, you will soon stop performing and the risk is that you will get sick or get sacked. Either way, your financial problems may get worse.

19.7.1.4 Rest, relaxation and sleep

It seems so simple that it almost goes without saying. If you are tired you will feel grumpier, more emotional and more irritable. People who are deliberately deprived of sleep by torturers start suffering with depression and psychosis. We rest and sleep because we need to. So, try and build plenty of both into your schedule. Make sure that you take your allocation of leave, and try and spend time doing things you enjoy or with those whose company you enjoy while you are on leave.

19.7.1.5 Watch the chemicals

A little bit of caffeine keeps us on our toes, and a little bit of alcohol helps us relax (and actually increases life expectancy). Too much of either does the opposite. There is plenty of evidence that health workers overuse chemicals, whether alcohol, caffeine, nicotine or prescription drugs.

19.7.1.6 Eat well

Literally as well as metaphorically, you are what you eat. If you are on an unbalanced diet, or becoming overweight or underweight, you will lose your stamina and your effectiveness.

19.7.1.7 Exercise regularly

Exercise not only makes you fitter and live longer, it makes you feel better too. Exercise releases 'happy chemicals' such as endorphins and serotonins. Did you know that exercise is as effective as anti-depressants in the management of depression, and can now be prescribed by doctors in some parts of the world? So, get out and get fit. But remember, it's supposed to be healthy. If it causes muscle strains, ligament tears or heart-attacks, that defeats the object! So be sensible. Secondly, if it is painful and miserable, unless you are a masochist you won't enjoy it, so you'll stop doing it, feel guilty and probably eat more as a result. It doesn't have to hurt. Have fun!

19.7.1.8 Be with people

Remember the BBC study showing that loneliness is a potent cause of misery? You might be isolated. You may not have a broad circle of friends. But, however hard it might be, try and nurture relationships with others. Other people can make us feel appreciated, they can help us put things in perspective and they can offer a shoulder to cry on. Try and make friends both at work and out of work. Join a religious or community group that is meaningful to you. Form or join a support group. Get online. It is hard but it is worth it.

19.7.1.9 Look for wonder and meaning

You may have a religious faith. If so, nurture it. Pray, sing, read and worship. If you do not, look at the stars or at a baby or at a flower and rediscover a sense of wonder and amazement at the hugeness and infinite connectedness of all things. Whoever or whatever your God or your belief, keep things in perspective. 'Don't tell your God how big your storm is; tell your storm how big your God is'.

19.7.2 Strengthening your environment

With heavy workloads and rushed environments, it is easy to focus only on the patients. But teams, just like individuals, have to be honest and realistic about their limits and be able to set boundaries. Teams need time for themselves as well as for patients. Remember the evidence that dysfunctional teams split and are a major cause of stress and burnout in children's palliative care. You and your managers need to invest a significant proportion of your work time building and supporting your team. This is difficult for us to get our heads round when we have been trained to think that the only 'real work' is face-to-face patient work. But, if we don't do this, our teams will be less functional and our patient care will suffer.

19.7.2.1 Personal objectives, appraisal and review

We need to know what is expected of us. We need to know our objectives, and we need proper feedback from colleagues and from line-managers. Without all of these, we will flounder, our boundaries won't be clear, we will keep making the same mistakes over and over and we will miss opportunities to develop. You should have a clear job description, a clear knowledge of your objectives, formal feedback from colleagues and a regular appraisal or review. If you don't have these things, it is important to ask your manager for them so that you know what the expectations and boundaries of your job are. If you are a manager, make sure that you ensure your team-members have all of these. If you have these things in place and they are not helpful, try and discuss the issues with your manager and/or ask someone else to help you review your performance.

19.7.2.2 Make sure that you have adequate supervision

Feeling out of your depth or unsure of your direction is frightening and unsettling. Children's palliative care is stressful enough without having to deal with that as well. Regular supervision, one-to-one or as a team, provides a system for talking through difficult cases, sharing problems, sifting solutions and planning the way forward. If you don't have this, as a professional it is your duty to try and set it up. If you cannot do it formally, try and set up a group informally. See Appendix 19.1 on clinical supervision for more information.

19.7.2.3 Team support meetings

We all struggle in children's palliative care from time to time, and at other times the lights are all green and we seem to fly through. If you can meet regularly with colleagues, the chances are different members will be at different stages, and those who are flying can support those who are struggling. What goes around comes around, and soon the team will develop a sense of group responsibility and trust for each other. See Appendix 19.2. on how to set up a team support group.

19.7.3 Strengthen your organization

If you are a practical person, this one might appeal to you. Remember the importance of role-clarity, boundaries and work-life balance. Do you have a clear job description and contract? Do they accurately reflect what you are doing? Do you have clear breaks? Can you get away on time? Are managers overly-critical? Do you have an unfair burden of on-call or weekend work? If there are problems in any of these areas, speak to your manager. If you are the manager, explain to yourself why these are important – you are not superman/wonderwoman!

19.8 **If you think you might be burning out**

It might be that, despite all the above, you are still feeling a bit stressed or a bit burnt out. If so, you need to remember your health or social care training and turn your diagnostic and therapeutic skills on yourself. You need to do three things:

1. **Diagnose yourself**: Assess yourself. Check out where you are. Do a personal audit of your personality, your circumstances, your team and your organization. Speak to someone that knows you and who will be honest or speak to a health adviser. To paraphrase Bob Marley, if we don't know where we are coming from, how will we know where we are going to?

2. **Write a management plan**: Once you have assessed what the issues are, prioritize them and plan your management approach for each. But remember, Rome wasn't built in a day. So, pick out the most important things and address those first. Plan what steps you are going to take and when you are going to take them.

3. **Treat**: Planning is no use unless we put the plan into action. This bit might be particularly hard if you are a bit burnt out (remember resistance to change is an early feature). But no-one is going to change your life for you. You need to act if you are to change.

19.8.1 **Diagnose yourself: audit and assess**

There are a number of things you can assess to work out where you are. Here are some of them:

19.8.1.1 **Burnout inventory**

Do you think you are a bit burnt out? If so, try checking properly. There are a number of inventories (questionnaires) that you can fill out. The most thoroughly validated is the Maslach inventory, but you need to buy that. However, the one we have created below should act well as a basic screen.

Instructions: For each question, tick in the column that most applies, then score yourself below.

Count how many ticks you put in the column labelled 'sometimes or often'. If it is less than 5, you are probably doing *ok*. If it is between 6 and 10, you need to watch out. You may be burning out.

Table 19.1 Burnout inventory

Question	Never or rarely	Sometimes or often
Do you feel that your job is not giving you the sense of satisfaction that you need?		
Are you feeling run down or drained of energy?		
Are other problems or people at work annoying you more than they used to?		
Do you find it harder to be sympathetic with the problems of others than you used to?		
Do you feel your colleagues don't appreciate or understand you properly?		
Do you feel that there is no one you can talk to?		
Does thinking about your work make you feel negative?		
Do you sense that you should be achieving more?		
Does the pressure to improve or succeed more at work get to you?		
Do you get the feeling you are working in the wrong place or the wrong job?		
Do you find yourself getting easily frustrated with parts or all of your job?		

Table 19.1 (continued) Burnout inventory

Question	Never or rarely	Sometimes or often
Does the sheer volume of work seem unmanageable for you?		
Do you feel there is not enough time to do all the things you need to do to carry out your job properly?		
Do you feel there is not enough time to plan your work?		
Are the politics or bureaucracy at work preventing you from getting on with your job in the way that you would like?		

If it is more than 10 you are at a high risk of burnout or may be already burnt out and should do something about it immediately.

19.8.1.2 The wheel of life

This is a way of assessing how balanced your life is. It is derived from the ancient Buddhist concept of the wheel of life. See below for an example, but you can draw your own. Each segment of the wheel represents one area of your life. Label the sections anything you like; but try and include all areas of your life that are important to you. Consider each section: How satisfied are you with all these areas of your life? Are you putting as much time, energy and attention into these areas as you would like? The centre of the wheel is 0 and means you are totally dissatisfied; the outer edge is 10 and represents full satisfaction and achievement. Which areas make you happy, satisfied and fulfilled? Which areas need improvement? Decide your degree of satisfaction from 0 to 10 and mark it on the relevant spoke. Now draw a line to join your degree marks together. How big and how balanced is your life? Is the wheel big, circular and even or small, irregular and bumpy? If it is the latter, perhaps it's not surprising that your life is bumpy and hard work.

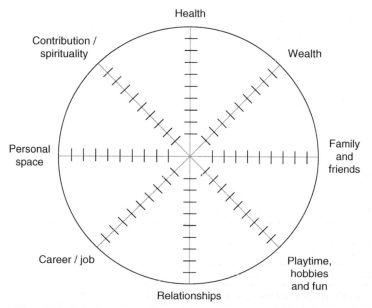

Fig. 19.1 The wheel of life.

19.8.1.3 Examine your relationship with yourself

Have you ever stopped to think what your own needs are? It's not that you need to become maudlin or introspective. Just a simple list of those things you need to keep going will do. Think of it like a check-list for a service for a vehicle. Write a list of what you need to keep yourself on the road, and then score how well you are doing on each. Think of practical ones (food, sleep, relationships, sex, exercise) as well as 'existential' ones (what kind of a person am I, which values do I rate most highly, what kind of person do I want to be and how do I want to be remembered?). Try writing an epitaph for yourself as others would write it, and then ask yourself if it says the kind of things about you that you would value the most. If not, now is the time to change.

19.8.1.4 Understand your personality

There are a number of tools you can use to analyze your personality type, what kind of things are likely to stress you the most, and what strategies for coping are most likely to be successful. You can pay to do these formally, or use free online (shorter but not so well validated) tools such as Myers-Briggs or Belbin. Check out these websites for more information:

◆ http://www.humanmetrics.com/cgi-win/JTypes2.asp

◆ https://team-belbin.com/

19.8.1.5 Audit your job satisfaction

Identify those aspects of your work duties and office environment which are presently satisfying, enjoyable or rewarding, and also look for things that are frustrating or downright demotivating. In the table below (adapted from Open Door Coaching)[26] we have put together some questions that might help you work out how satisfied you are with your work. Please circle the appropriate response after each item. 1 = strongly disagree; 2 = no opinion; 3 = strongly agree. To determine your score, total off all numbers you have circled. The highest possible score is 51; lowest is 17.

Table 19.2 Job satisfaction inventory

1. I like my current job.	1	2	3
2. I am clear about my career direction and life purpose.	1	2	3
3. It is easy for me to set goals for myself.	1	2	3
4. I usually attain the goals I set.	1	2	3
5. I have no fears about changing jobs.	1	2	3
6. I think of myself as a successful person.	1	2	3
7. I have high self-esteem.	1	2	3
8. Once I decide to make a change in my life, I usually move ahead and do so without making excuses or procrastinating.	1	2	3
9. I view change as a healthy occurrence.	1	2	3
10. The work environment in my current job meets all of my needs.	1	2	3
11. I know exactly which career field I want to enter (or in which I want to stay).	1	2	3
12. I understand what motivates me to work, and I make job choices based on those factors.	1	2	3
13. I understand the inner needs that I feel a job should fulfill.	1	2	3

Table 19.2 (continued) Job satisfaction inventory

14. My inner needs are fulfilled through my work.	1	2	3
15. I know the signs that tell me when it is time for me to change jobs or careers.	1	2	3
16. I enjoy nearly all of the tasks performed in my job.	1	2	3
17. My job allows me to satisfy my personal values and fulfill my personal goals as I do the work.	1	2	3

Scoring:

- 40–51 High level of satisfaction
- 27–39 Medium level of satisfaction
- <27 Low level of satisfaction

19.8.1.6 Keep a stress diary

If you are finding your job stressful but are not sure why, or are having difficulty pinning down the exact issues, you might find it useful to keep a stress diary. Try and fill it in every day and record an entry for every stressful event that you experience, however small. Each time you make an entry try and record the time and date, what triggered the stress, what the fundamental causes might be (being as honest and objective as you can) and how stressed or relaxed you feel just now (use a scale if you like). Then, record what you did at the time, how well your reaction worked to reduce your stress and how you would act if you could turn the clock back and do it again. Finally, evaluate how well you did. After a few weeks, sit down for a couple of hours and look to see whether common themes emerge. Are there particular issues that stress you, particular people or particular times of day? Do your reactions make things better or worse? What could you do differently? Are you still feeling stressed, or have things moved on?

19.8.2 Prioritize and plan

19.8.2.1 Setting goals and objectives

The problem with getting stressed is it makes us more obsessed with work and ever less likely to stand back, take a deep breath and remind ourselves what is important to us in life. Before we can plan how to tackle our stress, we need to remind ourselves what is most important to us. Then, we need to set life goals or objectives.

Try and answer the following questions:

- What do I want to do and achieve?
- Where do I want to go?
- What kind of a person am I or do I want to become?
- What do I want to be remembered for?

19.8.2.2 Analyse your audits

Ok, so you have reminded yourself where you want to be in life, and you have analyzed where you actually are. Now you need to start planning and prioritizing. Write a list of those issues or areas that seem to be stressing you the most. Remember to think broadly: include your personal factors, your personality type, team factors, organizational factors and environmental factors. Choose those areas that are stressing you the most and that you have most chance of changing.

Prioritize the list from the top priority to the lowest, and decide with yourself which ones you are going to tackle first. But please note that this step is usually easier if you can do it with someone else. It is often hard to be objective about yourself. Try to choose someone whose opinion you trust and who will be honest. It might be a friend or family member, it might be your supervisor or mentor at work.

19.8.3 Act

So, by now you should have identified where you want to go, where you are and what the biggest issues are. Now it is time to act. Of course we cannot cover all your possible options, but here are a few suggestions about things you could do to improve your resilience and make you more likely to survive and thrive in the world of children's palliative care.

19.8.3.1 Strengthening yourself

People are not fixed. Unlike leopards, we *can* change our spots (although admittedly it gets harder as we get older). We can understand ourselves better and we can change our lives so that we live more constructively and healthily. This might be something you are able to do yourself, but often this is something that is much easier to do with someone else's support. You have a variety of options:

- **Counselling and support:** If you are one of the many 'wounded healers', you may well feel that some of the traumas or losses that you suffered are unresolved. If so, you might benefit from formal counselling to discuss, come to terms with and learn from your experiences. This might not be for everyone (remember talking treatments don't help all personality types) but they do help some. The important thing is that you should not feel ashamed. In fact, your experiences actually can make you a more empathic and more effective healer than someone whose life has been plain-sailing, as long as you can come to terms with them and allow yourself to be 'good enough'. You may not have easy access to counselling, but there are many religious organizations, NGOs and voluntary organizations in Africa who should be able to help. You might prefer to speak one to one, but group work with other health workers can be very powerful and also help you to realize that you are not weird, different or alone, but actually probably one of the silent majority.

- **Mentoring and coaching:** These also involve talking, but with less emphasis on the past and with more emphasis on the future. Mentoring and coaching help us to identify problem areas, remember our values and life-goals and set plans for moving forward. Mentoring can happen at work, and we can all be both mentors and mentees (although ideally we should get some training). There are plenty of online-resources for people wanting to be mentored and to learn how to mentor.

19.8.4 If things have gone too far

Hopefully, if you use some of the tactics suggested above, you may find that your resilience strengthens and your work stress reduces enough so that you can start thriving rather than just surviving again. However, you may find that, despite all this, things are still not working for you. If this applies to you, there are two more questions you should ask yourself. These are as follows:

(1) Am I unwell?

(2) Am I in the right job?

It may simply be that you are in the wrong job. If so, you need to think seriously about changing. Or it may be that you have become unwell. You might be feeling at the end of your tether, too stressed or too anxious to address things systematically or simply too low or depressed to bother. You might be drinking too much, or taking addictive medications or drugs. If so, you are not alone. Many others are in your position now, and many have been. You can recover but you probably need help. Here are some of your options.

19.9 **Am I unwell?**

19.9.1 **Depression and anxiety**

Depression and anxiety disorders are very common. Remember that 25% of UK doctors are suffering with them at any one time. If you add alcoholism and other substance abuse, the figure is even higher. If you have become unwell, you should seek help. If you think you might be depressed, try completing the brief questionnaires that we have put together for you below.

Depression questions		
	Always or as much as before	**Never or less than before**
Do you feel you still have the energy and 'zip' that you used to?		
Do you still enjoy the things you used to?		
Do you still have an interest in the way you look?		
Do you feel you can still laugh and see the funny side of things?		
Do you sleep well?		
Do you feel cheerful?		

Count how many ticks you have in the column labelled 'never or less than before'. If you have ticked less than 2, you are probably fine. If you have ticked 3 or 4, you may be bordering on depression. If you have ticked 5 or 6, you are probably depressed and should seek help.

Anxiety questions		
	Never or only sometimes	**Often or almost always**
Do you feel tense?		
Do you get anxious sensations like racing heart, butterflies in the stomach, chest tightness or sweaty palms?		
Do you get the feeling that something bad is going to happen to you or those you love?		
Do you feel agitated or unable to be still?		
Do you get worrying thoughts or ruminations running over and over in your mind?		
Do you feel like you might be about to panic?		
Do you feel you are unable to relax?		

Count how many ticks you have in the column labelled 'often or almost always'. If you have ticked fewer than 3, you are probably fine. If you have ticked 4 or 5, you may be bordering on anxiety. If you have ticked 6 or 7 you are probably suffering with an anxiety disorder and should seek help.

19.9.2 Substance abuse and addictions

Are you concerned that you might be addicted to alcohol or drugs (either prescription drugs or street drugs)? Do you get anxious at the thought of not being able to drink or take drugs? Do you feel bad if you go too long between drinks or doses? Do you feel guilty about how much you are drinking or dosing? These are all signs that you have moved beyond using alcohol or other drugs for harmless enjoyment or relaxation, and you have become addicted. Try using the adapted CAGE questionnaire below. If the answer to any of the following questions is yes, you are almost certainly addicted. If so, you need to seek help.

---

1. Have you ever felt you should **C**ut down on your drinking/drug-taking?

2. Have people **A**nnoyed you by criticizing your drinking/drug-taking?

3. Have you ever felt bad or **G**uilty about your drinking/drug taking?

4. Have you ever had a drink/drugs first thing in the morning to steady your nerves or get rid of a hangover (**E**ye-opener)?

Fig. 19.2 Adapted CAGE questionnaire[27].

If you are suffering from anxiety, depression or substance abuse, it is very difficult to pull yourself back just by carrying on and hoping for the best. So don't try and be superman or wonderwoman. Seek medical help and consider counselling and/or drug treatment. Be honest with your manager (or with yourself if you are the manager). You almost certainly need to take a break, either as complete sickness leave or at least as a transfer to a different work while you recover. The service probably won't fall apart without you and, if it does, that is probably a sign that it was not a healthy service to start with. Remember, even if you worked every hour of every day, you would hardly scratch the surface of human suffering. So, be honest and real with yourself. You owe it to your patients, your colleagues, your family and yourself to get healthy and stay healthy.

19.9.3 Am I in the right job?

If you are not unwell (and here you need to be very, very honest with yourself otherwise you are going to make a bad decision and end up back at square one), and if you have tried some or all of the tips suggested in the sections above to strengthen yourself, your team and your organization, then you probably need to decide whether you are in the right job or even in the right career. It may be that you have come to the conclusion that children's palliative care simply isn't for you. It may be that you don't enjoy it, that you don't feel you are achieving what you want, or that it is simply too painful. The conclusion is hard to avoid: you should leave and find a different pathway which suits you better.

There are downsides to change. You may be left without a job, although health workers are so scarce in Africa that the chances are you will find another. It may be that you will lose some of the benefit of the experience you have already gained, but a lot of that experience will be transferable, even if you leave caring professions altogether. You might fear that you will have to drop down the ladder and rejoin a different profession or discipline with people younger than you and with lower salaries. You may feel a sense of failure that you have had to quit.

However, if you have been honest in your audit and assessment of yourself and your situation, you will have only come to this decision because the benefits of leaving are greater than the benefits of staying. Doing nothing and putting up with it is likely to result in your becoming increasingly stressed, bitter or withdrawn. Your performance will probably decline and you may well end up being forced out anyway. If you do decide to change, and as long as you have been honest with yourself and faced up to your part in the process, you will have been able to use your experience for personal growth. Remember the glass is half-full not half-empty. In losing your past you are gaining a new and hopefully much happier future.

19.10 **Conclusion**

Perhaps it would be good to finish with a quote from Nomfundo Walasa, in 'Life without violence: Women and men together'[28].

'There is a cost to caring. Anyone working in a context where human trauma and tragedy is the focus of attention, risks developing what has become known as 'compassion fatigue'; they experience a change in their interaction with the world, themselves, and their family. Or they may experience burnout which brings with it emotional exhaustion, depersonalisation (where they feel emotionally hardened and distanced from others) and a reduced sense of personal accomplishment. Along with this comes feelings of depression and anxiety. In order to care effectively in the context of HIV/ AIDS in Africa, as people working at a grassroots level, we need to take care of ourselves. This means recognising our limits, knowing when to say 'No', recognising when we need to take a break, and most importantly, continuously prioritising our well being. One way of doing this is to consciously challenge ourselves with the following question:*
How do I take care of myself:

- *Emotionally*
- *Spiritually*
- *Physically*
- *Socially*

The challenge is not only on a personal level, but also organisationally. The onus is on each of us to take care of, not only ourselves, but also of one another. Africa's primary resource in the face of crisis lies in the people. In strengthening ourselves, we nurture the strength to help others'.

Notes

1 Professor Ed Diener, University of Illinois. Available online at BBC Website. Http://News.Bbc.Co.Uk/2/ Hi/Programmes/Happiness_Formula/4785402.Stm
2 Foxhall, Zimmerman, Standley & Ben. (1990). A Comparison of frequency and sources of nursing job stress perceived by intensive care, hospice and medical-surgical nurses. *Journal of Advanced Nursing, 15*, 577–84.
3 Bene & Foxhall. (1991). Death anxiety and job stress in hospice and medical-surgical nurses. *Hospice Journal, 7*, 25–31.
4 Woolley, Stein, Forrest & Baum. (1989). Staff stress and job satisfaction at a children's hospice. *Archives of Disease in Childhood, 64*, 114–8.
5 Amery, J. & Lapwood, S. (2004). A study into the educational needs of children's hospice doctors. *Palliative Medicine, 18*(8), 727–33.

6 Ramirez, A., Addington-Hall, J. & Richards, M. (1998). ABC of Palliative Care: The Carers. *BMJ, 316*, 208–11.

7 British Medical Association. (1998). *The Misuse of Alcohol and Other Drugs by Doctors*. BMA, London.

8 Maslach, C. & Leiter, P. (1997). *Areas of Worklife: A Structured Approach to Organizational Predictors of Job Burnout*. (p. 17). Jossey-Bass Publishers, San Francisco.

9 Burnout, Patient.co.uk. Available online at http://www.patient.co.uk/showdoc/40002118/

10 Kirwan M. & Armstrong, D. (1995). Investigation of burnout in a sample of British general practitioners. *British Journal of General Practice. 45*(394), 259–60.

11 Costa, P.T., Somerfield, M.R. & Mccrae, R.R. (1996). *Handbook of Coping*. (Chapter 3, pp. 44–61).

12 Barter, S. (1997). Social work students with personal experience of sexual abuse: Implications for diploma in social wok programme providers. *Social Work Education, 16*(2), 113–32.

13 Vachon M.L.S. (1987). *Occupational Stress in The Care of The Critically Ill, The Dying and The Bereaved*. Hemisphere Press, New York.

14 Selwyn, P.A. (1998). *Surviving The Fall*. Yale University Press, New Haven.

15 Alexander, D. & Richie, E. (1990). Stressors and dealing with the terminal patient. *Journal of Palliative Care, 6*(3), 28–33.

16 Papadatou, D. (2006). Healthcare provider's responses to the death of a child. *Oxford Textbook of Palliative Care for Children*. Oxford University Press, Oxford.

17 Gabbard, G.O. (1985). The Role of Compulsiveness in The Normal Physician. *JAMA, 254*, 2926–9.

18 Gabbard, G.O. & Menninger, R.W. (1988). *Medical Marriages*. American Psychiatric Press, Washington, DC.

19 Lazarus, R.S. & Folkman, S. (1984). *Stress, Appraisal, and Coping*. Springer, New York.

20 Taylor, F. (2005). Will you burn out? *BMJ Career Focus, 331*, Gp220.

21 Vachon, M. (2005). The Stress of Caregivers. In Doyle, Hanks, Cherny & Calman (Eds) *Oxford Textbook of Palliative Medicine* (3rd Edition). (Chapter 14, p. 919) Oxford University Press, Oxford.

22 Hale, C.J., Hannum, J.W. & Espelage, D.L. (2005). Social support and physical health: The importance of belonging. *Journal of American College Health, 53*, 276–84.

23 Winnicot, D.W. (1990). The theory of the parent–infant relationship in the maturational process and the facilitating environment. (p. 37). Karnac Books, London.

24 Papadatou, D. (2006). Healthcare providers' responses to the death of a child. *Oxford Textbook of Palliative Care for Children*. Oxford University Press, Oxford.

25 Amery And Lapwood (See Iv).

26 Dunwoodie & Auret. (2007). Psychological morbidity and burnout in palliative care doctors in Western Australia. *Internal Medicine Journal, 37*(10), 693–8(6).

27 Open Door Coaching. Available online at www.opendoorcoaching.com. Copyright © 2003 Marcia Bench And Career Coach Institute; Reprinted with permission.

28 Ewing, J.A. (1984). Detecting alcoholism: The CAGE questionaire. *Journal of the American Medical Association, 252*, 1905–7.

29 Norwegian Church Aid. (2004). Writing in life without violence: women and men together.

30 Bond, M. & Holland, S. (1998). *Skills of Clinical Supervision for Nurses*. (pp. 11–42). Open University Press, UK.

Appendix 1: Clinical supervision

Clinical supervision, either individually or in groups, is an exceptionally good way of getting not only supervision, but support and teaching as well. If you can, try and set up supervision for yourself. If you cannot find one person, try and form your own group and supervise each other. Clinical supervision is 'regular, protected time for facilitated, in depth reflection on practice'[29]. The objectives of clinical supervision are to:

- maintain and promote standards of care
- safeguard practice
- empower the health worker
- develop skills and knowledge
- support practice
- improve communication
- enable the individual to develop emotional awareness
- enhance effectiveness
- improve questioning skills
- increase job satisfaction
- quality assurance
- motivate workforce
- enhance retention and recruitment
- develop and maintain a challenging and stimulating environment
- promote the organization's credibility.

It is not:

- overt and autocratic managerial supervision
- individual performance review or appraisal
- hierarchical in nature
- whistle blowing
- direct assessment or judgement of an individual's practice
- a statutory requirement (although it is felt to be fundamental in keeping abreast of the constantly changing environment of health care).

The ground rules are confidentiality, mutual respect, trust, honesty, participation, timekeeping and enjoyment!

How to go about it

Set up a group of 3–8 people. Agree in advance who will be chairperson. The role of the chairperson is to make sure that all of the tasks of supervision are met in the time available, to make sure that everyone gets a chance to speak, and to ensure that the ground rules are kept. Rotate the chair otherwise the chairperson never gets to benefit from the sessions.

Also, agree in advance who will bring a case. Unlike a general support group (where anything can be discussed), supervision should be based upon a specific case, although discussion of that case can act as a springboard for discussion of clinical, emotional, organizational or any other type of issue. Usually this means an issue that has 'touched' you because it was challenging, moving, frustrating or complex.

Set aside an hour or so, make sure that you keep time and use the following process:

(1) Remind yourselves of ground rules and time (chairperson).

(2) Present the case (presenter).

(3) Describe what happened (presenter with clarifying questions from the group). This presentation should be facts only (no feelings, reflections or emotions at this stage). What happened by who to whom in what order and when.

(4) Describe how it felt to be the carer in that case (presenter with clarifying questions from the group). Describe how you felt, how you behaved, and how you reflected.

(5) Analysis of the case (whole group): decide what issues the case raised and prioritize and agree which issues you want to talk about today (usually one or two only). Think broadly: the issues might be clinical, emotional, behavioural, about the team, about the organization, about the community, about ethics and morality, about law or anything else.

(6) Evaluation (whole group): What was good and bad about the experience and what else could you have done?

(7) Action plan (chairperson): If it arose again what would you do? What have you learnt and what needs to be done immediately, soon and in the long term? Be specific. Agree exactly and write this down.

Gibbs reflective cycle

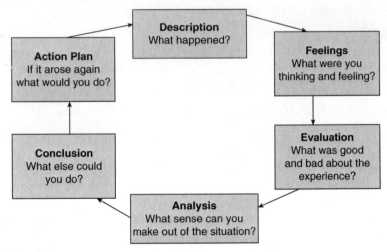

Fig. 19.3 Gibbs cycle.

Appendix 2: Setting up a support group

Support groups provide a useful forum for people to share their experiences, access information and increase understanding about a common problem. Here are useful guidelines to help you set up your own support group.

What is the focus of the group?

You need to decide on a clear focus for the group. You will be more successful if you offer a group with a specific focus such as 'confidential and closed group to allow health workers at XX to discuss personal and emotional issues arising out of patient care' as opposed to a more general group with an undefined focus.

Ask yourself:

- What is the problem?
- Who needs support?
- Who should attend?
- What would you like to achieve?

An accessible venue and appropriate time

Choose a venue which is central. If you cannot find a suitable public venue, you could decide to have your meetings at members' homes. Choose a time that would suit most members. It may be necessary to provide childcare facilities.

Getting your group together

Once you have decided on a focus, you need to recruit members. Advertise in places where you think like-minded colleagues may see.

Decide on the size of the support group

The size of a support group is important. If your group is too big, some members will never have the opportunity to contribute. Rather split the group into two more manageable groups. If the group is too small, there is a chance that your group will dissolve due to absenteeism and dropout.

Your first meeting

Use the first meeting to find out what people would like to gain from the group. Your group will be more successful if you take these issues into account.

Agree ground rules

Is the group open (i.e. people can come and go) or closed (i.e. it is for specific people who commit to come to all sessions for an agreed period)? How many times will you meet and how often? Is it *ok* to cry or express emotion? What will you do if emotions get too hot (agree a cooling off plan)? What will you do if members need more help than the group can offer? Who is out there that you can turn to? Will you bring in guest speakers or coordinators?

Share the responsibility

Don't take on all the responsibility. You will soon feel overburdened. Elect a coordinator for each meeting and rotate this so that everyone gets a turn to coordinate and a turn to be part of the group. Apart from preventing burnout, sharing of responsibility will also give more people the chance to become involved in the group.

Prevent drop out

Many support groups stop functioning due to lack of interest. Keep your members active and interested by covering a range of issues.

Ask for advice

Contact other support groups for advice on what worked well for them.

Adapted from Ilse Pauw, Health24.com

Section 6

Children's palliative care formulary for Africa

Chapter 20

Formulary

Justin Amery and Sat Jassal

20.1 Notes on drug treatment in children[1]

There are some basic rules of prescribing for children. These are as follow:

- Use only when they are necessary.
- Always balance the potential benefit versus potential risk of drug treatment.
- Make sure to discuss the treatment options carefully with the child and the child's carer.

20.1.1 Taking medicines to best effect

Compliance/adherence to treatment is often a problem in children, especially where the child cannot see an immediate benefit. There are factors which make compliance/adherence less likely and these are:

- difficulty in taking the medicine (e.g. inability to swallow the medicine);
- unattractive formulation (e.g. unpleasant taste);
- purpose of medicine not clear;
- perceived lack of efficacy;
- real or perceived side effects;
- carers' or child's perception of the risk and severity of side effects may differ from that of the prescriber;
- ambiguous instructions for administration;
- frequent administration.

Tips for improving compliance/adherence are as follows:

- Make sure that you include the child in the discussion about the medicine: make it clear why the medicine will help, and point out those symptoms which are troubling the child that the medicine will make better.
- Explain that medicines might take time to work and so the need to be patient.
- Use palatable formulations where possible: you might need to mix it with small quantities of food, but not too much because the full dose might not be taken.
- Although small children (less than five) usually prefer liquid formulation, older children can often be taught to manage tablets or capsules, which have no taste.
- Think about using the rectal route in babies and smaller children.
- Avoid intramuscular routes wherever possible: they are painful.

20.1.2 **Children's response to drugs**

Children, and particularly neonates, differ from adults in their response to drugs. Their metabolic rates vary with age. Children's livers and kidneys are less mature and less able to handle drugs in early life; but conversely may become better able than adults in later childhood. This means that drug doses in children are not simply fractions of adult doses calculated as a proportion of body weight. So, for example, a neonate needs significantly less morphine per kg body weight than an adult, but a 4-year-old will need significantly more.

Special care is needed in the neonatal period (first 28 days of life) and doses should always be calculated with care; the risk of toxicity is increased by a reduced rate of drug clearance and differing target organ sensitivity.

For most drugs the adult maximum dose should not be exceeded. For example if the dose is 8 mg/kg (max. 300 mg), a child of 10 kg body weight should receive 80 mg but a child of 40 kg body weight should receive 300 mg (rather than 320 mg).

Most drugs can be administered at slightly irregular intervals during the day. Some drugs, e.g. antimicrobials, are best given at regular intervals. Some flexibility should be allowed in children to avoid waking them during the night. For example, the night-time dose may be given at the parent's bedtime.

20.2 **Principles of effective morphine prescribing**

- Give immediate release morphine 4 hourly (6 hourly in neonates or in patients with impaired renal function).
- Start at low dose (as per chart below).
- Increase the dose in 30–50% steps (usually after a minimum of two doses) until pain control is achieved.
- If available, convert the immediate release morphine dose to the equivalent 12 hourly sustained release morphine dose by adding the previous days total morphine requirement (regular and breakthrough doses) and dividing by 2.
- Give the last immediate release morphine dose with the first sustained release dose to ensure full analgesic cover.
- Always prescribe immediate release morphine PRN (at a dose equivalent to 4 hourly dose of morphine) to cover breakthrough pain. If breakthrough pain occurs regularly increase the sustained release morphine dose by 30–50%.
- There is no dose limit in terminal illness, any chronic illness not just terminal.
- If you have facilities, switch to parenteral opioid only when the child is unable to take oral medication.

20.3 **Equivalent dose of opioids**

Opioid drugs can be used interchangeably fairly simply, using the conversion table below. The exception for this is methadone. See the individual entry for this in Section 20.4 below.

20.4 **CPC formulary**

The following drug doses are sourced from the UK British National Formulary for Children (BNFC)[3], the Rainbows Symptom Control Guide[4] or the Hospice Africa Uganda 'Blue Book'[5]. The doses given are a guide only. Where possible, we have used the BNFC as a guide. The BNFC

Table 20.1 Opioid equivalent doses[2]

Oral opioid		Subcutaneous infusion of opioid				Opioid by patch	
Dose in mg per 24 hours		Syringe driver dose in mg per 24 hours				Dose in mcg/hr 72 hourly patches	
Morphine	Oxycodone	Morphine	Diamorphine	Oxycodone	Alfentanil	Fentanyl	Buprenorphine
	½ oral morphine dose	½ oral morphine dose	1/3 oral morphine dose	½ oral oxycodone dose	1/10 diamorphine equivalent	See manufacturers' charts for equivalence – reproduced here	
20	10	10	5	5	N/A	N/A	N/A
40	20	20	15	10	2	12	35
90	45	45	30	20	3	25	52.5
180	90	90	60	45	6	50	105
280	140	140	90	70	9	75	140
360	180	Use alfentanil	120	90	12	100	N/A

is updated annually and for the latest guidelines readers should consult the current edition at www.bnfc.org. Different countries have different licencing policies, so readers should consult their own national formularies where available. In CPC we often use drugs or doses that are not licenced. Where drugs and doses are not licenced in the BNFC, this is noted in the table. Prescribers must take ultimate responsibility for the drugs and doses they prescribe.

You must always double check doses with your own departmental guide or local formulary. Please also check with your local formulary for cautions, contraindications, side effects and risks of prescribing in pregnancy.

Aciclovir	**Herpes simplex treatment**
	By mouth
	Child 1 month–2 years: 100 mg 5 times daily, usually for 5 days (longer if new lesions appear during treatment or if healing incomplete); dose doubled if immunocompromised or if absorption impaired
	Child 2–18 years: 200 mg 5 times daily, usually for 5 days (longer if new lesions appear during treatment or if healing incomplete); dose doubled if immunocompromised or if absorption impaired
	By intravenous infusion
	Neonate
	20 mg/kg every 8 hours for 14 days (21 days if CNS involvement)
	Child 1–3 months with disseminated herpes simplex: 20 mg/kg every 8 hours for 14 days (21 days if CNS involvement)
	Child 3 months–12 years: 250 mg/m^2 every 8 hours usually for 5 days, dose doubled if CNS involvement (given for up to 21 days) or if immunosuppressed
	Child 12–18 years: 5 mg/kg every 8 hours usually for 5 days, dose doubled if CNS involvement (given for up to 21 days) or if immunosuppressed
	Note: to avoid excessive dose in obese patients parenteral dose should be calculated on the basis of ideal weight for height
	Herpes simplex prophylaxis in the immunocompromised
	By mouth
	Child 1 month–2 years: 100–200 mg 4 times daily
	Child 2–18 years: 200–400 mg 4 times daily
	Chickenpox and herpes zoster infection
	By mouth
	Child 1 month–12 years: 20 mg/kg (max. 800 mg) 4 times daily for 5 days
	Child 12–18 years: 800 mg 5 times daily for 7 days
	By intravenous infusion
	Neonate: 10–20 mg/kg every 8 hours for at least 7 days
	Child 1–3 months: 10–20 mg/kg every 8 hours for at least 7 days
	Child 3 months–12 years: 250 mg/m^2 every 8 hours usually for 5 days, dose doubled if immunocompromised
	Child 12–18 years: 5 mg/kg every 8 hours usually for 5 days, dose doubled if immunocompromised
	Note: to avoid excessive dose in obese patients parenteral dose should be calculated on the basis of ideal weight for height

Table (continued)

	Attenuation of chickenpox if varicella–zoster immunoglobulin not indicated

By mouth

Child 1 month–18 years: 10 mg/kg 4 times daily for 7 days starting 1 week after exposure

Amitriptyline | **Neuropathic pain in palliative care**

By mouth

Child 2–12 years: initially 200–500 micrograms/kg (max. 25 mg) once daily at night, increased if necessary; max. 1 mg/kg twice daily on specialist advice

Child 12–18 years: initially 10–25 mg once daily at night, increased gradually if necessary to usual dose 75 mg at night; higher doses on specialist advice

Amoxicillin | **Susceptible infections including urinary-tract infections, sinusitis, *haemophilus influenzae* infections**

By mouth

Neonate under 7 days: 30 mg/kg (max. 62.5 mg) twice daily; dose doubled in severe infection

Neonate 7–28 days: 30 mg/kg (max. 62.5 mg) three times daily; dose doubled in severe infection

Child 1 month–1 year: 62.5 mg three times daily; dose doubled in severe infection

Child 1–5 years: 125 mg three times daily; dose doubled in severe infection

Child 5–18 years: 250 mg three times daily; dose doubled in severe infection

By intramuscular injection

Child 1 month–18 years: 30 mg/kg every 8 hours (max. 500 mg every 8 hours)

By intravenous injection or infusion

Neonate under 7 days: 30 mg/kg every 12 hours; dose doubled in severe infection

Neonate 7–28 days: 30 mg/kg every 8 hours; dose doubled in severe infection

Child 1 month–18 years: 20–30 mg/kg (max. 500 mg) every 8 hours; dose doubled in severe infection (max. 4 g daily)

Uncomplicated community-acquired pneumonia, invasive salmonellosis

By mouth

Child 1 month–1 year: 125 mg three times daily

Child 1–5 years: 250 mg three times daily

Child 5–18 years: 500 mg three times daily

By slow intravenous injection or by intravenous infusion

Neonate under 7 days: 50 mg/kg every 12 hours

Neonate 7–28 days: 50 mg/kg every 8 hours

Child 1 month–18 years: 30 mg/kg every 8 hours; dose doubled in severe infection (max. 4 g daily)

Listerial meningitis (in combination with another antibacterial), group B streptococcal infection, enterococcal endocarditis

By intravenous infusion

Neonate under 7 days: 50 mg/kg every 12 hours; dose may be doubled in meningitis

Neonate 7–28 days: 50 mg/kg every 8 hours; dose may be doubled in meningitis

Child 1 month–18 years: 50 mg/kg every 4–6 hours (max. 2 g every 4 hours)

(continued)

	Otitis media
	By mouth
	Child 1 month–18 years: 40 mg/kg daily in three divided doses (max. 3 g daily in three divided doses)
Amphotericin	**Severe invasive and/or systemic candidal or fungal infections**
	By intravenous infusion
	There are different preparations of amphotericin which each have different dosing instructions. The reader should check the product information for the preparation they have available locally
Asilone®	**For indigestion and acid reflux**
	By mouth
	Child 12–18 years: 5–10 mL after meals and at bedtime or when required up to four times daily
Baclofen	**For dystonia**
	By mouth
	Child 1–10 years: 0.75–2 mg/kg daily or 2.5 mg four times daily increased gradually according to age to maintenance:
	Child 1–2 years: 10–20 mg daily in divided doses
	Child 2–6 years: 20–30 mg daily in divided doses
	Child 6–10 years: 30–60 mg daily in divided doses
	Child 10–18 years: 5 mg three times daily increased gradually; max. 2.5 mg/kg or 100 mg daily
	By intrathecal injection
	Child 4–18 years: initial test dose 25 micrograms over at least 1 minute via catheter or lumbar puncture, increased in 25 microgram steps (not more often than every 24 hours) to max. 100 micrograms to determine appropriate dose then dose-titration phase, most often using infusion pump (implanted into chest wall or abdominal wall tissues) to establish maintenance dose (ranging from 24 micrograms to 1.2 mg daily in children under 12 years or 1.4 microgram daily for those over 12 years) retaining some spasticity to avoid sensation of paralysis
Benzyl benzoate	Apply over whole body and repeat the following day (without washing). Wash off after a further 24 hours. It is irritant and other drugs (such as malathion or permethrin) should be used if available. If benzyl benzoate is used it should be diluted to minimize risk of irritation, although this reduces efficacy. Not recommended for children in the UK, but often used in Africa where no other options are available
Benzylpenicillin (Penicillin G)	**Mild to moderate susceptible infections (including throat infections, otitis media, pneumonia, cellulitis, neonatal sepsis)**
	By intramuscular injection or by slow intravenous injection or infusion (intravenous route recommended in neonates and infants)
	Preterm neonate and neonate under 7 days: 25 mg/kg every 12 hours; dose doubled in severe infection
	Neonate 7–28 days: 25 mg/kg every 8 hours; dose doubled in severe infection
	Child 1 month–18 years: 25 mg/kg every 6 hours; increased to 50 mg/kg every 4–6 hours (max. 2.4 g every 4 hours) in severe infection

	Endocarditis (combined with another antibacterial if necessary)
	By slow intravenous injection or infusion
	Child 1 month–18 years: 25 mg/kg every 4 hours, increased if necessary to 50 mg/kg (max. 2.4 g) every 4 hours
	Meningitis, meningococcal disease
	By slow intravenous injection or infusion
	Preterm neonate and neonate: 75 mg/kg every 8 hours
	Child 1 month–18 years: 50 mg/kg every 4–6 hours (max. 2.4 g every 4 hours)
	Note: Important. If bacterial meningitis and especially meningococcal disease is suspected, give a single injection of benzylpenicillin by intravenous injection (or by intramuscular injection) before transferring the patient urgently to hospital. Suitable doses are: Infant under 1 year 300 mg; Child 1–9 years 600 mg, 10 years and over 1.2 g. In penicillin allergy, cefotaxime may be an alternative; chloramphenicol may be used if there is a history of anaphylaxis to penicillins
	Treatment or prevention of neonatal group B streptococcus infection
	By slow intravenous injection or infusion
	Preterm neonate and neonate under 7 days: 50 mg/kg every 12 hours
	Neonate 7–28 days: 50 mg/kg every 8 hours
Bethanechol	Not licensed in children. Unlicensed use 0.1 – 0.25 mg/kg up to max. of 25 mg three times daily before food. Not licenced for use in children in the UK
Bisacodyl	**Constipation**
	(tablets act in 10–12 hours; suppositories act in 20–60 minutes)
	By mouth
	Child 4–10 years: 5 mg at night
	Child 10–18 years: 5–10 mg at night; increased if necessary (max. 20 mg)
	By rectum (suppository)
	Child 2–10 years: 5 mg in the morning
	Child 10–18 years: 10 mg in the morning
Buprenorphine	**Moderate to severe pain**
	By sublingual administration
	Child body weight 16–25 kg: 100 micrograms every 6–8 hours
	Child body weight 25–37.5 kg: 100–200 micrograms every 6–8 hours
	Child body weight 37.5–50 kg: 200–300 micrograms every 6–8 hours
	Child body weight over 50 kg: 200–400 micrograms every 6–8 hours
	By intramuscular or by slow intravenous injection
	Child 6 months–12 years: 3–6 micrograms/kg every 6–8 hours, max. 9 micrograms/kg
	Child 12–18 years: 300–600 micrograms every 6–8 hours
	Patches: (a total daily morphine dose of 40 mg is equivalent to 35 mcg/hour patches). Patches are available from Napp in 5 micrograms/hour; 10 micrograms/hour and 20 micrograms/hour for 7 days. They are also available in 35 micrograms/hour; 52.5 micrograms/hour and 70 micrograms/hour for 96 hours
	When starting, analgesic effect should *not* be evaluated until the system has been worn for *72 hours* (to allow for gradual increase in plasma-buprenorphine concentration)—if necessary, dose should be adjusted at 3-day intervals using a patch of the next strength or 2 patches of the same strength (applied at *same time* to avoid confusion). Maximum two patches can be used at any one time. Not licenced for use in children in the UK

(continued)

Carbachol	**Urinary retention (secondary to morphine)** *Subcutaneously* Child 1–5: 75 micrograms three times daily Child 5–12: 150 micrograms three times daily Child 12–18: 250 micrograms three times daily. Not licenced for use in children in the UK
Carbamazepine	**Partial and generalized tonic–clonic seizures, neuropathic pain, some movement disorders** *By mouth* Child 1 month–12 years: initially 5 mg/kg at night or 2.5 mg/kg twice daily, increased as necessary by 2.5–5 mg/kg every 3–7 days; usual maintenance dose 5 mg/kg two to three times daily; doses up to 20 mg/kg daily have been used Child 12–18 years: initially 100–200 mg one to two times daily, increased slowly to usual maintenance dose 200–400 mg two to three times daily; in some cases doses up to 1.8 g daily may be needed *By rectum* Child 1 month–18 years: use approx. 25% more than the oral dose (max. 250 mg) up to four times daily
Ceftazidime	**Infections due to sensitive Gram-positive and Gram-negative bacteria** *By intravenous injection or infusion* Neonate under 7 days: 25 mg/kg every 24 hours; dose doubled in severe infection and meningitis Neonate 7–21 days: 25 mg/kg every 12 hours; dose doubled in severe infection and meningitis Neonate 21–28 days: 25 mg/kg every 8 hours; dose doubled in severe infection and meningitis Child 1 month–18 years: 25 mg/kg every 8 hours; dose doubled in severe infection, febrile neutropenia and meningitis (max. 6 g daily)
Ceftriaxone	**Infections due to sensitive Gram-positive and Gram-negative bacteria** *By intravenous infusion over 60 minutes* Neonate: 20–50 mg/kg once daily *By deep intramuscular injection, by intravenous injection over 2–4 minutes or by intravenous infusion* Child 1 month–12 years: body weight under 50 kg: 50 mg/kg once daily; up to 80 mg/kg daily in severe infections and meningitis; doses of 50 mg/kg and over by intravenous infusion only. Body weight 50 kg and over: dose as for child 12–18 years Child 12–18 years: 1 g daily; 2–4 g daily in severe infections and meningitis; intramuscular doses over 1 g divided between more than one site; single intravenous doses above 1 g by intravenous infusion only
Chloramphenicol	**Severe infections such as septicaemia, meningitis and epiglottitis** *By intravenous injection* Neonate up to 14 days: 12.5 mg/kg twice daily Neonate 14–28 days: 12.5 mg/kg two to four times daily *By mouth or by intravenous injection or infusion* Child 1 month–18 years: 12.5 mg/kg every 6 hours; dose may be doubled in severe infections such as septicaemia, meningitis and epiglottitis providing plasma-chloramphenicol concentrations are measured and high doses reduced as soon as indicated *Note*: Check dosage carefully; overdosage can be fatal

Table (continued)

Chlorpromazine	**Relief of acute psychosis or delirium**
	By deep intramuscular injection

Child 1–6 years: 500 micrograms/kg every 6–8 hours (max. 40 mg daily)

Child 6–12 years: 500 micrograms/kg every 6–8 hours (max. 75 mg daily)

Child 12–18 years: 25–50 mg every 6–8 hours

Nausea and vomiting

By mouth

Child 1–6 years: 500 micrograms/kg every 4–6 hours; max. 40 mg daily

Child 6–12 years: 500 micrograms/kg every 4–6 hours; max. 75 mg daily

Child 12–18 years: 10–25 mg every 4–6 hours

By deep intramuscular injection

Child 1–6 years: 500 micrograms/kg every 6–8 hours; max. 40 mg daily

Child 6–12 years: 500 micrograms/kg every 6–8 hours; max. 75 mg daily

Child 12–18 years: initially 25 mg then 25–50 mg every 3–4 hours until vomiting stops

Cholestyramine	**Pruritus associated with liver disease (trial for 3 days only, if o effect try alternative treatment); diarrhoea associated with small bowel disease or radiation**

By mouth

Child 1 month–1 year : 1 g once daily in a suitable liquid, adjusted according to response; total daily dose may alternatively be given in 2–4 divided doses (max. 9 g daily)

Child 1–6 years : 2 g once daily in a suitable liquid, adjusted according to response; total daily dose may alternatively be given in 2–4 divided doses (max. 18 g daily)

Child 6–12 years : 4 g once daily in a suitable liquid, adjusted according to response; total daily dose may alternatively be given in 2–4 divided doses (max. 24 g daily)

Child 12–18 years : 4–8 g once daily in a suitable liquid, adjusted according to response; total daily dose may alternatively be given in 2–4 divided doses (max. 36 g daily)

Counselling: Other drugs should be taken at least 1 hour before or 4–6 hours after cholestyramine to reduce possible interference with absorption

Clonazepam	**All forms of epilepsy**

By mouth

Child 1 month–1 year: initially 250 micrograms at night for four nights, increased over 2–4 weeks to usual maintenance dose of 0.5–1 mg at night (may be given in three divided doses if necessary)

Child 1–5 years: initially 250 micrograms at night for four nights, increased over 2–4 weeks to usual maintenance of 1–3 mg at night (may be given in three divided doses if necessary)

Child 5–12 years: initially 500 micrograms at night for four nights, increased over 2–4 weeks to usual maintenance dose of 3–6 mg at night (may be given in three divided doses if necessary)

Child 12–18 years: initially 1 mg at night for four nights, increased over 2–4 weeks to usual maintenance dose of 4–8 mg at night (may be given in 3–4 divided doses if necessary)

Cloxacillin	Not licenced for use in children in UK

(continued)

Table (continued)

Co-danthramer	**Constipation**
	Capsules, co-danthramer 25/200 (dantron 25 mg, poloxamer '188' 200 mg).
	By mouth
	Child 6–12 years: 1 capsule at night
	Child 12–18 years: 1–2 capsules at night
	Strong capsules, co-danthramer 37.5/500 (dantron 37.5 mg, poloxamer '188' 500 mg).
	By mouth
	Child 12–18 years: 1–2 capsules at night
Co-danthrusate	**Constipation**
	By mouth
	Child 6–12 years: 1 capsule at night
	Child 12–18 years: 1–3 capsules at night
Codeine phosphate	**Mild to moderate pain**
	By mouth or by rectum or by subcutaneous injection or by intramuscular injection
	Neonate: 0.5–1 mg/kg every 4–6 hours
	Child 1 month–12 years: 0.5–1 mg/kg every 4–6 hours, max. 240 mg daily
	Child 12–18 years: 30–60 mg every 4–6 hours, max. 240 mg daily
Co-trimoxazole	**Treatment of susceptible infections** (dose expressed as co-trimoxazole)
	By mouth
	Child 6 weeks–12 years: 24 mg/kg twice daily or
	Child 6 weeks–6 months: 120 mg twice daily
	Child 6 months–6 years: 240 mg twice daily
	Child 6–12 years: 480 mg twice daily
	Child 12–18 years: 960 mg twice daily
	By intravenous infusion
	Child 6 weeks–18 years: 18 mg/kg every 12 hours; increased in severe infection to 27 mg/kg (max. 1.44 g) every 12 hours
	Treatment of *Pneumocystis jiroveci*/*Pneumocystis carinii* (*P. carinii*) infections
	By mouth or by intravenous infusion
	Child 1 month–18 years: 60 mg/kg every 12 hours for 14 days; total daily dose may alternatively be given in three to four divided doses
	Note: Oral route preferred
	Prophylaxis of *Pneumocystis jiroveci* *Pneumocystis carinii* (*P. carinii*) infections
	By mouth
	Child 1 month–18 years: 450 mg/m^2 (max 960 mg) twice daily for three days of the week (either consecutively or on alternate days)
	Note: Dose regimens may vary, consult local guidelines

Table (continued)

Cyclizine	**Nausea and vomiting of known cause; nausea and vomiting associated with vestibular disorders and palliative care** *By mouth or by intravenous injection over 3–5 minutes* Child 1 month–6 years: 0.5–1 mg/kg up to three times daily; max. single dose 25 mg Child 6–12 years: 25 mg up to three times daily Child 12–18 years: 50 mg up to three times daily *By rectum* Child 2–6 years: 12.5 mg up to three times daily Child 6–12 years: 25 mg up to three times daily Child 12–18 years: 50 mg up to three times daily *By continuous intravenous or subcutaneous infusion* Child 1 month–2 years: 3 mg/kg over 24 hours Child 2–5 years: 50 mg over 24 hours Child 6–12 years: 75 mg over 24 hours Child 12–18 years: 150 mg over 24 hours
Dantrolene	**Chronic severe spasticity of voluntary muscle** *By mouth* Child 5–12 years: initially 500 micrograms/kg once daily; after 7 days increase to 500 micrograms/kg/dose three times daily; every 7 days increase by further 500 micrograms/kg/dose until satisfactory response; max. 2 mg/kg three to four times daily (max. total daily dose 400 mg) Child 12–18 years: initially 25 mg once daily; increase to three times daily after 7 days; every 7 days increase by further 500 micrograms/kg/dose until satisfactory response; max. 2 mg/kg three to four times daily (max. total daily dose 400 mg)
Dexamethasone	**Inflammatory and allergic disorders** *By mouth* Child 1 month–18 years: 10–100 micrograms/kg daily in one to two divided doses, adjusted according to response; up to 300 micrograms/kg daily may be required in emergency situations *By intramuscular injection or slow intravenous injection or infusion* Child 1 month–12 years: 100–400 micrograms/kg daily in one to two divided doses; max. 24 mg daily Child 12–18 years: initially 0.5–24 mg daily **Cerebral oedema associated with malignancy** *By intravenous injection* Child under 35 kg body weight: initially 20 mg, then 4 mg every 3 hours for 3 days, then 4 mg every 6 hours for 1 day, then 2 mg every 6 hours for 4 days, then decrease by 1 mg daily Child over 35 kg body weight: initially 25 mg, then 4 mg every 2 hours for 3 days, then 4 mg every 4 hours for 1 day, then 4 mg every 6 hours for 4 days, then decrease by 2 mg daily **Bacterial meningitis** *By slow intravenous injection (as dexamethasone phosphate)* Child 2 months–18 years: 150 micrograms/kg every 6 hours for 4 days starting before or with first dose of antibacterial

(continued)

Diamorphine	**Acute or chronic pain** *By mouth* Child 1 month–12 years: 100–200 micrograms/kg (max. 10 mg) every 4 hours as necessary Child 12–18 years: 5–10 mg every 4 hours as necessary *By intravenous administration* Neonate (ventilated): initially by intravenous injection over 30 minutes, 50 micrograms/kg then by continuous intravenous infusion, 15 micrograms/kg/hour Neonate (non-ventilated): by continuous intravenous infusion 2.5–7 micrograms/kg/hour Child 1 month–12 years: by continuous intravenous infusion 12.5–25 micrograms/kg/hour *By intravenous injection* Child 1–3 months: 20 micrograms/kg every 6 hours as necessary Child 3–6 months: 25–50 micrograms/kg every 6 hours as necessary Child 6–12 months: 75 micrograms/kg every 4 hours as necessary Child 1–12 years: 75–100 micrograms/kg every 4 hours as necessary Child 12–18 years: 2.5–5 mg every 4 hours as necessary *By continuous subcutaneous infusion* Child (any age): 20–100 micrograms/kg/hour *By subcutaneous or by intramuscular injection* Child 12–18 years: 5 mg every 4 hours as necessary **Acute pain in an emergency setting, short painful procedures** *Intranasally* Child 3–18 years: 100 micrograms/kg
Diazepam	**Status epilepticus, febrile convulsions, convulsions caused by poisoning** *By intravenous injection over 3–5 minutes* Neonate: 300–400 micrograms/kg repeated after 10 minutes if necessary Child 1 month–12 years: 300–400 micrograms/kg repeated after 10 minutes if necessary Child 12–18 years: 10–20 mg repeated after 10 minutes if necessary *By rectum (as rectal solution)* Neonate: 1.25–2.5 mg repeated after 10 minutes if necessary Child 1 month–2 years: 5 mg repeated after 10 minutes if necessary Child 2–12 years: 5–10 mg repeated after 10 minutes if necessary Child 12–18 years: 10 mg repeated after 10 minutes if necessary **Dystonia (muscle spasm) in cerebral spasticity or in postoperative skeletal muscle spasm** *By mouth* Child 1–12 months: initially 250 micrograms/kg twice daily Child 1–5 years: initially 2.5 mg twice daily Child 5–12 years: initially 5 mg twice daily Child 12–18 years: initially 10 mg twice daily; max. total daily dose 40 mg **Tetanus** *By intravenous injection* Child 1 month–18 years: 100–300 micrograms/kg repeated every 1–4 hours *By intravenous infusion (or by nasoduodenal tube)* Child 1 month–18 years: 3–10 mg/kg over 24 hours, adjusted according to response

Table (continued)

Diclofenac	**For mild to moderate pain, fever and inflammatory diseases**

For mild to moderate pain, fever and inflammatory diseases

By mouth or by rectum

Child 6 months–18 years: 0.3–1 micrograms/kg (max. 50 mg) three times daily

Postoperative pain

By rectum

Child 6–18 years: 0.5–1 mg/kg (max. 75 mg) twice daily for max. 4 days; total daily dose may alternatively be given in three divided doses

By intravenous infusion or deep intramuscular injection into gluteal muscle

Child 2–18 years: 0.3–1 mg/kg once or twice daily for max. 2 days (max. 150 mg daily)

Dihydrocodeine

Moderate to severe pain

By mouth or by intramuscular injection or by subcutaneous injection

Child 1–4 years: 500 micrograms/kg every 4–6 hours

Child 4–12 years: 0.5–1 mg/kg (max. 30 mg) every 4–6 hours

Child 12–18 years: 30 mg (max. 50 mg by intramuscular or deep subcutaneous injection) every 4–6 hours

Docusate

Constipation

By mouth

Child 6 months–2 years: 12.5 mg three times daily (use paediatric oral solution)

Child 2–12 years: 12.5–25 mg three times daily (use paediatric oral solution)

Child 12–18 years: up to 500 mg daily in divided doses

Note: Oral preparations act within 1–2 days; response to rectal administration usually occurs within 20 minutes; recommended doses may be exceeded on specialist advice

Domperidone

Nausea and vomiting

By mouth

Body weight up to 35 kg; 250–500 micrograms/kg three to four times daily; max. 2.4 mg/kg in 24 hours

Body weight 35 kg and over: 10–20 mg three to four times daily, max. 80 mg daily

By rectum

Body weight 15–35 kg; 30 mg twice daily

Body weight over 35 kg: 60 mg twice daily

Fentanyl

For breakthough pain

By transmucosal application

(lozenge with oromucosal applicator available as 200 micrograms, 400 micrograms, 600 micrograms, 800 micrograms)

Child 2–18 years (over 10 kg body weight) 15–20 micrograms/kg as a single dose; max. dose 400 micrograms

For chronic pain

By transdermal route

(Patches available 12 micrograms/hour for 72 hours), 25 micrograms/hour for 72 hours, 50 micrograms/hour for 72 hours, 75 micrograms/hour for 72 hours, 100 micrograms/ hour for 72 hours

A total 24 hour dose of 40 mg morphine is equivalent to one 12 micrograms/ hour patch.

Child 2–16 years: previously treated with strong opioid analgesic, initial dose based on previous 24-hour opioid requirement (see above)

(continued)

Table (continued)

	Child 16–18 years: child not previously treated with strong opioid analgesic, one '12' or '25 micrograms/hour' patch replaced after 72 hours. Child previously treated with strong opioid analgesic, initial dose based on previous 24-hour opioid requirement\

Dose adjustment

When starting, evaluation of the analgesic effect should *not* be made before the system has been worn for *24 hours* (to allow for the gradual increase in plasma–fentanyl concentration)—previous analgesic therapy should be phased out gradually from time of first patch application; if necessary dose should be adjusted at 72-hour intervals in steps of 12–25 micrograms/hour. More than one patch may be used at a time for doses greater than 100 micrograms/hour (but applied at *same time* to avoid confusion)—consider additional or alternative analgesic therapy if dose required exceeds 300 micrograms/hour (*important:* it may take up to 25 hours for the plasma–fentanyl concentration to decrease by 50%—replacement opioid therapy should be initiated at a low dose and increased gradually). In view of the long duration of action, children who have had severe side effects should be monitored for up to 24 hours after patch removal

Fluconazole

Mucosal candidiasis (except genital)

By mouth or by intravenous infusion

Neonate under 2 weeks: 3–6 mg/kg on first day then 3 mg/kg every 72 hours

Neonate 2–4 weeks: 3–6 mg/kg on first day then 3 mg/kg every 48 hours

Child 1 month–12 years: 3–6 mg/kg on first day then 3 mg/kg (max. 100 mg) daily for 7–14 days in oropharyngeal candidiasis (max. 14 days except in severely immunocompromised patients); for 14–30 days in other mucosal infections (e.g. oesophagitis, candiduria, non-invasive bronchopulmonary infections)

Child 12–18 years: 50 mg daily (100 mg daily in unusually difficult infections) given for 7–14 days in oropharyngeal candidiasis (max. 14 days except in severely immunocompromised patients); for 14–30 days in other mucosal infections (e.g. oesophagitis, candiduria, non-invasive bronchopulmonary infections)

Vaginal candidiasis and candidal balanitis

By mouth

Child 16–18 years: a single dose of 150 mg

Tinea pedis, corporis, cruris, pityriasis versicolor and dermal candidiasis

By mouth

Child 1 month–18 years: 3 mg/kg (max. 50 mg) daily for 2–4 weeks (for up to 6 weeks in tinea pedis); maximum duration of treatment is 6 weeks.

Invasive candidal infections (including candidaemia and disseminated candidiasis) and cryptococcal infections (including meningitis)

By mouth or by intravenous infusion

Neonate under 2 weeks: 6–12 mg/kg every 72 hours, treatment continued according to response (at least 8 weeks for cryptococcal meningitis)

Neonate 2–4 weeks: 6–12 mg/kg every 48 hours, treatment continued according to response (at least 8 weeks for cryptococcal meningitis)

Child 1 month–18 years: 6–12 mg/kg (max. 800 mg) daily, treatment continued according to response (at least 8 weeks for cryptococcal meningitis)

Prevention of fungal infections in immunocompromised patients

By mouth or by intravenous infusion:

Neonate under 2 weeks: according to extent and duration of neutropenia, 3–12 mg/kg every 72 hours

Neonate 2–4 weeks: according to extent and duration of neutropenia, 3–12 mg/kg every 48 hours

Child 1 month–18 years: according to extent and duration of neutropenia, 3–12 mg/kg (max. 400 mg) daily; 12 mg/kg (max. 800 mg) daily if high risk of systemic infections, e.g. following bone marrow transplantation; commence treatment before anticipated onset of neutropenia and continue for 7 days after neutrophil count in desirable range

Flucloxacillin	**Infections due to beta-lactamase-producing staphylococci; adjunct in pneumonia, impetigo, cellulitis**

By mouth

Neonate under 7 days: 25 mg/kg twice daily

Neonate 7–21 days: 25 mg/kg three times daily

Neonate 21–28 days: 25 mg/kg four times daily

Child 1 month–2 years: 62.5–125 mg four times daily

Child 2–10 years: 125–250 mg four times daily

Child 10–18 years: 250–500 mg four times daily

By intramuscular injection

Child 1 month–18 years: 12.5–25 mg/kg every 6 hours (max. 500 mg every 6 hours)

By slow intravenous injection or by intravenous infusion

Neonate under 7 days: 25 mg/kg every 12 hours; may be doubled in severe infection

Neonate 7–21 days: 25 mg/kg every 8 hours; may be doubled in severe infection

Neonate 21–28 days: 25 mg/kg every 6 hours; may be doubled in severe infection

Child 1 month–18 years; 12.5–25 mg/kg every 6 hours (max. 1 g every 6 hours); may be doubled in severe infection

Fluoxetine	**Major depression**

By mouth

Child 8–18 years: 10 micrograms once daily increased after 3 weeks if necessary, max. 20 micrograms once daily (exceptionally, up to 40 micrograms once daily)

Note: Long duration of action. Consider the long half-life of fluoxetine when adjusting dosage (or in overdosage)

Folic acid	**Folate supplementation in neonates**

By mouth

Neonate: 50 micrograms once daily or 500 micrograms once weekly

Megaloblastic anaemia due to folate deficiency

By mouth

Neonate: initially 500 micrograms/kg once daily for up to 4 months; maintenance 500 micrograms/kg every 1–7 days

Child 1 month–1 year: initially 500 micrograms/kg once daily (max. 5 mg) for up to 4 months; maintenance 500 micrograms/kg (max. 5 mg) every 1–7 days

Child 1–18 years: 5 mg daily for 4 months; maintenance 5 mg every 1–7 days

(continued)

Table (continued)

	Haemolytic anaemia; metabolic disorders

By mouth

Child 1 month–12 years: 2.5–5 mg once daily

Child 12–18 years: 5–10 mg once daily

Foscarnet **CMV retinitis**

By intravenous infusion

Child 1 month–18 years: induction 60 mg/kg every 8 hours for 2–3 weeks then maintenance 60 mg/kg daily, increased to 90–120 mg/kg if tolerated; if retinitis progresses on maintenance dose, repeat induction regimen

Mucocutaneous herpes simplex infection

By intravenous infusion

Child 1 month–18 years: 40 mg/kg every 8 hours for 2–3 weeks or until lesions heal

---

Furosemide **Oedema**

By mouth

Neonate: 0.5–2 mg/kg every 12–24 hours (every 24 hours if post-menstrual age under 31 weeks)

Child 1 month–12 years: 0.5–2 mg/kg two to three times daily (every 24 hours if post-menstrual age under 31 weeks); higher doses may be required in resistant oedema; max. 12 mg/kg daily, not to exceed 80 mg daily

Child 12–18 years: 20–40 mg daily, increased in resistant oedema to 80 mg daily or more

By slow intravenous injection

Neonate: 0.5–1 mg/kg every 12–24 hours (every 24 hours if post-menstrual age under 31 weeks)

Child 1 month–12 years: 0.5–1 mg/kg (max. 4 mg/kg) repeated every 8 hours as necessary

Child 12–18 years: 20–40 mg repeated every 8 hours as necessary; higher doses may be required in resistant cases

By continuous intravenous infusion

Child 1 month–18 years: 0.1–2 mg/kg/hour (following cardiac surgery, initially 100 micrograms/kg/hour, doubled every 2 hours until urine output exceeds 1 mL/kg/hour)

Note: For administration by mouth tablets may be crushed and mixed with water or injection solution diluted and given by mouth

For intravenous injection give over 5–10 minutes at a usual rate of 100 micrograms/kg/minute (not exceeding 500 micrograms/kg/minute), max. 4 mg/minute; for intravenous infusion dilute with sodium chloride 0.9% intravenous infusion to a concentration of 1–2 mg/mL—glucose solutions unsuitable (infusion pH must be above 5.5)

Ganciclovir **Life-threatening or sight-threatening cytomegalovirus infections in immunocompromised patients**

By intravenous infusion

Child 1 month–18 years: initially (induction) 5 mg/kg every 12 hours for 14–21 days for treatment or for 7–14 days for prevention; for maintenance dose, see below

Maintenance (for patients at risk of relapse of retinitis)

By intravenous infusion

Child 1 month–18 years: 6 mg/kg daily on 5 days per week or 5 mg/kg daily until adequate recovery of immunity; if retinitis progresses initial induction treatment may be repeated

Table (continued)

Gaviscon® Infant	**Dyspepsia and Gastro-oesophageal reflux**
	By mouth
	Neonate body weight under 4.5 kg: 1 'dose' (half dual-sachet) mixed with feeds (or water, for breast-fed infants) when required (max. six times in 24 hours)
	Neonate body weight over 4.5 kg: two 'doses' (1 dual-sachet) mixed with feeds (or water, for breast-fed infants) when required (max. six times in 24 hours)
	Child 1 month–2 years: body weight under 4.5 kg – dose as for neonate
	Body–weight over 4.5 kg – two 'doses' (1 dual-sachet) mixed with feeds (or water, for breast-fed infants) when required (max. six times in 24 hours)
Gaviscon® Advance	Child 2–12 years: 2.5–5 mL after meals and at bedtime (under medical advice only)
	Child 12–18 years: 5–10 mL after meals and at bedtime
	These prepartions are not yet available in Africa, but may become so
Gentamicin	**Septicaemia, meningitis and other CNS infections, biliary-tract infection, acute pyelonephritis, endocarditis, pneumonia in hospital patients, adjunct in listerial meningitis**
	Multiple daily dose regimen by intramuscular or by slow intravenous injection over at least 3 minutes
	Child 1 month–12 years: 2.5 mg/kg every 8 hours
	Child 12–18 years: 2 mg/kg every 8 hours
	Once daily dose regimen (not for endocarditis or meningitis) by intravenous infusion
	Child 1 month–18 years: initially 7 mg/kg, then adjusted according to serum-gentamicin concentration
	Pseudomonal lung infection in cystic fibrosis
	By slow intravenous injection over at least 3 minutes or by intravenous infusion
	Child 1 month–18 years: 3 mg/kg every 8 hours
	By inhalation of nebulized solution
	Child 1 month–2 years: 40 mg twice daily
	Child 2–8 years: 80 mg twice daily
	Child 8–18 years: 160 mg twice daily
	Bacterial ventriculitis and CNS infection (supplement to systemic therapy)
	By intrathecal or intraventricular injection, seek specialist advice
	Neonate: seek specialist advice
	Child 1 month–18 years: 1 mg daily (increased if necessary to 5 mg daily)
	Note: only preservative-free, intrathecal preparation should be used
Glycerin/glycerol	**Constipation**
	By rectum
	Child 1 month–1 year: 1-g suppository as required
	Child 1–12 years: 2-g suppository as required
	Child 12–18 years: 4-g suppository as required
Glycopyrronium	**Control of upper airways secretion and hypersalivation**
	By mouth
	Child 1 month–18 years: 40–100 micrograms/kg three to four times daily, adjusted according to response

(continued)

Table (continued)

Griseofulvin	**Dermatophyte infections where topical therapy has failed or is inappropriate**
	By mouth
	Child 1 month–12 years: 10 mg/kg (max. 500 mg) once daily or in divided doses; in severe infection dose may be doubled, reducing when response occurs
	Child 12–18 years: 500 mg once daily or in divided doses; in severe infection dose may be doubled, reducing when response occurs
	Tinea capitis caused by *Trichophyton tonsurans*
	By mouth
	Child 1 month–12 years: 15–20 mg/kg (max. 1 g) once daily or in divided doses
	Child 12–18 years: 1 g once daily or in divided doses
Haloperidol	**Management of psychomotor agitation or delirium**
	Child 2–12 years: initially 12.5–25 micrograms/kg twice daily, adjusted according to response to max. 10 mg daily. Child 12–18 years initially 0.5–3 mg two to three times daily or 3–5 mg two to three times daily in severe delirium
	Nausea and vomiting in palliative care
	By mouth
	Child 12–18 years: 1.5 mg once daily at night, increased to 1.5 mg twice daily if necessary; max. 5 mg twice daily
	By continuous intravenous or subcutaneous infusion
	Child 1 month–12 years: 25–85 micrograms/kg over 24 hours
	Child 12–18 years: 1.5–5 mg over 24 hours
Hyoscine butylbromide	**Symptomatic relief of gastro-intestinal or genito-urinary disorders characterized by smooth muscle spasm**
	By mouth
	Child 6–12 years: 10 mg three times daily
	Child 12–18 years: 20 mg four times daily
	Excessive respiratory secretions and bowel colic in palliative care
	By mouth
	Child 1 month–2 years: 300–500 micrograms/kg (max. 5 mg) three to four times daily
	Child 2–5 years: 5 mg three to four times daily
	Child 5–12 years: 10 mg three to four times daily
	Child 12–18 years: 10–20 mg three to four times daily
	By intramuscular or intravenous injection
	Child 1 month–4 years: 300–500 micrograms/kg (max. 5 mg) three to four times daily
	Child 5–12 years: 5–10 mg three to four times daily
	Child 12–18 years: 10–20 mg three to four times daily
Hyoscine hydrobromide	**Motion sickness**
	By mouth
	Child 3–4 years: 75 micrograms 20 minutes before the start of journey, repeated if necessary; max. 150 micrograms in 24 hours
	Child 4–10 years: 75–150 micrograms 30 minutes before the start of journey, repeated every 6 hours if required; max. three doses in 24 hours
	Child 10–18 years: 150–300 micrograms 30 minutes before the start of journey, repeated every 6 hours if required; max. three doses in 24 hours

Table (continued)

	By topical application
	Child 10–18 years: apply 1 patch (1 mg) to the hairless area of skin behind ear 5–6 hours before journey; replace if necessary after 72 hours, siting replacement patch behind the other ear
	Excessive respiratory secretions
	By mouth or by sublingual administration
	Child 2–12 years: 10 micrograms/kg, max. 300 micrograms four times daily
	Child 12–18 years: 300 micrograms four times daily
	By transdermal route
	Child 1 month–3 years: 250 micrograms every 72 hours (quarter of a patch)
	Child 3–10 years: 500 micrograms every 72 hours (half a patch)
	Child 10–18 years: 1 mg every 72 hours (one patch)
	By subcutaneous injection or intravenous injection
	Child 1 month–18 years: 10 micrograms/kg (max. 600 micrograms) every 4 to 8 hours
	By subcutaneous injection or intravenous infusion
	1.5 to 2.5 micrograms/kg per hour (no age range specified).
	Care should be taken to avoid the discomfort of a dry mouth.
Ibuprofen	**Mild to moderate pain, pain and inflammation of soft-tissue injuries, pyrexia**
	By mouth
	Child 1–3 months: 5 mg/kg three to four times daily preferably after food
	Child 3–6 months: 50 mg three times daily preferably after food; in severe conditions up to 30 mg/kg daily in three to four divided doses
	Child 6 months–1 year: 50 mg three to four times daily preferably after food; in severe conditions up to 30 mg/kg daily in three to four divided doses
	Child 1–4 years: 100 mg three times daily preferably after food; in severe conditions up to 30 mg/kg daily in three to four divided doses
	Child 4–7 years: 150 mg three times daily preferably after food; in severe conditions up to 30 mg/kg in three to four divided doses; max. 2.4 g daily
	Child 7–10 years: 200 mg three times daily preferably after food; in severe conditions up to 30 mg/kg in three to four divided doses; max. 2.4 g daily
	Child 10–12 years: 300 mg three times daily preferably after food; in severe conditions up to 30 mg/kg in three to four divided doses; max. 2.4 g daily
	Child 12–18 years: 200–400 mg three to four times daily preferably after food; increased if necessary to max. 2.4 g daily
	Pain and inflammation in rheumatic disease including juvenile idiopathic arthritis
	By mouth
	Child 3 months–18 years (and body weight over 5 kg): 30–40 mg/kg daily in three to four divided doses preferably after food; in systemic juvenile idiopathic arthritis up to 60 mg/kg daily, max 2.4 g daily; (unlicenced), in four to six divided doses
Imipramine	**Irritable bladder, insomnia, neuropathic pain**
	By mouth
	Child 6–8 years: 25 mg at bedtime
	Child 8–11 years: 25–50 mg at bedtime
	Child 11–18 years: 50–75 mg at bedtime

(continued)

Table (continued)

Ketamine	**Prior to invasive or painful procedures**
	By intravenous injection
	Child 1 month–18 years: 1–2 mg/kg as a single dose
	Oral for Pain
	0.1–0.3 mg/kg/hr (max. 1.5 mg/kg/hr)
	Not licenced route in the UK. These are anecdotal dosing instructions only.
Ketoconazole	**Systemic mycoses that cannnot be treated with other antifungals (including histoplasmosis, blastomycosis, coccidioidomycosis, paracoccidioidomycosis); skin, hair and mucosal mycoses that cannot be treated with other antifungals (including dermatophytoses, pityrosporum folliculitis, cutaneous candidiasis, chronic mucocutaneous candidiasis, oropharyngeal and oesophageal candidiasis)**
	By mouth
	Child body weight 15–30 kg: 100 mg once daily
	Child body weight over 30 kg: 200 mg once daily, increased if response inadequate to 400 mg once daily
	Note: Treatment continued until symptoms have cleared and cultures negative (usually for 4 weeks in dermatophytoses, 2–3 weeks for oral and cutaneous candidiasis, 1–2 months for hair infections)
Lactulose	**Constipation**
	(May take up to 48 hours to act)
	By mouth
	Child 1 month–1 year: 2.5 mL twice daily, adjusted according to response
	Child 1–5 years: 5 mL twice daily, adjusted according to response
	Child 5–10 years: 10 mL twice daily, adjusted according to response
	Child 10–18 years: initially 15 mL twice daily, adjusted according to response
	Hepatic encephalopathy
	By mouth
	Child 12–18 years: 30–50 mL three times daily; adjust dose to produce 2–3 soft stools per day
Levomepromazine	**Restlessness and confusion in palliative care**
	By continuous subcutaneous infusion
	Child 1–12 years: 0.35–3 mg/kg over 24 hours
	Child 12–18 years: 12.5–200 mg over 24 hours
	Nausea and vomiting in palliative care
	By continuous intravenous or subcutaneous infusion
	Child 1 month–12 years: 100–400 micrograms/kg over 24 hours
	Child 12–18 years: 5–25 mg over 24 hours
Lorazepam	**Status epilepticus**
	By slow intravenous injection or by rectum or by sublingual administration
	Neonate: 100 micrograms/kg as a single dose, repeated once after 10 minutes if necessary
	Child 1 month–12 years: 100 micrograms/kg (max. 4 mg) as a single dose, repeated once after 10 minutes if necessary
	Child 12–18 years: 4 mg as a single dose, repeated once after 10 minutes if necessary

Mecysteine	**Reduction of sputum viscosity**
	By mouth
	Child 5–12 years: 100 mg three times daily
	Child 12–18 years: 200 mg four times daily for 2 days, then 200 mg three times daily for 6 weeks, then 200 mg twice daily
Methadone	**Severe pain not responding to other treatment**
	Note: pharmacokinetics of methadone are complicated. A single dose of methadone is marginally more potent than *morphine*. With repeated doses, methadone is several times more potent. It is also longer acting. Starting doses are therefore different to maintenance doses. Read guidance below carefully
	Oral starting dose
	0–12 years: 0.2 mg/kg as a single dose
	13 years plus: 5–10 mg as a single dose
	Not licenced route in the UK. These are anecdotal dosing instructions only
	IV or SC starting dose
	0–12 years: 0.1 mg/kg as a single dose
	13 years plus: 5–10 mg as a single dose
	Calculation of maintenance doses
	Give single doses every 4–12 hours PRN for 48 hours. After 48 hours calculate total dose of methadone given over 48 hours. Divide this figure by four to give 12 hourly dose.
	Methadone titration from morphine (or morphine equivalent)
	(from www.palliativedrugs.com)
	Note: 'Start low and go slow'.
	1. Stop morphine abruptly. *Do not reduce morphine progressively*
	2. Prescribe a dose of methadone that is 1/10th of the 24 oral morphine dose the child was on (or the morphine equivalent if the patient was on a different strong opioid). In any event, prescribe an initial maximum of 30 mg.
	3. Prescribe this same dose every 3 hours *as required*
	4. On day 6, calculate the total methadone dose *over the previous 48 hours only*, and divide this by 4 to give a regular 12 hourly dose
	5. Allow prn doses for breakthrough on top of this regular 12 hourly dose (a prn dose should be half the 12 hourly dose)
	6. Increase the 12 hourly dose by one-third *every 4–6 days* until prn medication is no longer needed
Metoclopramide	**Severe intractable vomiting of known cause, vomiting associated with radiotherapy and cytotoxics, aid to gastro-intestinal intubation, as a prokinetic in neonates**
	By mouth, by intramuscular injection or by intravenous injection over 1–2 minutes
	Neonate: 100 micrograms/kg every 6–8 hours (by mouth or by intravenous injection only)
	Child 1 month–1 year and body weight up to 10 kg: 100 micrograms/kg (max. 1 mg) twice daily
	Child 1–3 years and body weight 10–14 kg: 1 mg two to three times daily
	Child 3–5 years and body weight 15–19 kg: 2 mg two to three times daily
	Child 5–9 years and body weight 20–29 kg: 2.5 mg three times daily
	Child 9–15 years and body weight 30–60 kg: 5 mg three times daily
	Child 15–18 years and body weight over 60 kg: 10 mg three times daily
	Note: Daily dose of metoclopramide should not normally exceed 500 micrograms/kg

(continued)

Table (continued)

Miconazole	**Prevention and treatment of oral and intestinal fungal infections**

By mouth

Neonate: (oral fungal infections only) 1 mL two to four times daily smeared around the mouth after feeds

Child 1 month–2 years: 2.5 mL twice daily in the mouth after food; retain near lesions before swallowing

Child 2–6 years: 5 mL twice daily in the mouth after food; retain near lesions before swallowing

Child 6–12 years: 5 mL four times daily in the mouth after food; retain near lesions before swallowing

Child 12–18 years: 5–10 mL four times daily in the mouth after food; retain near lesions before swallowing

Note: Treatment should be continued for 48 hours after lesions have healed.

Oral gel for localized lesions

Child 6–18 years: smear small amount on the affected area with clean finger four times daily for 5–7 days (orthodontic appliances should be removed at night and brushed with gel); continue treatment for 48 hours after lesions have healed

Midazolam	**Seizures**

By buccal or intranasal administration

(Do not use nasal route unless buccal route is unavailable as it causes nasal stinging)

Neonate: 300 micrograms/kg as a single dose

Child 1–6 months: 300 micrograms/kg (max. 2.5 mg), repeated once if necessary

Child 6 months–1 year: 2.5 mg, repeated once if necessary

Child 1–5 years: 5 mg, repeated once if necessary

Child 5–10 years: 7.5 mg, repeated once if necessary

Child 10–18 years: 10 mg, repeated once if necessary

By intravenous administration

Neonate: initially by intravenous injection 150–200 micrograms/kg followed by continuous infusion of 1 microgram/kg/minute (increased by 1 microgram/kg/minute every 15 minutes until seizure controlled; max. 5 micrograms/kg/minute)

Child 1 month–18 years: initially by intravenous injection 150–200 micrograms/kg followed by continuous intravenous infusion of 1 microgram/kg/minute (increased by 1 microgram/kg/minute every 15 minutes) until seizure controlled; max. 5 micrograms/kg/minute

Sedation

SC or IV infusion (not licenced route)

Loading dose 0.15 micrograms/kg. Maintenance dose 50–300 micrograms/kg/hour.

Intranasal: 200–300 micrograms/kg/single dose (do not use nasal route unless buccal route is unavailable as it causes nasal stinging)

Buccal

300 micrograms/kg/single dose (start with 300 micrograms/kg, ideally with supervision for first dose).

Table (continued)

Morphine	**Pain**

By subcutaneous injection or by intramuscular injection

Neonate: initially 100 micrograms/kg every 6 hours, adjusted according to response

Child 1–6 months: initially 100–200 micrograms/kg every 6 hours, adjusted according to response

Child 6 months–2 years: initially 100–200 micrograms/kg every 4 hours, adjusted according to response

Child 2–12 years: initially 200 micrograms/kg every 4 hours, adjusted according to response

Child 12–18 years: initially 2.5–10 mg every 4 hours, adjusted according to response

By intravenous injection over at least 5 minutes

Neonate: initially 50 micrograms/kg every 6 hours, adjusted according to response

Child 1–6 months: initially 100 micrograms/kg every 6 hours, adjusted according to response

Child 6 months–12 years: initially 100 micrograms/kg every 4 hours, adjusted according to response

Child 12–18 years: initially 2.5 micrograms every 4 hours, adjusted according to response

By intravenous injection and infusion

Neonate: initially by intravenous injection (over at least 5 minutes) 25–100 micrograms/kg then by continuous intravenous infusion 5–40 micrograms/kg/hour, adjusted according to response

Child 1–6 months: initially by intravenous injection (over at least 5 minutes) 100–200 micrograms/kg then by continuous intravenous infusion 10–30 micrograms/kg/hour, adjusted according to response

Child 6 months–12 years: initially by intravenous injection (over at least 5 minutes) 100–200 micrograms/kg then by continuous intravenous infusion 20–30 micrograms/kg/hour, adjusted according to response

Child 12–18 years: initially by intravenous injection (over at least 5 minutes) 2.5–10 mg then by continuous intravenous infusion 20–30 micrograms/kg/hour, adjusted according to response

By mouth or by rectum

Child 1–12 months: initially 80–200 micrograms/kg every 4 hours, adjusted according to response

Child 1–2 years: initially 200–400 micrograms/kg every 4 hours, adjusted according to response

Child 2–12 years: initially 200–500 micrograms/kg (max. 20 mg) every 4 hours, adjusted according to response

Child 12–18 years: initially 5–20 mg every 4 hours, adjusted according to response

By continuous subcutaneous infusion

Child 1–3 months: 10 micrograms/kg/hour

Child 3 months–18 years: 20 micrograms/kg/hour

Naloxone	Reversal of respiratory and CNS depression following opioid overdose

By intramuscular injection

Neonate: 200 micrograms (60 micrograms/kg) as a single dose at birth

By intravenous or subcutaneous injection

Neonate: 10 micrograms/kg, repeated every 2–3 minutes if required

Reversal of opioid-induced respiratory depression

(continued)

Table (continued)

	By intravenous injection Neonate: 5–10 micrograms/kg, repeated every 2–3 minutes if required Child 1 month–12 years: 5–10 micrograms/kg; if response inadequate, give a subsequent dose of 100 micrograms/kg (max. 2 mg) Child 12–18 years: 1.5–3 micrograms/kg; if response inadequate, give subsequent doses of 100 micrograms every 2 minutes **By continuous intravenous infusion** Neonate: 5–20 micrograms/kg/hour, adjusted according to response Child 1 month–18 years: 5–20 micrograms/kg/hour, adjusted according to response
Naproxen	**Pain and inflammatory disorders** *By mouth* Child 1 month–18 years: 5 mg/kg twice daily; in severe disease, 10–15 mg/kg twice daily for short-term use only (max. 1 g daily)
Nystatin	**Treatment of intestinal candidiasis** *By mouth* Neonate:100 000 units four times daily after feeds Child 1 month–12 years: 100 000 units four times daily; immunocompromised children may require higher doses (e.g. 500 000 units four times daily) Child 12–18 years: 500 000 units four times daily; doubled in severe infection **Oral and perioral fungal infections** Neonate:100 000 units four times daily after feeds Child 1 month–18 years:100 000 units four times daily after food *Note*: Treatment is usually given for 7 days, and continued for 48 hours after lesions have healed.
Octreotide	**Bleeding from oesophageal or gastric varices** *By continuous intravenous infusion* Child 1 month–18 years: 1 microgram/kg/hour, higher doses may be required initially; when no active bleeding reduce dose over 24 hours; usual max. 50 micrograms/hour
Omeprazole	**Gastro-oesophageal reflux disease, acid-related dyspepsia, treatment of duodenal and benign gastric ulcers, prophylaxis of acid aspiration,** *By mouth* Neonate: 700 micrograms/kg once daily, increased if necessary after 7–14 days to 1.4 mg/kg; some neonates may require up to 2.8 mg/kg once daily Child 1 month–2 years: 700 micrograms/kg once daily, increased if necessary to 3 mg/kg (max. 20 mg) once daily Child body weight 10–20 kg: 10 mg once daily, increased if necessary to 20 mg once daily (in severe ulcerating reflux oesophagitis, max. 12 weeks at higher dose) Child body weight over 20 kg: 20 mg once daily, increased if necessary to 40 mg once daily (in severe ulcerating reflux oesophagitis, max. 12 weeks at higher dose) *By intravenous injection over 5 minutes or by intravenous infusion* Child 1 month–12 years: initially 500 micrograms/kg (max. 20 mg) once daily, increased to 2 mg/kg (max. 40 mg) once daily if necessary Child 12–18 years: 40 mg once daily

Table (continued)

Ondansetron	**Prevention and treatment of chemotherapy- and radiotherapy-induced nausea and vomiting**

By slow intravenous injection or by intravenous infusion

Child 1–12 years: 5 mg/m^2 immediately before chemotherapy (max. single dose 8 mg), then either repeat every 8–12 hours during chemotherapy and for at least 24 hours afterwards or give by mouth

Child 12–18 years: 8 mg immediately before chemotherapy, then either repeated every 8–12 hours during chemotherapy and for at least 24 hours afterwards or give by mouth

By mouth following intravenous administration

Child 1–12 years: 4 mg every 8–12 hours for up to 5 days

Child 12–18 years: 8 mg every 8–12 hours for up to 5 days

Oxybutynin — **Urinary frequency, urgency and incontinence, neurogenic bladder instability**

By mouth

Child 2–5 years: 1.25–2.5 mg two to three times daily

Child 5–12 years: 2.5–3 mg twice daily, increased to 5 mg two to three times daily

Child 12–18 years: 5 mg two to three times daily, increased if necessary to max. 5 mg four times daily

By intravesical instillation

Child 2–18 years: 5 mg two to three times daily

Oxycodone — **Moderate to severe pain in palliative care**

By mouth

Child 1 month–12 years: initially 200 micrograms/kg (up to 5 mg) every 4–6 hours, dose increased if necessary according to severity of pain

Child 12–18 years: initially 5 mg every 4–6 hours, dose increased if necessary according to severity of pain

Paracetamol — **Pain, pyrexia**

By mouth

Neonate over 32 weeks post-menstrual age: 20 mg/kg as a single dose then 10–15 mg/kg every 6–8 hours as necessary; max. 60 mg/kg daily in divided doses

Child 1–3 months: 30–60 mg every 8 hours as necessary; for severe symptoms 20 mg/kg as a single dose then 15–20 mg/kg every 6–8 hours; max. 60 mg/kg daily in divided doses

Child 3–12 months: 60–120 mg every 4–6 hours (max. four doses in 24 hours); for severe symptoms 20 mg/kg every 6 hours (max. 90 mg/kg daily in divided doses) for 48 hours (or longer if necessary and if adverse effects ruled out) then 15 mg/kg every 6 hours

Child 1–5 years: 120–250 mg every 4–6 hours (max. four doses in 24 hours); for severe symptoms 20 mg/kg every 6 hours (max. 90 mg/kg daily in divided doses) for 48 hours (or longer if necessary and if adverse effects ruled out) then 15 mg/kg every 6 hours

Child 6–12 years: 250–500 mg every 4–6 hours (max. four doses in 24 hours); for severe symptoms 20 mg/kg (max. 1 g) every 6 hours (max. 90 mg/kg daily in divided doses, not to exceed 4 g) for 48 hours (or longer if necessary and if adverse effects ruled out) then 15 mg/kg every 6 hours; max. 4 g daily

Child 12–18 years: 500 mg every 4–6 hours (max. four doses in 24 hours); for severe symptoms 0.5–1 g every 4–6 hours (max. four doses in 24 hours)

(continued)

Table (continued)

	By rectum
	Neonate over 32 weeks post-menstrual age: 30 mg/kg as a single dose then 20 mg/kg every 8 hours as necessary; max. 60 mg/kg daily in divided doses
	Child 1–3 months: 30–60 mg every 8 hours as necessary; for severe symptoms 30 mg/kg as a single dose then 20 mg/kg every 8 hours; max. 60 mg/kg daily in divided doses
	Child 3–12 months: 60–125 mg every 4–6 hours as necessary (max. four doses in 24 hours); for severe symptoms 40 mg/kg as a single dose then 20 mg/kg every 4–6 hours (max. 90 mg/kg daily in divided doses) for 48 hours (or longer if necessary and if adverse effects ruled out) then 15 mg/kg every 6 hours
	Child 1–5 years: 125–250 mg every 4–6 hours as necessary (max. four doses in 24 hours); for severe symptoms 40 mg/kg as a single dose then 20 mg/kg every 4–6 hours (max. 90 mg/kg daily in divided doses) for 48 hours (or longer if necessary and if adverse effects ruled out) then 15 mg/kg every 6 hours
	Child 5–12 years: 250–500 mg every 4–6 hours as necessary (max. four doses in 24 hours); for severe symptoms 40 mg/kg (max. 1 g) as a single dose then 20 mg/kg every 6 hours (max. 90 mg/kg daily in divided doses) for 48 hours (or longer if necessary and if adverse effects ruled out) then 15 mg/kg every 6 hours
	Child 12–18 years: 500 mg every 4–6 hours (max. four doses in 24 hours); for severe symptoms 0.5–1 g every 4–6 hours; max. 4 g daily in divided doses
	By intravenous infusion over 15 minutes
	Child body weight 10–50 kg: 15 mg/kg every 4–6 hours; max. 60 mg/kg daily
	Child body weight over 50 kg: 1 g every 4–6 hours; max. 4 g daily
Paraldehyde	**Status epilepticus**
	By rectum
	Neonate: 0.4 mL/kg (max. 0.5 mL) as a single dose
	Child 1–3 months: 0.5 mL as a single dose
	Child 3–6 months: 1 mL as a single dose
	Child 6 months–1 year: 1.5 mL as a single dose
	Child 1–2 years: 2 mL as a single dose
	Child 2–5 years: 3–4 mL as a single dose
	Child 5–18 years: 5–10 mL as a single dose
	Note: Administration – for rectal administration, dilute 1 part paraldehyde with nine parts sodium chloride 0.9% (some centres mix paraldehyde with an equal volume of olive oil or sunflower oil instead)
	Note: Do not use paraldehyde if it has a brownish colour or an odour of acetic acid. Avoid contact with rubber and plastics
Phenobarbitone/ phenobarbital	**All forms of epilepsy except absence seizures**
	By mouth or by intravenous injection
	Neonate: initially 20 mg/kg by slow intravenous injection then 2.5–5 mg/kg once daily either by slow intravenous injection or by mouth; dose and frequency adjusted according to response

Table (continued)

	By mouth
	Child 1 month–12 years: initially 1–1.5 mg/kg twice daily, increased by 2 mg/kg daily as required; usual maintenance dose 2.5–4 mg/kg once or twice daily
	Child 12–18 years: 60–180 mg once daily
	Status epilepticus
	By slow intravenous injection
	Neonate: initially 20 mg/kg then 2.5–5 mg/kg once or twice daily
	Child 1 month–12 years: initially 20 mg/kg then 2.5–5 mg/kg once or twice daily
	Child 12–18 years: initially 20 mg/kg (max. 1 g) then 300 mg twice daily
Phenytoin	**All forms of epilepsy except absence seizures**
	By intravenous injection (over 20–30 minutes) and by mouth
	Neonate: initial loading dose by slow intravenous injection 18 mg/kg then by mouth 2.5–5 mg/kg twice daily adjusted according to response and plasma–phenytoin concentration (usual max. 7.5 mg/kg twice daily)
	By mouth
	Child 1 month–12 years: initially 1.5–2.5 mg/kg twice daily, then adjusted according to response and plasma–phenytoin concentration to 2.5–5 mg/kg twice daily (usual max. 7.5 mg/kg twice daily or 300 mg daily)
	Child 12–18 years: initially 75–150 mg twice daily then adjusted according to response and plasma–phenytoin concentration to 150–200 mg twice daily (usual max. 300 mg twice daily)
	Status epilepticus, acute symptomatic seizures associated with trauma or neurosurgery
	By slow intravenous injection or infusion (with blood pressure and ECG monitoring)
	Neonate: initially 18 mg/kg as a loading dose then 2.5–5 mg/kg twice daily
	Child 1 month–12 years: initially 18 mg/kg as a loading dose then 2.5–5 mg/kg twice daily
	Child 12–18 years: initially 18 mg/kg as a loading dose then up to 100 mg three to four times daily
Phosphate enema	**Constipation**
(sodium acid phosphate 12.8 g, sodium phosphate 10.24 g, purified water 128 mL)	*By rectum*
	Child 3–7 years: 45–65 mL once daily
	Child 7–12 years: 65–100 mL once daily
	Child 12–18 years: 100–128 mL once daily
Phytomenadione	**Neonatal hypoprothrombinaemia or vitamin K deficiency bleeding**
(Vitamin K_1)	*By intravenous injection*
	Neonate: 1 mg repeated 8 hourly if necessary
	Neonatal biliary atresia and liver disease
	By mouth
	Neonate: 1 mg daily

(continued)

Table (continued)

Prednisolone	**Inflammatory disorders** *By mouth* Child 1 month–18 years: initially 1–2 mg/kg once daily (usual max. 60 mg daily), then reduced after a few days if appropriate **Adjunctive therapy in severe pneumocystis infections associated with HIV infection** *By mouth* 2 mg/kg (max. 80 mg daily) for 5 days
Promethazine	**Night sedation and insomnia (short-term use)** *By mouth* Child under 2 years: not recommended Child 2–5 years: 15–20 mg at bedtime Child 5–10 years: 20–25 mg at bedtime Child 10–18 years: 25 mg at bedtime increased to 50 mg if necessary **Sedation** *By mouth or by slow intravenous injection or by deep intramuscular injection* Child 1 month–12 years: 0.5–1 mg/kg (max. 25 mg) four times daily, adjusted according to response Child 12–18 years: 25–50 mg four times daily, adjusted according to response **Nausea and vomiting** *By mouth* Child 2–5 years: 5 mg at bedtime on night before travel, repeat following morning if necessary Child 5–10 years: 10 mg at bedtime on night before travel, repeat following morning if necessary Child 10–18 years: 20–25 mg at bedtime on night before travel, repeat following morning if necessary
Pyrimethamine	**Toxoplasmosis (in combination with sulfadiazine and folinic acid)** Loading dose 2 mg/kg/day (max 50 mg) for 2 days then maintenance, 1 mg/kg/day (max 25 mg) plus sulfadiazine 50 mg/kg every 12-hours plus folinic acid 5–20 mg three times weekly. Treat until 1–2 weeks beyond resolution of signs and symptoms
Ranitidine	**Reflux oesophagitis, benign gastric and duodenal ulceration, other conditions where gastric acid reduction is beneficial** *By mouth* Neonate: 2 mg/kg three times daily but absorption unreliable; max. 3 mg/kg three times daily Child 1–6 months: 1 mg/kg three times daily; max. 3 mg/kg three times daily Child 6 months–3 years: 2–4 mg/kg twice daily

Table (continued)

	Child 3–12 years: 2–4 mg/kg (max. 150 mg) twice daily; increased up to 5 mg/kg (max. 300 mg) twice daily in severe gastro-oesophageal reflux disease
	Child 12–18 years: 150 mg twice daily or 300 mg at night; increased if necessary, to 300 mg twice daily or 150 mg four times daily for up to 12 weeks in moderate to severe gastro-oesophageal reflux disease
Salbutamol	**Acute asthma** *By aerosol inhalation* 2–10 puffs as required, ideally through spacer device *Nebulized solution inhalation* 2.5–5 mL of 1 mg/1 mL as required
Senna	**Constipation** *By mouth* Child 6–12 years: 1–2 tablets at night (or in the morning if preferred) Child 12–18 years: 2–4 tablets at night (or in the morning if preferred)
Sodium citrate (rectal)	**Constipation** *By rectum* Child 3–18 years: 5 mL as a single dose
Sodium valproate	**All forms of epilepsy** *By mouth or by rectum* Neonate: initially 20 mg/kg once daily; usual maintenance dose 10 mg/kg twice daily Child 1 month–12 years: initially 5–7.5 mg/kg twice daily; usual maintenance dose 12.5–15 mg/kg twice daily (up to 30 mg/kg twice daily in infantile spasms; monitor clinical chemistry and haematological parameters if dose exceeds 20 mg/kg twice daily) Child 12–18 years: initially 300 mg twice daily increased in steps of 200 mg daily at 3-day intervals; usual maintenance dose 0.5–1 g twice daily; max. 1.25 g twice daily *Note: If switching from oral therapy to intravenous therapy, the intravenous dose should be the same as the established oral dose* *By intravenous injection over 3–5 minutes* Neonate: 10 mg/kg twice daily Child 1 month–18 years: 10 mg/kg twice daily *By continuous intravenous infusion* Child 1 month–12 years: initially 10 mg/kg by intravenous injection then by continuous intravenous infusion 20–40 mg/kg daily Child 12–18 years: initially 10 mg/kg by intravenous injection then up to max. 2.5 g daily by continuous intravenous infusion Administration: for rectal administration, sodium valproate oral solution may be given rectally and retained for 15 minutes (may require dilution with water to prevent rapid expulsion). For intravenous injection, may be diluted in glucose 5% or sodium chloride 0.9%. For continuous intravenous infusion, dilute injection solution with glucose 5% or sodium chloride 0.9%

(continued)

Table (continued)

Sodium picosulphate	**Constipation**
	By mouth
	Child 1 month–4 years: 250 micrograms/kg (max. 5 mg) at night
	Child 4–10 years: 2.5–5 mg at night
	Child 10–18 years: 5–10 mg at night
	Note: the onset of action 6–12 hours; recommended doses may be exceeded on specialist advice.
Sulfadiazine	See under pyrimethamine
Sulfamethoxazole	See under Co-trimoxazole
Temazepam	**Premedication and sedation for clinical procedures**
	By mouth
	Child 1–12 years: 1 mg/kg (max. 30 mg) 1 hour before surgery
	Child 12–18 years: 20–30 mg 1 hour before surgery
Thioridazine	**For vomiting**
	By mouth
	Child 2–12 years: 0.5 mg/kg to 3.0 mg/kg per day in divided doses (twice or three times per day)
	Not licenced for children in the UK
Tramadol	**Moderate to severe pain**
	By mouth
	Child 12–18 years: 50–100 mg not more often than every 4 hours; total of more than 400 mg daily not usually required
	By intramuscular injection or by intravenous injection (over 2–3 minutes) or by intravenous infusion
	Child 12–18 years: 50–100 mg every 4–6 hours
Tranexamic Acid	**Bleeding**
	By mouth
	Child 1 month–18 years: 15–25 mg/kg (max. 1.5 g) two to three times daily
	By intravenous injection over at least 10 minutes
	Child 1 month–18 years: 10 mg/kg (max. 1 g) two to three times daily
	By continuous intravenous infusion:
	Child 1 month–18 years: 45 mg/kg over 24 hours
Triclofos	**Night sedation**
	By mouth
	Child 1 month–1 year: 25–30 mg/kg at night
	Child 1–5 years: 250–500 mg at night
	Child 6–12 years: 0.5–1 g at night
	Child 12–18 years: 1–2 g at night
	Sedation for painless procedures
	By mouth
	Child 1 month–18 years: 30–50 mg/kg (max. 2 g) 45–60 minutes before procedure; higher doses up to 100 mg/kg (max. 2 g) may be used but respiratory monitoring is required

Table (continued)

Vancomycin	**Infections due to Gram-positive bacteria including osteomyelitis, septicaemia and soft-tissue infections**
	By intravenous infusion
	Neonate 29-35 weeks post-menstrual age: 15 mg/kg every 12 hours
	Neonate over 35 weeks post-menstrual age: 15 mg/kg every 8 hours
	Child 1 month–18 years: 15 mg/kg every 8 hours (maximum daily dose 2 g), adjusted according to plasma concentration
Varicella-zoster immunoglobulin (Vzig)	**Herpes varicella zoster prophylaxis**
	Note: as soon as possible – not later than 10 days after exposure
	By deep intramuscular injection
	Neonate: 250 mg
	Child 1 month–6 years: 250 mg
	Child 6–11 years: 500 mg
	Child 11–15 years: 750 mg
	Child 15–18 years: 1 g
	Give second dose if further exposure occurs more than 3 weeks after first dose
Vitamin A supplementation	**Vitamin A deficiency**
	By mouth
	Neonate: 5000 units daily
	Child 1 month–1 year: 5000 units daily with or after food
	Child 1–18 years: 10 000 units daily with or after food
Vitamin K	See phytomenadione above
Whitfield's ointment (benzoic acid 6%, salicylic acid 3%, in emulsifying ointment)	**Superficial fungal infections**
	Topical
	Child 1 month–18 years: apply twice daily

20.5 **Formula for making oral morphine from powder**

(As prepared at *Hospice Uganda Pharmacy*)[i]

20.5.1 **Morphine solution for oral use 50 mg in 5 mL**

Ingredients

(1) Morphine sulphate powder BP 50 g

(2) Parabene[ii] concentrate 50 mL

(3) Freshly boiled and cooled water 5000 mL

Method

(1) Tare the balance.

(2) Weigh the morphine powder and transfer to a clean bucket.

(3) Make a paste by adding a small amount of water.

(4) Gradually add water to approximately ¾ of the final volume.

(5) Transfer the solution into a calibrated measuring jug.

(6) Measure the parabene concentrate and gradually add it to the morphine solution whilst stirring until fully dissolved (NB parabene is poorly soluble in water; at least ¾ of the final volume of solution is needed to dissolve the parabene).

(7) If the solution is to be used for dispensing add five drops of red food colouring and stir thoroughly[iii].

(8) Make up to the final volume with water and stir thoroughly.

(9) Check the final product.

(10) Transfer to a suitable clean container (e.g. 5 L clean jerry can) and label (see below).

(11) Transfer 100 mL of morphine solution to individual clean bottles and label for dispensing to individual patients (see below).

Label for the jerry can

Expiry Date:	*1 year from the date of manufacture*
Prepared by:	
Expiry storage conditions:	Store in a cool dark place
Final product checked by (Pharmacist/certified technician)	
Date	

---

[i] This solution has a shelf life of three months and is useful for work where we have a high turnover of morphine and patients are seen on average weekly at home. See 3b for solution made up at Joint Medical Store with a shelf life of one year.

[ii] Parebene comes as a powder: to be made up to a solution (see Pharmacopoeia) or as below:

[iii] We suggest different colours for different strengths: e.g. green for 5 mg/5 mL, red for 50 mg/5 mL

Label for individual patient bottles

KEEP OUT OF REACH OF CHILDREN

Oral Morphine Solution 5 mg/5ml

Batch number: Date of manufacture:

Expiry date:

Pharmacy Department, Hospice Uganda,

PO Box 7757, Kampala.

Notes

1 Adapted from *BNF for Children 2007*. (2007). BMJ Publishing Group Ltd, RPS Publishing, and RCPCH Publications Ltd.

2 Cancer Care Alliance Palliative Care Guidelines for the End of Life. Available online at http://www.cancercarealliance.nhs.uk/

3 Paediatric Formulary Committee. (2008). BNF for Children. London: BMJ Publishing Group, RPS Publishing, and RCPCH Publications.

4 Jassal, S.S. (2006). *Basic Symptom Control in Paediatric Palliative Care – The Rainbows Children's Hospice Guidelines* (6th Edition) (Available free for download at Http://Www.Act.Org.Uk/Content/View/100/1/)

5 Merriman, A. (2006). *Pain and Symptom Control in The Cancer and/or Aids Patient in Uganda and Other African Countries* (4th Edition). Hospice Africa Uganda, Kampala ISBN 9970-830-01-0.

Further reading

A clinical guide to supportive and palliative care for HIV/AIDS in Sub-Saharan Africa
A comprehensive textbook with an extensive list of resources of all kinds.
Available online at www.fhssa.org/i4a/pages/Index.cfm?pageID=3361. Order a CD-ROM: info@
hospiceafrica.or.ug

Basic Symptom Control in Paediatric Palliative Care
The Rainbows Children's Hospice Guidelines here: The manual, *Basic Symptom Control in
Paediatric Palliative Care: the Rainbows Children's Hospice Guidelines,* now in its seventh year, and
used by doctors and nurses throughout the world, is the only resource which provides comprehensive guidelines for treating a wide range of symptoms experienced by children with life-limiting
or complex health conditions. As well as being an 'industry bible' for professionals, the manual
has also been prepared for the use of parents who are caring for a terminally ill child. It has been
written by Dr. Satbir Singh Jassal, GP and Medical Director at Rainbows Children's Hospice and
is a collaboration from 27 leading paediatric and palliative care contributors from around the
world.

Cancer pain relief: guide to opioid availability
WHO document giving clinical information on pain relief but also guidelines on introducing
opioid use to governments. Short version online: www.medsch.wisc.edu/painpolicy/publicat/
cprguid.htm Order: bookorders@who.int

HIV, health and your community
A guide to setting up HIV programmes including home-based care, with advice on writing proposals
and training others. Available online at: www.hesperian.org/mm5/merchant.mvc?Store_Code=
HB&Screen=PROD&Product_ Code=B200. Order: hesperian@hesperian.org

Hospice information
A service promoting palliative care work around the world by providing information on existing
services and national associations, educational resources, advocacy, funding and how to start up
a new service. Also produces a free e-newsletter and a magazine, and manages an up-to-date
database of training courses, seminars and vacancies in the sector. Run by Help the Hospices in
association with St. Christopher's Hospice; Hospice Information enables easy access to wider
resources offered by these two organizations.
Available online at: www.hospiceinformation.info; e-mail for guidance and information: info@
hospiceinformation.info

IAHPC manual (International Association for Hospice and Palliative Care)
A user-friendly online manual covering all aspects of palliative care.
Available online at: www.hospicecare.com/manual/IAHPCmanual.htm

Introducing palliative care by Robert Twycross
An excellent basic textbook of palliative care which has recently been updated.
Published by Radcliffe Medical Press, Oxford. Available in India at low cost from The Institute of Palliative Medicine, Medical College, Calicut, Kerala, India. Email: pain@vsnl.com
Available in Africa at low cost from: Wits Palliative – training, PO Box 212, Pimville, 1808, Soweto, South Africa. Email: palliative.training@wits.ac.za

Oxford Textbook of Palliative Care for Children (Hardcover) by Ann Goldman, Richard Hain, Stephen Liben Oxford University Press; 1 edition (January 2006)
This book is the first authoritative, systematic and comprehensive text to define the increasingly important and evolving specialty of paediatric palliative care. The Oxford Textbook of Palliative Care for Children is about the care of children for whom cure of their underlying disease is not possible. It encompasses the physical management of symptoms such as pain and nausea, as well as social issues such as accessing appropriate education and funding, emotional issues such as techniques for communication, and spiritual issues such as feelings of guilt and isolation.

Pain and symptom control in the cancer and/or AIDS patient in Uganda and other African countries
A more detailed guide to symptom control produced by Hospice Africa, Uganda, but usable all over the world. It contains a section on ARTs in palliative care. Available online at: www.hospiceafrica.or.ug/redesign/docs/bluebk40506.pdf Order: info@hospiceafrica.or.ug

Palliative care toolkit: Improving care from the roots up by Dr Vicky Lavy, Dr Charlie Bond and Ruth Wooldridge for Help the Hospices and the Worldwide Palliative Care Alliance.
This is a practical manual to equip, empower and encourage health workers in resource-limited settings to integrate palliative care into their work and their communities. It brings holistic and 'can do' approach to delivering care for those suffering with life-limiting diseases and is an important contribution to increasing the spread of palliative care globally. Hard copies of the toolkit and CD ROMs have been produced. If you are interested in distributing the toolkit in resource-limited settings; please contact c.morris@helpthehospices.org.uk.
For individuals based in non-resource-limited settings, the toolkit costs £10. Contact info@hospiceinformation.info for more information.

Palliativedrugs.com
An online formulary containing information about all drugs used in palliative care. A large selection of palliative care books can be ordered through the website. Available online at: www.palliativedrugs.com

Red Cross guide to setting up CHBC programmes
Contains useful principles and planning tools. Available online at: www.ifrc.org/cgi/pdf_pubs.pl?health/hivaids/hbc.pdf

Teaching-aids at Low Cost (TALC)
A charity providing free and low-cost health care books and accessories on a wide range of topics.
To order free resources from their catalogue, contact by: Email: info@talcuk.org
Post: TALC, PO Box 49, St Albans, Herts, AL1 5TX, UK. Available online at: www.talcuk.org/index.htm

When Children Die: Improving palliative and end-of-life care for children and their families
Committee on Palliative and End-of-Life Care for Children and Their Families. Board on Health Sciences Policy
Marilyn J. Field and Richard E. Behrman, Editors. Institute of Medicine of The National Academies. The National Academies Press. Washington, DC. Available online at: **www.nap.edu**

WHO integrated management of adult and adolescent illness (IMAI)
Five practical, easy-to-use booklets: Palliative care – a handy, portable guide to symptom control; Caregiver booklet – helpful instructions for family and volunteer caregivers; Chronic care with ART and prevention – how to prescribe ARTs; General principles of good chronic care – guidelines for health workers; Acute care – guidelines on management of common illnesses. Available online at: www.who.int/3by5/publications/documents/imai/en/ Order free hard copies: imaimail@who.int

WHO New guide on palliative care services for people living with advanced cancer: Palliative Care: (Cancer control: knowledge into action: WHO guide for effective programmes; Module 5).
The WHO's first guide on planning palliative care services for people living with advanced stages of cancer. The guide, which is based on consultations with more than 70 leading cancer experts in the world, has identified highly effective low-cost public health models to care for terminally ill cancer patients, especially in developing countries. It is available online at: www.who.int/cancer/media/FINAL-PalliativeCareModule.pdf

Index

abdominal pain 120, 212
abdominal splash 138
abscesses 211
abuse 242, 295, 322
acceptance 272
aciclovir 156, 185, 197, 198, 221, 222, 380
acidosis 337, 339
aclometasone dipropionate 192
acute heart failure 128
acute necrotizing gingivitis 211
addiction 98, 368
adherence 296–7, 377
adolescents 289–304
  adherence problems 296–7
  carers 297
  communication 292
  development 289–92
  disclosure 297
  dying 299–300
  grief 251, 254
  illness experience 292–3
  peer relationships 290, 293, 299, 301
  poor care 293–4
  psychosocial challenges 294
  sexual abuse 295
  sexuality 291–2
  wills 301
adrenalin, topical 338–9
African Children's Palliative Care Charter 4–5
agitation 176–7, 212, 215, 338
AIDS, see HIV/AIDS
airway obstruction 337
alcohol 296, 360, 368
alfentanil 379
allocation of resources 318
aloe 165
alternative goodbyes 260
aluminium chloride hexahydrate 200
Ama's story 239
amitriptyline 118, 200, 218, 243, 381
amoxicillin 143, 202, 220, 381
amphotericin 156, 222, 382
amphotericin B 184, 185, 222
ampicillin 143, 220
anaemia 143
analgesics 114, 115–18
anger 28–9, 236, 261, 293
angular stomatitis 156
animals 330
ano-genital ulceration 214
anorexia 212, 213
antacids 131
anthraquinones 165
anticipatory grief 255–6
anticonvulsants 114, 118

antidepressants 114, 243
antiemetics 160–1
antiflatulents 131
antihistamines 160, 218
antimicrobials 143
antiretroviral therapy (ART) 118, 172, 180,
    212, 216–18
  discontinuation 219–20
  pharmacology 216
antispasmodics 119
anxiety 120, 176, 212, 243, 262, 367–8
aphthous stomatitis 156
appraisal 361
artificial feeding 339–40
artificial hydration 150
ascorbic acid 144
asilone 382
aspiration 129, 337
aspirin 115
assertiveness 356
assessment 79–88, 93, 95
  aims 81
  community 229
  dehydration 151–2
  eating problems 134–5
  end of life care 332–3
  family 83, 84, 85, 235
  framework 82–4
  malnutrition 137–9
  neurological 172–5
  pain 99, 100–5
  principles 81–2
  process 84–8
  respiratory 125–6
  spirituality 277–9
  urinary system 201
Association for Children's Palliative Care
    (ACT) 4, 80–1
assumptions 18–19
asthma 128
atopic dermatitis 193
autonomy 298, 308
avoidance 22, 256
awareness contexts 21–2

baclofen 119, 131, 187, 382
bacterial meningitis 183, 184, 222
bacterial pneumonia 220
bad death 328
bad news 23–6, 331
barriers to communication 16–17
bed sores 338
behavioural development 83
belief 276–7, 281–2, 313–14, 356
beneficience 313, 315

benzodiazepines 114, 119, 121, 127, 128, 177, 178, 218, 243, 335, 337, 338
benzyl benzoate 195, 221, 382
benzyl penicillin 382–3
bereavement 250
  dysfunctional 260–2
  support 254–60
bereavement tree 264, 267–9
best interests 313, 314
beta blockers 218
betamethasone dipropionate 192
betamethasone valerate 192
bethanechol 202, 383
bisacodyl 165, 383
bladder irritability 204
blame 236, 261
bleeding
  GI 130, 162–3
  massive 338–9
blistering lesions 197–8
blood glucose 139
blood smear 139, 183
blood transfusion 141, 143
blue-band margarines 165
blue nails 199
body, seeing after death 259
body image 293, 298, 299
body language 15
boils 195, 196
bone pain 119, 212
book corner 52
bowel obstruction 164
box construction 56
brain imaging 179
bran 165
breaking bad news 23–6, 331
breakthrough pain 336, 347
breathlessness 126–8, 212, 214
bronchiectasis 220
bronchospasm 128
buprenorphine 116, 336, 379, 383
Burkitt's lymphoma 172
burnout 352, 353–4, 356, 358
Burnout Inventory 362–3
Buscopan 132, 337, 347

cachexia 135–6
CAGE questionnaire 368
calculation of value 315
cancer
  adherence problems 296–7
  breathlessness 126, 127
  cachexia 135
  disease trajectory 328–9
  dysphagia 157
  head and neck 172, 181
  malnutrition 136
  mouth problems 155
  neurological problems 171–2
  pain 107–9
  prognostication 329
  seizures 177
  skin problems 189

candidiasis 156, 157, 158, 211, 213, 222
capacity 311
capillary refill time 151
carbachol 202, 384
carbamazepine 118, 180, 217, 384
carers
  adolescents 297
  malnutrition prevention 148
  pain assessment 103
  young 33
caries 156, 211
cascara 165
castor oil 165
catastrophic haemoptysis 129, 130
catheterization 203–4
cauda equina compression (CEC) 182–3
CD4 cells 209
ceftazidime 220, 384
ceftriaxone 184, 220, 222, 384
cellulitis 199, 211
cerebral infection 176
challenge 352
change 358
charcoal 199
Charter for Bereaved Children 250
checklists 59, 66–77, 334, 340–1
chest infections 220–1
chest pain 211, 212
chest X-ray 140
chickenpox 222
child abuse 242, 295, 322
child development 38–9
  play and 43–4
  spirituality 275–6
child-friendly environment 21
child protection 322
children's will 264
chills 212
chloral hydrate 218
chloramphenicol 143, 184, 222, 384
chloroquine 218
chlorpromazine 131, 385
choices 258, 333
choking 131
cholestyramine 169
chronic heart failure 128
chronic respiratory disease 135
chunks 25
cigarette smoke 217
cimetidine 200, 217
ciprofloxacin 168, 217
circles of support 229
cisapride 218
clarithromycin 217
clinical assessment 87
clinical supervision 361, 371–2
cliques 358
clobetasol propionate 192
clobetasone butyrate 192
clonazepam 385
clotrimazole 195, 196, 213
co-trimoxazole 158, 168, 218
clotting disorders 130

cloxacillin 195, 198, 220, 385–6
cloxacin 221
CMV infection 184, 222
CMV retinitis 184, 222
CNS infections 222
coaching 366
co-danthramer 386
co-danthrusate 386
codeine 116
codeine linctus 129
codeine phosphate 129, 386
cognition 174, 210
cognitive development 38, 63–4, 290
cold hands and feet 138, 139
colicky abdominal pain 120
collusion 22–3
communication 11–35, 218–20
    adolescents 292
    end of life 330–1
    ethics 319–20
    pre-bereavement 255
community 228–31
community assessment 229
community circles of support 229
community resources 84
compassion fatigue 356, 369
competence 308–9
compliance 377
concepts 42
condylomata accuminata 197
confusion 173
congestive heart failure 141, 143
conjunctive faith 275
connection 20, 352
consciousness 138, 173
consent 23, 219, 308, 311
consequences 313, 315–17
constipation 150, 165–7, 214, 338
contact dermatitis 193
control 258, 293, 300, 333, 357
convulsions 215
coping 28, 114, 354–9
cor pulmonale 128
corticosteroids 119, 182–3
co-trimoxazole 143, 158, 168, 220, 221, 386
cough 128–9, 212, 214
cough ladder 129
cough suppressants 129
counselling
    cardiotoxicity 218
    children 243–4
    epilepsy 179–80
    for health care workers 366
critical learning periods 39–40
cryptococcal meningitis 183, 184, 222
cryptococcus 185, 222
cryptosporidium 211, 214
CSF 180
CT scan 180
culture 18
cutting and pasting 56
cyanosis 126
cyclizine 160, 161, 162, 347, 387

CYP inducers 217
CYP inhibitors 217, 218
cytochrome P450 (CYP) system 216–17

Daktarin oral gel 156, 158
dancing 57
dantrolene 187, 387
dantron 165
day care programme 49–51
death 257–8
    after-death practices 258–60
    approaches 284–7
    bad death 328
    beliefs and practices 281–2
    children's understanding 12–15
    good death 257, 282, 327–8
    rituals 251–2
    see also bereavement
death rattle 131–2, 337
decision-making 307–19
deep breathing 111
defence mechanisms 293
dehydration 139, 140–1, 150–3
delirium 150, 176–7, 215
dementia 172, 174
denial 22–3, 255, 293
dental caries 156, 211
dental pain 157
depression 212, 215, 243, 299, 367–8
Derian House pain diary 105–6
dermatitis 215
developmental delay 172, 180, 210
developmental milestones 61–6
developmental stages 38
development checklists 59, 66–77
dexamethasone 119, 158, 182, 347, 387
diamorphine 116, 129, 347, 379, 388
diarrhoea 138, 139, 167–9, 212, 214
diazepam 119, 127, 128, 178, 187, 335, 336, 338, 388
diclofenac 115, 389
difficult conversations 20–9
difficult questions 29–31
diflucortolone valerate 192
digoxin 128
dihydrocodeine 117, 389
dilemmas 320–2
diltiazem 217
dioctyl sodium 165
disclosure 26–8, 297
disease trajectory 328–9
distancing 19
distraction 110–11
distressing terminal events 334–5
diuretics 128, 141, 143
Doctrine of Double Effect (DDE) 315–16
docusate 165, 389
domperidone 131, 158, 160, 161, 162, 389
double effect 315–16
drama 245
drawing 56
dreamcatcher 262, 266
dreams 278
drug abuse 360, 368

drug compatibility 347
drug doses 378
drug interactions 216–18
dry skin 193
duties 313, 314–15
dying
  adolescents 299–300
  children's understanding 12–15
  patterns of 328–9
dysfunctional bereavement 260–2
dysphagia 157–8, 213
dyspnoea 126–8, 212, 214
dystonia (muscle spasm) 119, 185–7
dystonic pain 211
dysuria 201

eating problems 134–5
ecthyma 198
eczema 199
education 27, 83, 148, 231, 298–9
EEG 179, 186
eicosapentaenoic acid (EPA) 135
electrolyte balance 140–1
emergencies
  seizures 178
  spinal cord compression 182–3
emotional development 41, 64–5, 83, 290
emotional reactions 19, 240–1, 312
employment 84
encephalopathies 180–1
end of life care 327–44
  assessment 332–3
  care plan 341–3
  checklists 334, 340–1
  communication 330–1
  management plan 334
  symptom control 334–40
enlightenment 275
environment 21, 357, 361
EPA 135
epilepsy 177, 179, 186
epistaxis 339
Erikson, E. 40
erythroderma 199
erythromycin 195, 217, 218, 221
ethambutol 184, 222
ethical competencies 309–10
ethical issues 218–20, 305–24
ethionamide 184, 218, 222
euthanasia 316, 321–2
examination
  children 87–8
  neurological 174–5
exercise 360
explanation 21, 84
extended family 232

F-75 142, 144, 145, 146
F-100 142, 144, 145, 147
Faces pain scale 99, 102
facts 312
faecal softeners 165
faeces 139
  manual evacuation 166

faith 274–5
family 232–8
  adolescents 290
  assessment 83, 84, 85, 235
  end of life care 333
  pain assessment 103
  problems facing 236
  roles 233
  subgroups 233
  supporting 233, 236–8
  theory 232
  types 232–3
family bonds 233
family conference 235–6
family record 263, 300–1
family systems 232
family trees 233–4
fatigue 212, 213
fear 19, 20, 256, 357, 358
feeding 133–54
  artificial 339–40
feet 138, 139, 173, 210, 212
fentanyl 117, 336, 379, 389–90
fever 125, 212, 215
finance 230–1, 236, 294
finger tip units (FTU) 191
fish oils 135
fixed drug eruption 199
FLACC scale 105
flucloxacillin 198, 221, 391
fluconazole 156, 158, 184, 185, 196, 217, 222, 390
fluid administration 152–3
fluocinolone acetonide 192
fluoxetine 217, 391
fluticasone valerate 192
focal neurological signs 173
folic acid 144, 147, 391
folinic acid 185, 222
folliculitis 194, 195
forgiveness 272, 279
formula diets 142, 144, 145, 146
formulary 377–409
foscarnet 184, 222, 392
Fowler, J. W. 274
frangipani milk 197, 215
frequency 201
Freud, S. 40
fun 359–60
functional abilities 86
funerals 251, 259
fungal infections 195, 196
fungal meningitis 183
fungating tumours 198–9
furosemide 143, 337, 392
furuncles 195, 196

gabapentin 118
gag reflex 159
gait 174–5
gamma benzene hexachloride 195, 221
ganciclovir 184, 222, 392
gastric stasis 161
gastritis 161
gastroenteritis 214

gastrointestinal bleeding 130, 162–3
gastrointestinal symptoms 155–70, 210
gaviscon 393
genograms 233–4
gentamicin 143, 169, 220, 393
gentian violet 158, 196
Gibbs reflective cycle 372
gingivitis 211, 214
glucose 140
glycerin/glycerol 393
glyceryl trinitrate 166
glycopyrrollate 347
glycopyrronium 393
goals 358, 365
'goodbyes', alternative 260
good death 257, 282, 327–8
good-enough health worker 356
Graseby syringe driver 345–6
grief 236, 250–4
   anticipatory 255–6
griseofulvin 196, 221, 394
ground-nut oil 165
guided imagery 112–13
guilt 236, 261

haematuria 201, 204–5
haemoglobin 139
haemoptysis 129–30
haemorrhage 338–9
Hallpike's test 175
haloperidol 131, 160, 161, 162, 177, 217, 218, 336,
   338, 347, 394
handprints 263
hands 138, 139, 173, 210, 212
happiness 351–2
harm 19
headache 173, 211, 212
head and neck cancers 172, 181
'healing' 273
health 83
heart failure 128, 135
hepatosplenomegaly 211
herpes simplex 156, 185, 198, 214, 222
herpes zoster 197, 221
hiccup 131
Hippocratic Oath 314
HIV/AIDS 207–224
   adherence problems 296–7
   adolescents 294
   ART, see antiretroviral therapy
   breathlessness 126, 127, 214
   cachexia 135
   cardiomyopathy 210
   challenges facing palliative care 209
   chest infection 220–1
   communication 218–20
   cough 128, 214
   delirium and agitation 176, 215
   diarrhoea 167, 214
   disclosure 26–8
   dysphagia 157, 213
   effects on children in Africa 208
   ethics 218–20
   facts and figures 1–2, 208
   GI system 210
   kidneys 210
   malnutrition 136
   meningitis 183
   mother-to-child transmission (MTCT) 208
   mouth problems 155, 214, 222
   neurological problems 171–2, 210, 222
   opportunistic infections 210, 220–2
   pain 106, 107–9, 211–12, 213
   pathology 209–10
   poor prognosis indicators 219–20
   prevalence of symptoms 211
   psychosocial issues 210–11
   respiratory system 210
   seizures 177
   skin problems 189, 215, 221–2
   symptom management 213–15
   symptom prevalence 211–12
HIV encephalopathy 119, 172, 180, 210
HIV enteropathy 210
HIV pneumonia 128
holding environment 358
holistic care 79, 80, 81, 89, 298
Home Based Care (HBC) programmes 230
home-work boundaries 358
honey 199
hope 272
hostility 236
housing 84, 230
hydration 133–54
hydrocortisone 192
hydrocortisone 17-butyrate 192
hyoscine 160, 336
hyoscine butylbromide 120, 132, 168, 337, 347, 394
hyoscine hydrobromide 161, 347, 394–5
hyperhidrosis 199–200
hyperventilation 125
hypnosis 112
hypodermoclysis 153
hypoglycaemia 139, 140, 337
hypothermia 138, 139, 140
hypoxaemia 337
hypoxia 176, 177, 186

ibuprofen 115, 395
identity 83, 293
illness, children's understanding 12–15
imipramine 200, 395
immune reconstitution 209
immunization 149
immunosuppression 184–5, 209
impetigo 198, 221
income 84
incontinence 201
individuative-reflective faith 275
infestations 185, 194
informed consent 23, 219, 308, 311
initiation ceremonies 291
insomnia 243
International Children's Palliative Care Network
   (ICPCN) charter 4–5
intestinal obstruction 163–4
intracranial pressure 119, 162, 175, 177, 183
intravenous rehydration 141, 152

intuitive-projective faith 274
iron 147
irritable bladder 204
isoniazid 184, 217, 222
isphagula 165
itchy skin 193
itraconazole 196, 217
IV lines 153

job satisfaction 352–3, 364–5
joint pain 212
justice 318–19

kangaroo technique 140
Kaposi's sarcoma 197, 199, 211
ketamine 181, 396
ketoconazole 195, 196, 217, 221, 396
ketorolac 347
ketosis 339
kidney, HIV-related nephropathy 210
know your limits 360
kwashiorkor 136

lactitol 165
lactulose 165, 396
lamotrigine 180
language 15–16, 30
language development 42, 62–3
laughter 360
laxatives 165
Lazarus effect 218
left ventricular failure 337
legal issues 305–24
levomepromazine 160, 161, 162, 177, 347, 396
lidocaine 158
life-limiting illness 14–15, 26–8, 292–4
life-satisfaction 351–2
lifestyle 359–61
life-sustaining treatments (LSTs) 320
lignocaine 121
liver
  cirrhosis 135
  enlargement/tenderness 138
  failure 141, 337
Liverpool Care Pathway 341–3
local anaesthetics 114, 121
local community 228
loin pain 201
lorazepam 119, 121, 178, 338, 396
lower respiratory tract infection 125
low mood 243
lumbar puncture 183
lymphocytic interstitial pneumonitis 128, 221
lymphoma 172, 181

macrolides 218
macronutrient malnutrition 136
magnesium salts 165
magnesium sulfate solution 141
magnesium trisilicate 161
malabsorption 135, 136, 214
malnutrition 136–49
  assessment 137–9

causes 136
discharge 148–9
follow-up 137, 149
initial treatment 136, 140–6
investigation 139–40
rehabilitation 136, 146–9
stages of treatment 136–7
WHO classification 137
management planning 88–92, 334, 362
mannitol 165
manual evacuation 166
marasmus 136
massive bleeding/haemorrhage 338–9
meaning 272, 352, 360–1
mecysteine 397
memory box/book 245, 262–3, 300
memory of pain 98
meningitis 172, 183–4, 211, 222
mental health problems 353
mental state 139
mentoring 366
metabolic disorders 215, 337
methadone 114, 116, 181, 218, 397
methylcellulose 165
methylprednisolone aceponate 192
metoclopramide 131, 158, 160, 161, 347, 397
metronidazole 168, 169, 195, 198, 217
miconazole 221, 398
micralax enema 398
micronutrient malnutrition 136
midazolam 121, 178, 179, 335, 338, 347, 398
Miracle Paint 198
mobility 182, 185, 187
molluscum contagiosum 196
mometasone furoate 192
monoparesis 174
moral development 65
morphine 115–16, 127, 128, 129, 202, 335, 336, 399
  making oral morphine from powder 408–9
  prescribing principles 117–18, 378, 379
mother-to-child transmission (MTCT) 208
motor development 61
mourning 250
mouth 155–6, 211, 214, 222
muscle pain 212
muscle relaxation 111–12
muscle spasm (dystonia) 119, 185–7
music 56, 245
mutual pretence 21, 22
mycobacterium avium intracellulare (MAI) 211
Mycobutin 218
mythic-literal faith 274

nalidixic acid 168
naloxone 399–400
naproxen 400
narrative therapy 245
nasogastric feeding 142
nausea and vomiting 158–62, 212, 213
needs 82–4
neonates 105, 378
nerve (neuropathic) pain 107, 118, 181, 211
neural tumours 172, 181

neurological symptoms 171–88
  assessment 172–5
  examination 174–5
  history 172–3
  symptom clusters 173–4
neuropathic pain 107, 118, 181, 211
nifedipine 131
nitrous oxide 121, 181
nociceptive pain 107
nodules 196–7
noisy secretions 131–2, 337
non-maleficience 313, 315
non-opioid analgesics 115
non-steroidal anti-inflammatory drugs (NSAIDS)
  114, 115, 119
non-verbal communication 20
Norwegian scabies 194
nuclear family 232
numbness 212
numerical rating scale 103
nutritional rehabilitation 147
nystatin 156, 158, 222, 400

objectives 365
ocreotide 400
oedema 125, 137, 138
oesophageal candidiasis 157, 211, 213
oesophagitis 161
omega-3 fish oils 135
omeprazole 158, 161, 217, 400
ondansetron 160, 161, 162, 401
opioids 98, 114, 115–18, 181
  equivalent doses 378
  patches 336
  side effects 117
opportunistic infections 172, 184–5, 210, 220–2
optimism 356
oral candidiasis 156, 157, 158, 222
oral care 155–6
oral rehydration salts (ORS) 140
orbital syndrome 181
organizational factors 357–8, 361
orphans 208, 210, 227–8
orthopnoea 125
otitis media 211
outdoor play 54–5, 57
over-feeding 135
overwhelmed care worker 355
oxybutynin 204, 401
oxycodone 379, 401
oxygen 127, 128

packed-cell volume 139, 143
packed red cells 143
pain 97–124
  assessment 99, 100–5
  cancer 107–9
  classification 107
  diaries 105–6
  end of life 335–6
  extent of problem in Africa 106
  flow sheets 105–6
  hands and feet 173, 210, 212

HIV/AIDS 106, 107–9, 211–12, 213
  myths 97–100
  non-pharmacological management 110–14
  pharmacological management 114–18
  practical approach to management 121–2
  principles of management 109–10
  total pain 109–10
  WHO pain ladder 114–15
painting 55
palliative care
  five steps 80
  need for 1–3
papular pruritic eruptions 194–5
papules, non-itchy 196–7
paracetamol 114, 115, 156, 220, 401–2
paraldhyde 178, 402
paraparesis 174
parasites 214
partings 262
patient-controlled analgesia 98
patterns of dying 328–9
paw-paw 165, 199
peace 273
peer relationships 290, 293, 299, 301
penicillin 220, 382–3
PEPSI-COLA assessment framework 91–2
perceptual development 62
perfect care worker 355–6
peripheral neuropathy 118, 172, 210
permanency planning 264
personality 354–5, 364
personal objectives 361
personal space 21
pethidine 116
petroleum jelly glycerine suppository 165
pets 330
phenobarbital 178, 217, 402–3
phenobarbitone 179, 338, 402–3
phenoxymethylpenicillin 198
phenytoin 118, 178, 180, 217, 403
phosphate enema 403
photosensitive drug reactions 199
phrases, useful 31–2
physical abuse 242
phytomenadione 403
Piaget, J. 38, 40
play 37–60
  child development 42–3
  facilitating and encouraging 44–9
  language 15–16
  malnutrition 148
  programmes 49
  setting up a play area 52–6
  specific activities 55–57
  theory 40–4
  types of 43
  ways of playing 42
play dough 57
play therapy 100, 244–5
pleural effusion 128
Pneumocystis carinii pneumonia (PCP) 221
pneumonia 128, 211, 220, 221
pneumothorax 128

podophyllin 197
polyethylene glycol 165
polyneuropathy 212
positive thinking 359
post-herpetic neuralgia 118, 215
post-nasal drip 129
prayers 280–1
pre-bereavement stage 255–7
prediction 315
prednisolone 119, 156, 217
prednisone 221
pregabalin 118
prescribing 377–8
pressure sores 150, 215
pretence 21, 22
prioritizing 365–6
privacy 298
problem list 90–2
problem of unforeseen consequences 315
problem solving skills 356
procedural pain 120–1
proctoclysis 153
prognostication 219–20, 328, 329–30
progressive multifocal leukoencephalopathy
    (PML) 180
promazine 131, 161, 162
promethazine 404
propantheline 200
propranolol 200
protozoal meningitis 183
proxy decision-makers 310, 312
pruritus 212
psoriasis 196, 199
psychological aspects 238–45, 291
psychosocial issues 210–11, 227–31, 294
psyllum 165
pulmonary embolism 337
pulse rate 138, 139
punishment 276, 279
purpose 352
pyrazinamide 222
pyridoxine 144
pyrimethamine 185, 222, 404

quinine 218

radial pulse 138, 139
radiculopathy 212
radiotherapy 119, 182
raised intracranial pressure (ICP) 119, 162, 175,
    177, 183
ranitidine 158, 161, 404
rash atlas 189
rationality 312
reconstituted family 232
record keeping 58–9
rectal examination 165
reflux 129
regression 180, 252
regret 236
rehabilitation 136, 146–9
rehydration 140–1
rejection 256, 299
relatedness 272

relationships 37, 39, 41, 42, 83
relaxation 240, 360
religion 272, 360–1
renal failure 150, 337
resilience 354–9
ReSoMal 140
resource allocation 318
resources 357, 358
respiratory panic 337
respiratory pattern 151
respiratory symptoms 125–32, 210
rest 360
restlessness, terminal 150, 338
retinoblastoma 172, 181
review 92, 361
rheumatoid arthritis 135
riboflavin 144
rifabutin 218
Rifadin 217
rifampicin 184, 222
rifampin 217
rights 313, 317
ringworm 221
risk taking 42
ritonavir 217
rituals 251–2, 280–1, 282
role clarity 357
role-play 245
Romberg's test 175
rule of threes 332

sadness 243, 250
salbutamol 221, 405
saliva 155
sarcoma 172, 181
    Kaposi's 197, 199, 211
scabies 194, 221
scaly patches and plaques 195–6
scapegoating 358
schooling 231, 294
seborrhoeic dermatitis 194, 195
secretions, noisy 131–2, 337
seizures 173, 177–80, 186, 337–8
selenium 136
selenium sulphide shampoo 195
self-blame 261
self-care 359–61
senna 165, 405
senna coffee 165
sensory polyneuropathy 210
separation 236, 256
septic shock 138, 139, 141
Septrin 217, 218
sexual abuse 242, 295
sexuality 291–2
sexually-transmitted diseases (STDs) 292
shingles 118, 211, 215
siblings 32, 236, 238
silver nitrate 205
sinusitis 211
sinus symptoms 212
skills 19, 174
skin 151, 189–200, 212, 215, 221–2
sleep 55, 243, 262, 360

SMART 79
social development 42, 64–5
social factors 290
social integration 84
social isolation 211, 293
social presentation 83
social relationships 83
social skills 356
social support 357
society 17
sodium citrate enema 398
sodium picosulfate 165, 405
sodium valproate 118, 180, 405
soft tissue pain 119
soft tissue sarcomas 172, 181
somatic pain 107, 211
sorbitol 165
sore mouth 156, 214
sorrow 261–2
spasticity 119
speaking to children 15–17
special investigations 88
spinal cord compression 174, 182–3, 202
spinal cord vascular myelopathy 210
spirituality 271–83
  assessment 277–9
  challenges 279–80
  development 65–6, 274–7
  needs 280–1
'splitting' teams 358
spoken language 16
SSRIs 243
staphylococcal infection 193, 194, 195, 220
status epilepticus 178–9
steroid creams 156, 190–2
steroids 119, 182–3
Stevens–Johnson syndrome 199
stigma 189, 236, 241, 256, 294
stomatitis 156
stool softeners 165
story telling 263, 300–1
streptomycin 184, 222
stress 239–40, 353, 354
stress diary 365
stridor 125, 127–8
subcutaneous drug administration 345–7
subcutaneous hydration 153
sub-groups 358
substance abuse 298, 360, 368
sucrose 140
sugar alcohols 165
sulfamethoxazole 217, 218
sulfadiazine 185, 222, 406
sulphamesoxazole 221, 406
sulphur ointment 195, 221
sunken eyes 138, 139
superman care type 355, 357
supervision 361, 371–2
support 231, 233, 236–8, 254–60, 357, 366
support groups 372–4
SVC obstruction 125, 337
sweating 199–200, 212, 215
swallowing 157–8, 213
symbols 150, 275

sympathetic pain 19
symptom control 213–15, 334–40
  four rules 95–6
synthetic-conventional faith 274
syringe driver 335–6, 345–6

team care 359–61
team support meetings 361
team working 358
Tegretol 217
temazepam 406
terbinafine 196
terfenadine 218
terminal restlessness 150, 338
thalamic pain 107
thiamine 144
thioridazine 406
thirst 138, 139, 152
thrush 214
thyroid malignancies 172, 181
tinea corporis/caput 196
tingling 212
tizanide 187
topical anaesthetics 121
topical steroids 156, 191–2
total pain 109–10
touch 21
touch visual pain (TVP) scale 103–5
toxic epidermal necrolysis 199
toxoplasmosis 185, 222
toys 44–8, 54–5
tradition 281, 282
trajectory of disease 328–9
tramadol 116, 406
tranexamic acid 338, 406
transcendence 273
trans-dermal opioid patches 336
transport 230
traumatic childhood events 355–6
triamcinolone acetonide 192
trichloracetic acid 197
triclofos 406
tricyclic antidepressants 118, 204, 218, 243
trigeminal neuralgia 181
trimethroprim 217, 221
trismus 157
trust 27
tuberculosis 221
tuberculosis skin test 140
tuberculous meningitis 183, 184, 222
tumours
  compression 119
  dysphagia 158
  fungating 198–9
TVP scale 103–5
typical day 85

understanding illness, death and dying 12–15
universalizing faith 275
universal precautions 339
upper airway bleeding 130
upper airway obstruction 127–8, 337
upper GI bleeding 130
urinary catheterization 203–4

urinary retention 202, 338
urinary symptoms 201–5
urinary system assessment 201
urinary tract infection 202
urine cultures 139
urine flow 138, 139

vaginal symptoms 212
vagus nerve irritation 131
valproate 118, 180, 406
values 313, 318
vancomycin 220, 407
varicella-zoster immune globulin (VZIG) 197,
    221, 407
verapamil 217
violence 242
viral meningitis 183
viral warts 197
visceral pain 107, 211
visual imagery 112–13
visual problems 212
vitamin A 143–4, 407
vitamin deficiencies 136, 143–4
vitamin K 339
vitamin K1 403
vomiting, *see* nausea and vomiting
Vygotsky, L. 41

walking 174–5
watery diarrhoea 139

weakness 174
weight loss 212, 213
Welfare of Children & Young People in Hospital 80
wheel of life 363
Whitfield's ointment 196, 221, 407
WHO
    classification of malnutrition 137
    pain ladder 114–15
whole blood 143
wholeness 273
wills 264, 301
Winston's Wish 250, 264
withdrawal 293
withholding/withdrawing treatment 150, 219–20,
    320–1, 331
wonderwoman care type 355, 357
Wong-Baker faces scale 99, 102
work overload 357
work-related stress 353, 354
worry dolls 262
wounded healer 355
Wow game 301–2
WPC Chunk method 25

yeast infections 195, 196
yoghurt 199
young carers 33

zinc 136, 168